Essential Endocrinology

FOURTH EDITION

Essential Endocrinology

Charles G.D. Brook

MA, MD, FRCP, FRCPCH
Emeritus Professor of Paediatric Endocrinology
University College London

Nicholas J. Marshall

BSc, MSc, PhD
Reader in Cellular Endocrinology
University College London

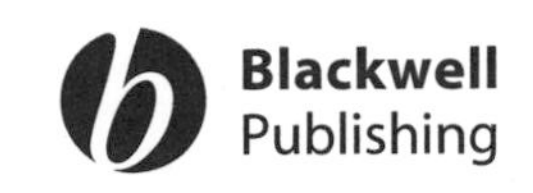

Editorial Offices:
Osney Mead, Oxford OX2 0EL
25 John Street, London WC1N 2BS
23 Ainslie Place, Edinburgh EH3 6AJ
350 Main Street, Malden
MA 02148-5018, USA
54 University Street, Carlton
Victoria 3053, Australia
10, rue Casimir Delavigne
75006 Paris, France

Other Editorial Offices:
Blackwell Wissenschafts-Verlag GmbH
Kurfürstendamm 57
10707 Berlin, Germany

Blackwell Science KK
MG Kodenmacho Building
7–10 Kodenmacho Nihombashi
Chuo-ku, Tokyo 104, Japan

Iowa State University Press
A Blackwell Science Company
2121 S. State Avenue
Ames, Iowa 50014–8300, USA

First published 1983
Reprinted 1984, 1985
Second edition 1988
Reprinted 1988
Japanese edition 1992
Indonesian edition 1993
Third edition 1996
Fourth edition 2001
Reprinted 2002, 2003

Set by Graphicraft Limited, Hong Kong
Printed and bound in Great Britain
by MPG Books Ltd, Bodmin, Cornwall

A catalogue record for this title
is available from the British Library

ISBN 0-632-05-615-0

Library of Congress
Cataloging-in-Publication Data

Brook, C. G. D. (Charles Groves Darville)
Essential endocrinology.—4th ed./
Charles G.D. Brook, Nicholas J. Marshall.
p. ; cm.
Includes index.
ISBN 0-632-05615-0
1. Endocrinology.
2. Endocrine Glands—Physiology.
I. Marshall, Nicholas J., 1944– II. Title.
[DNLM: 1. Endocrine Glands—
physiology. 2. Hormones—physiology.
WK 100 B871e 2001]
QP187 .B637—2001
612.4—dc21 00-140127

DISTRIBUTORS
Marston Book Services Ltd
PO Box 269
Abingdon, Oxon OX14 4YN
(*Orders*: Tel: 01235 465500
Fax: 01235 465555)

The Americas
Blackwell Publishing
c/o AIDC
PO Box 20
50 Winter Sport Lane
Williston, VT 05495-0020
(*Orders*: Tel: 800 216 2522
Fax: 802 864 7626)

Australia
Blackwell Science Pty Ltd
54 University Street
Carlton, Victoria 3053
(*Orders*: Tel: 3 9347 0300
Fax: 3 9347 5001)

For further information on
Blackwell Science, visit our website:
www. blackwell-science.com

Contents

Preface to the First Edition

This book is intended for those beginning to study endocrinology. The authors approach the subject from their different viewpoints, morphological, physiological, biochemical, pharmacological and clinical, and the text brings together these diverse views. It is based on the teaching given during the second year of the Basic Medical Sciences Course at The Middlesex Hospital Medical School, and we hope that it will appeal to medical students and those taking a science degree.

The opening chapter describes the underlying principles of modern endocrinology, at cellular, biochemical and physiological levels. The ensuing chapters are based on single glands or functional groups of glands. No attempt has been made to impose a rigid format on these chapters as each system lends itself to a slightly different emphasis. In general, however, in each chapter the introduction is an outline of the history of the subject, to provide an inkling of the basic, long established principles. Then the morphological and embryological basis for function is presented, and this leads on to the biochemical and physiological aspects. Clinical disorders are then considered from the viewpoint of the insight they give to the understanding of endocrine physiology. The link between basic endocrinology and clinical endocrinology is so close, that it seems very reasonable to do that, while attempting at the same time, to show that a knowledge of the scientific basis of endocrinology helps to explain the consequences of endocrine disease and the rationale of its treatment.

We would like to thank all those who contributed to this book. The authors have been very patient with us as we have brought together and edited the work of so many people and have striven to help the reader avoid the pitfalls of a multi-author book. The authors can justly claim credit for the virtues of this book, while the editors must accept responsibility for any faults that may be detected. Apart from authors, there are many to whom we are indebted. Dr Howard Jacobs very kindly advised in the writing on the chapter on reproductive endocrinology and many useful comments and suggestions were received from Professors J.F. Tait FRS, F. Hobbiger and E. Neil and Drs N.J. Marshall and P. Sanford on the chapters in their specialist fields. The many secretaries who contributed to the typing of manuscripts for this book are also gratefully acknowledged.

We hope that this book will stimulate its readers in endocrinology and that they will see how the various endocrine glands form a closely regulated, integrated system that is essential for homeostasis.

J.L.H. O'Riordan
P.G. Malan
R.P. Gould
Middlesex Hospital,
February 1982

Preface to the Fourth Edition

Since we prepared the last edition of this book, knowledge of the molecular aspects of hormone action and their associated endocrinopathies has inevitably expanded. Topics which had hitherto been in the realms of the research laboratory have matured into established concepts that now have a place in a basic text.

We have updated the book throughout, especially amplifying the sections on molecular mechanisms of hormone action in Chapter 2. For example, the descriptions of the intracellular phosphorylation cascades activated by a hormone such as insulin have been amplified. Molecular defects in such signalling pathways and their initiating receptors have also been related to clinical conditions explained by hormone resistance. We also show how the recently recognised key role played by StAR protein in steroid biosynthesis has resulted in a new understanding of congenital lipoid adrenal hyperplasia. In addition brief descriptions of the new hormone, leptin, and its actions as an appetite regulator are now included.

Our experience in using previous editions of this book as a teaching text has led us to expand the clinical case material and to include a new Appendix 3. The latter is designed to give students a palatable appreciation of the structure and functions of steroids.

We are grateful to many of our colleagues, and in particular Dr Tony Michael, Dr Barbara Whitehouse, Dr Gill Rumsby and Professor Mary Forsling, for very helpful comments and suggestions. We also acknowledge the skilled help of Blackwell Science in bringing our work to fruition.

C.G.D. Brook
N.J. Marshall

University College London
June 2001

CHAPTER 1

The Endocrine System

SUMMARY

The endocrine system co-ordinates the body's internal physiology, regulates its development throughout life, and helps it to adapt to nutritional and other external environmental changes. The system is based on a number of glands, which secrete hormones to act on target tissues. Hormones first interact with specific high-affinity receptors in or on the cells of target tissues. Receptor activation then initiates a cascade of linked biochemical reactions within the cell that produce the specific response.

Structurally there are three major groups of hormones, which are synthesized and secreted from endocrine cells in a tightly regulated manner. They comprise hormones derived from tyrosine, steroid hormones, which are cholesterol derivatives, and the much larger and more complex protein and glycoprotein hormones. After secretion, the less water-soluble hormones in particular are complexed with binding proteins in the blood. Very sensitive and hormonally specific immunoassays are used to measure the concentrations of hormones in the circulation. These assays contribute to the clinical management of patients with endocrine disorders, and have also helped greatly to define the feedback systems that regulate hormone synthesis and secretion.

INTRODUCTION

The endocrine and nervous systems constitute the two main control systems of the body, responsible for monitoring an animal's internal and external environments and making appropriate adaptive changes. The nervous system mediates its activity through nerves directly supplying the organs and structures concerned, while the endocrine system operates through chemical messengers (hormones). These may have actions related to their site of synthesis, or they may circulate in the blood to their respective target organs. The term 'hormone' was introduced in 1905 by Starling, and is derived from the Greek meaning 'to arouse' or 'to excite'—although it should be stressed that not all hormonal effects are stimulatory; some are inhibitory. Endocrine hormones are secreted into the circulation and therefore differ from exocrine hormones, which are secreted into ducts.

Unicellular and simple multicellular organisms cannot control their environment or insulate themselves from it. In humans, in whom there are about 10^{14} cells and 200 or more cell types, only a few cells are exposed to the outside world. Nevertheless, all the cells are affected directly or indirectly by external changes, and can survive only if the constancy of their environment is controlled. For this, the endocrine system is important. It responds to recurrent environmental changes, such as meals, and helps the organism to adapt to changing habits. It is also important for controlling development and growth, puberty and sexual maturation. Thus, the secretion of hormones, apart from maintaining the body's internal environment, can also induce important long-term changes in an organism's behaviour.

THE ROLE OF HORMONES

Hormones belong to a class of regulatory molecules synthesized in special cells. These cells may be collected into distinct endocrine glands, or may be found as single cells within some other organ, such as the gastrointestinal tract (Fig. 1.1, Table 1.1). From the cells that make them, hormones are released into the adjacent extracellular space (Fig. 1.2a, c), whence they enter a local blood vessel and circulate to their target cells. Some cells secrete hormones that act on themselves (autocrine hormones); some affect

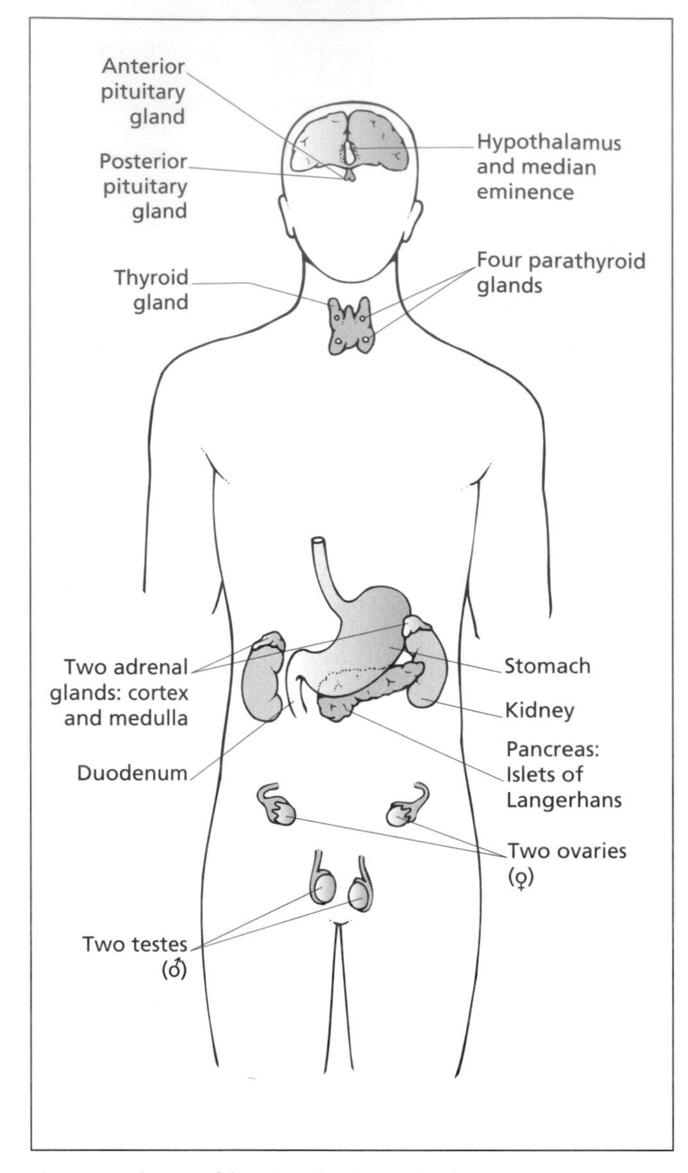

Figure 1.1 The sites of the principal endocrine glands.

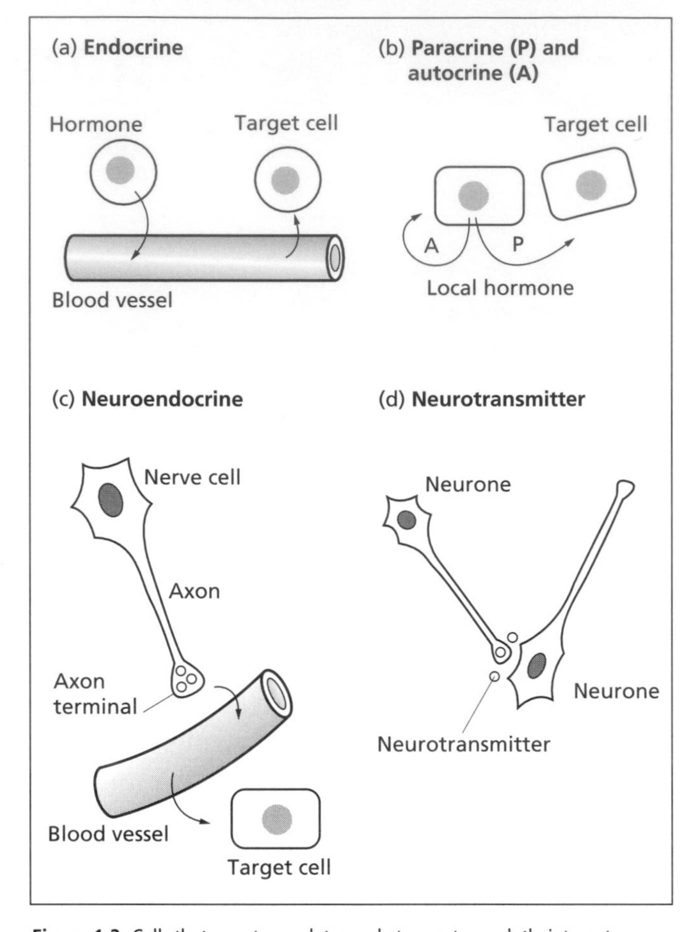

Figure 1.2 Cells that secrete regulatory substances to reach their target organs. (a) Endocrine cells secrete hormone into the blood vessel, where it is carried to the target cell. The target cell may be a considerable distance from the secreting cell, such as the anterior pituitary hormone, which acts, for example, on the thyroid. (b) Paracrine cells secrete local hormones that act on a nearby cell—for example, glucagon and somatostatin act on the adjacent pancreatic cells that secrete insulin. Some agents, such as prostaglandins and insulin-like growth factors, can act on the originating cell, and in this case they are described as exhibiting autocrine control. (c) Neuroendocrine cells secrete molecules from the neural axon terminals in response to some neural signal, and the hormone (e.g. epinephrine) is released into the bloodstream to travel to its target organ, such as the liver or adipose tissue. (d) Neurotransmitter cells secrete molecules from the axon terminals to activate adjacent neurones.

nearby cells without entering the bloodstream, and are called paracrine hormones (Fig. 1.2b). Paracrine and autocrine regulation may synergize with the initial stimulators, and thus amplify or prolong a response. Molecules secreted by neurones that excite or inhibit other neurones or muscle by means of synapses are called neurotransmitters (Fig. 1.2d). Sometimes, however, both neurotransmitters and hormones are secreted by neurones, thus forming the neuroendocrine system (Fig. 1.2c).

Hormones act by binding to specific receptors on the target-cell surface or within the cell. The result is a cascade of intracellular reactions, which frequently amplifies the original stimulus and leads ultimately to a final response. Some hormones have general importance in the body rather than acting on a specific target tissue. These include growth hormone (GH), underproduction of which leads to short stature in children, while overproduction causes gigantism. In adults, overproduction of GH causes acromegaly, with enlargement, for example, of the hands and feet and coarsening of the facial appearance. GH deficiency in adults results in a well-characterized syndrome of abnormal body composition (increased body fat and decreased lean body mass), muscle weakness, fatigue and lack of energy, drive and well-being. Thyroxine also

Table 1.1 The principal endocrine glands of the body and the hormones they produce.

Gland	Hormone	Molecular characteristics
Hypothalamus/median eminence	*Releasing and inhibiting hormones*: Thyrotrophin-releasing hormone Somatostatin Gonadotrophin-releasing hormone Corticotrophin-releasing hormone Growth hormone-releasing hormone	Peptides
	Prolactin-inhibiting factor (dopamine)	Biogenic amine
Anterior pituitary	Thyrotrophin or thyroid-stimulating hormone Luteinizing hormone Follicle-stimulating hormone	Glycoproteins
	Growth hormone Prolactin Adrenocorticotrophin	Proteins
Posterior pituitary	Vasopressin (antidiuretic hormone) Oxytocin	Peptides
Thyroid	Thyroxine and triiodothyronine	Tyrosine derivatives
	Calcitonin	Peptide
Parathyroid	Parathyroid hormone	Peptide
Adrenal cortex	Aldosterone and cortisol	Steroids
Adrenal medulla	Epinephrine and norepinephrine (formerly called adrenaline and noradrenaline)	Catecholamines
Stomach	Gastrin	Peptide
Pancreas (islets of Langerhans)	Insulin Glucagon Somatostatin	Proteins
Duodenum and jejunum	Secretin Cholecystokinin	Proteins
Ovary	Oestrogens and progesterone	Steroids
Testis	Testosterone	Steroid

acts on most tissues of the body, and the basal metabolic rate increases if it is present in excess and declines if there is a deficiency. Insulin acts on most, if not all, tissues, including the liver, muscle and adipose tissue, which implies that receptors for the hormone are widespread. The importance of insulin is illustrated by the fact that it is a key component for the maintenance of cells in tissue culture.

Many other hormones act only on one tissue: for example, thyrotrophin (thyroid-stimulating hormone, TSH), adrenocorticotrophin (adrenocorticotrophic hormone, ACTH) and gonadotrophins are secreted by the anterior pituitary and have specific target tissues—the thyroid gland, the adrenal cortex and the gonads, respectively.

Types of hormones

From the chemical standpoint, there are three groups of hormones: first, those derived from the amino acid tyrosine; secondly, peptide and protein hormones; and thirdly, steroid hormones.

Hormones derived from tyrosine

These include epinephrine (Fig. 1.3), which is secreted by the adrenal medulla, and norepinephrine, which can be produced in the adrenal medulla but is also produced at sympathetic nerve endings, where it acts as a neurotransmitter. Dopamine, another derivative of tyrosine, is a neurotransmitter that can also act as a hormone. It is released

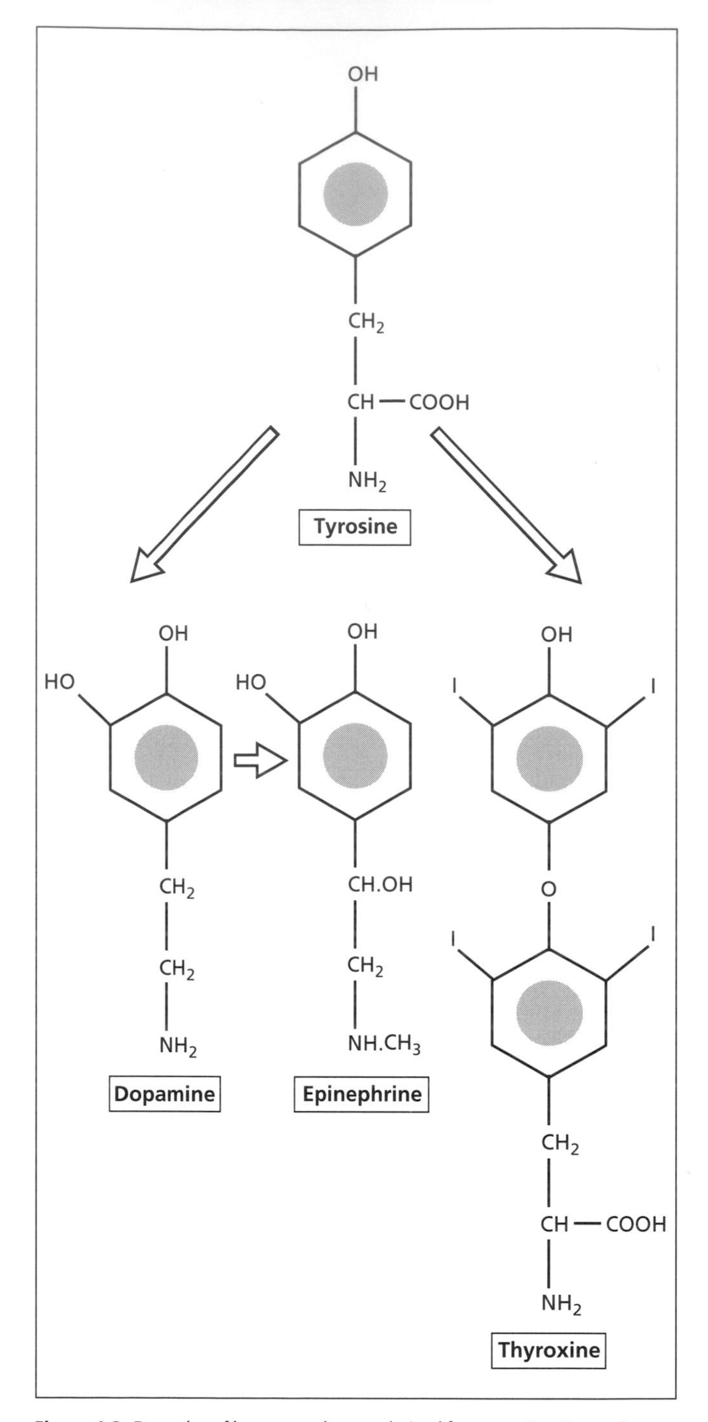

Figure 1.3 Examples of hormones that are derived from tyrosine. Dopamine exists as a hormone in its own right, but it also occurs as an intermediate in the synthesis from tyrosine of epinephrine and norepinephrine. Norepinephrine lacks the methyl group in the amino position of epinephrine. Triiodothyronine has only one of the two iodine atoms (I) present on the upper ring of thyroxine.

from the median eminence, and suppresses the secretion of prolactin (PRL) from the anterior pituitary. The thyroid hormones—thyroxine and triiodothyronine—each have two fused molecules of tyrosine; thyroxine has four iodine atoms attached to the amino acid rings, while triiodothyronine has three iodine atoms substituted in the two aromatic rings (see Chapter 5).

Protein and peptide hormones

These vary considerably in size. Thyrotrophin-releasing hormone (TRH), for example, which is secreted from the hypothalamus, has only three amino acid residues. Many of the hormones from the gastrointestinal tract—such as secretin from the duodenum and gastrin from the stomach—are larger, with up to 34 amino acids, while parathyroid hormone (PTH) is larger still, with 84. Ring structures linked by disulphide bridges are present in some hormones, including two from the pituitary gland—oxytocin and vasopressin (Fig. 1.4). Oxytocin is important for the contraction of the uterus in labour, and vasopressin regulates water excretion. Thus, they have very different physiological roles, even though they are structurally remarkably similar, with only small differences in their amino acid sequences. An intrachain disulphide bond to form a ring of seven amino acids at the amino terminus is also found in calcitonin, a hormone that can lower serum calcium.

Insulin may be regarded as a small protein or a large peptide; it consists of A-chains and B-chains linked by interchain disulphide bonds. Insulin is synthesized as a large precursor molecule (proinsulin) in a single chain (Fig. 1.8c). A section of the chain, called the connecting or C-peptide, is subsequently removed by enzymatic hydrolysis after the disulphide bonds have been formed, and the remaining two linked chains make up the insulin molecule. A number of other peptide hormones are synthesized in larger precursor forms that are modified prior to secretion (Fig. 1.8).

Some hormones are quite large proteins—for example, the glycoprotein hormones from the anterior pituitary, each of which has two peptide chains. The gonadotrophins, follicle-stimulating hormone (FSH) and luteinizing hormone (LH), and thyrotrophin (TSH) each have two chains, referred to as the α- and β-subunits. The two subunits are synthesized quite separately; the α-subunit in each is very similar, but the β-subunits are different and confer the biological specificities on the hormones. Within a given species, there may be considerable microheterogeneity of the structures of these hormones, so that a number of naturally occurring variants coexist. The variability of the glycoprotein hormones is largely due to differences in their carbohydrate composition, and the variants are referred to as isohormones or isoforms.

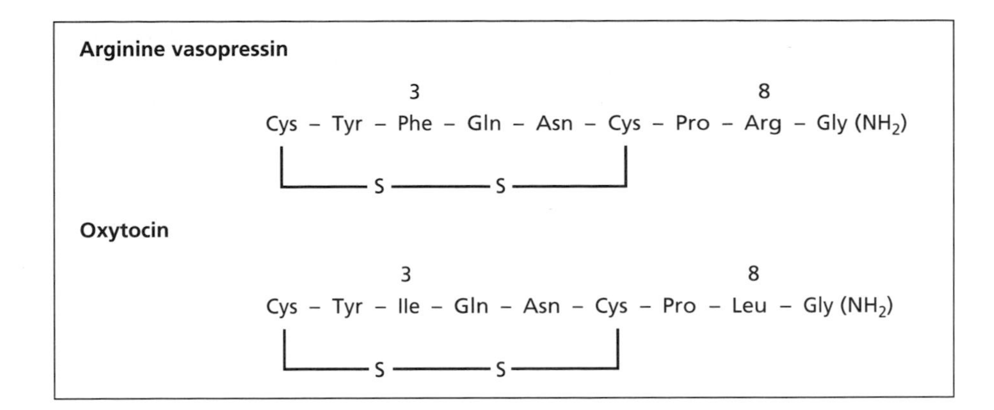

Figure 1.4 The structures of arginine vasopressin and oxytocin. The small differences in their chemical structure are indicated. These profoundly influence the physiological effects of the two hormones (see Chapter 3).

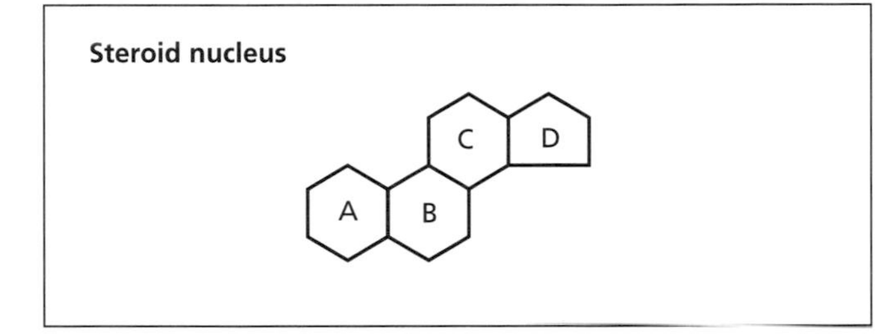

Figure 1.5 The ring identification system of the steroid nucleus. The carbon-numbering system used for steroids is shown in Appendix 3.

Steroid hormones

Steroids are a class of lipids derived from cholesterol. The letters used to denote the four rings of the steroid nucleus are shown in Fig. 1.5. The hormones include cortisol and aldosterone, which are produced by the adrenal cortex; testosterone, which comes from the testis; and progesterone and oestradiol, which come from the ovary. Steroid hormones affect carbohydrate metabolism, salt and water balance, and reproductive function. Small changes in the basic chemical structure cause dramatic changes in the physiological action of this group of hormones. Details of steroid structures are discussed in Appendix 3.

HORMONE BIOSYNTHESIS AND SECRETION

There are two principal types of cell that synthesize either peptide and protein hormones or steroid hormones. The cytological features that distinguish these two types of cell are illustrated in Fig. 1.6.

Peptides and proteins

Molecular biology of the synthesis of ribonucleic acid (RNA) and proteins

Protein or peptide hormone synthesis starts with the transcription of a gene, proceeds through translation of a messenger RNA (mRNA), and culminates in post-translational modification of the peptide or protein hormone.

In eukaryotic organisms, whose cells by definition have a true nucleus, the essential genetic information is contained in the deoxyribonucleic acid (DNA) of the chromosomes within the nucleus. Genes consist of lengths of DNA. Associated with the DNA in the nuclear chromatin are basic proteins, called histones, and other proteins, called nonhistone chromosomal proteins, some of which are likely to have regulatory roles in controlling gene expression. DNA carries genetic information in the form of a code of triplet sequences of nucleotides (bases) within the DNA strands. Before the triplet code can be transcribed to mRNA, the DNA containing the genes is attached to the nuclear matrix of the cell, and the DNA double helix is then parted in the region of the gene, after which it is transcribed by DNA-dependent RNA polymerase to yield mRNA (see, for example, Fig. 2.20e).

Each gene consists of a DNA sequence with a central region called the structural gene. On either side of the structural region, the gene has regulatory sequences, which define the circumstances under which the DNA segment will be transcribed into RNA (Fig. 1.7). The number and position of these regulatory sequences vary for individual genes, but tend to follow the common format outlined in Fig. 1.7.

'Upstream' from the start of transcription—that is, on the 5′ side of the structural gene—lies the promoter region, which regulates the binding of RNA polymerase and its associated factors. Counting of nucleotides in a gene sequence begins (Fig. 1.7) at the start of the structural gene, which is arbitrarily given the position number of 1. The promoter region lies within about 100 bases above the point at which transcription starts. Sequence conservation between different genes led to the recognition of promoter regions. They usually include a sequence similar to the thymidine–adenosine (TATA) box, which is a sequence of

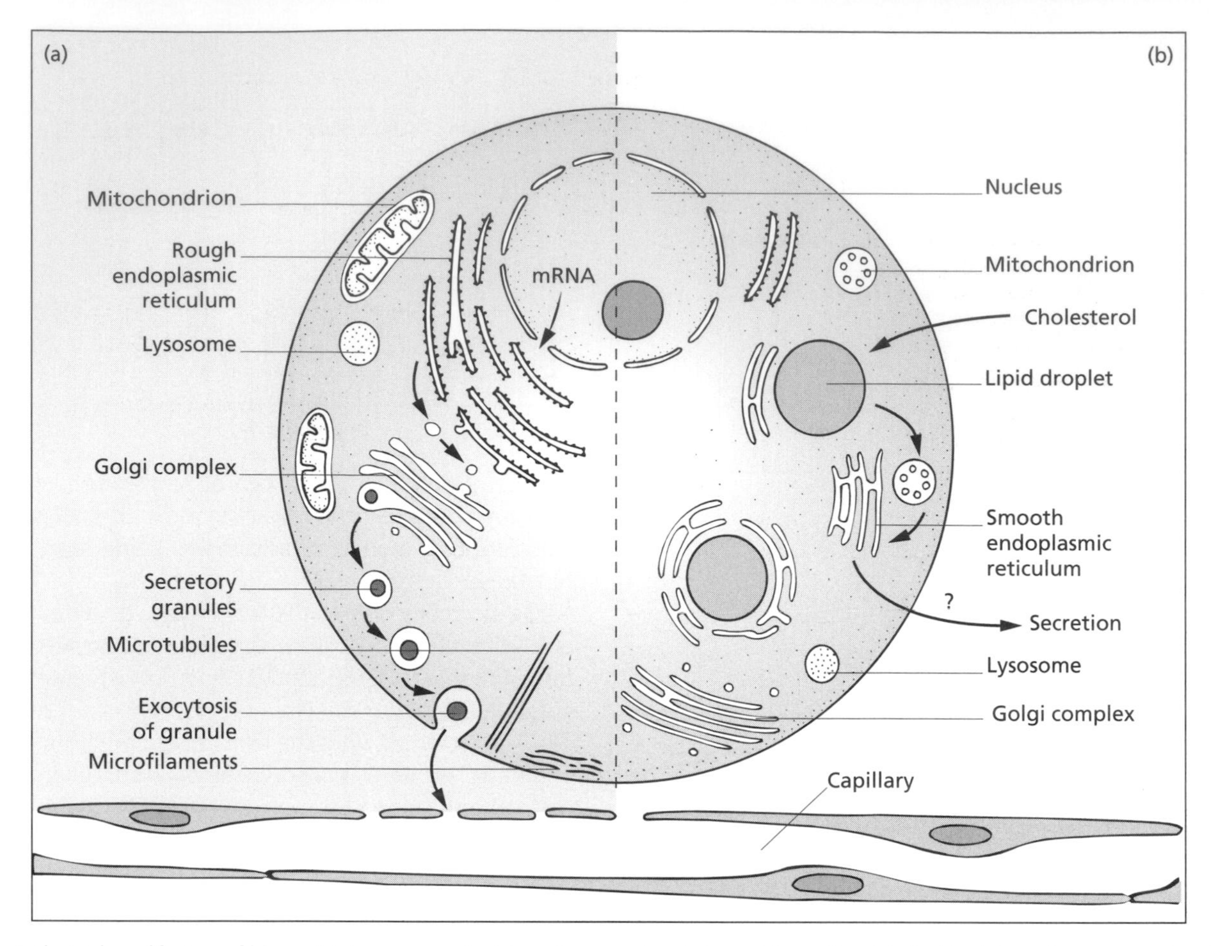

Figure 1.6 The cytological features of (a) a peptide hormone–synthesizing cell and (b) a steroid hormone–synthesizing cell. (a) Before synthesis of the peptide hormone starts, messenger ribonucleic acid (mRNA) leaves the nucleus and is translated on the ribosomes of the rough endoplasmic reticulum. The nascent protein (hormone) moves to the Golgi complex, where it may be further modified and packaged into secretory granules. The granules move to the cell membrane, with the involvement of microtubules and actin microfilaments. The granule membrane fuses with the plasma membrane, and granule (hormone) release through exocytosis occurs. The hormone then passes through the fenestrations of the capillary into the bloodstream. Lysosomes are involved in the removal of unwanted secretory granules (crinophagy) and cytoplasmic organelles. (b) Before steroid hormone synthesis, cholesterol enters the cell, and is stored as cholesterol esters in the lipid droplets until required. Cholesterol then moves to the mitochondria, where it is converted to pregnenolone. Pregnenolone is transported to the surrounding smooth endoplasmic reticulum, where it is transformed by a series of reactions into the appropriate steroid hormone (see Appendix 3). The mode of egress of the hormone from the cell is not certain.

seven bases found in prokaryotes (which do not contain a true nucleus). This is found about 30 bases before the start of transcription. Also associated with many genes are elements known as transcription-enhancers, in various positions within or around a gene. These sequences influence when transcription can occur, and they frequently control the tissue specificity of gene expression. The hormone-response elements for steroid and thyroid hormones are examples of such regions (see Figs 2.23 and 2.24).

The structural gene itself is made up of introns (also known as intervening sequences) and exons (for expressed sequence regions) (Fig. 1.7). Transcription of both the introns and exons of the structural gene gives a precursor called pre-mRNA. Post-transcriptional modification eliminates bases that were complementary to those of introns in the DNA sequence, and the exon-derived sequences are spliced together to give mature mRNA. Two other post-transcriptional events occur to mRNA: one is the capping of the 5′ end with a 7-methylguanosine residue, and the other involves the addition of a series of adenosine residues (A) to give a poly A tail at the 3′ end. Messenger RNA moves from the nucleus to the cytoplasm for translation of the message into peptide or protein hormones.

Translation of mRNA into a peptide hormone

Mature mRNA is transported from the cell nucleus and bound to ribosomes attached to the endoplasmic reticulum. This is a characteristic feature of protein-synthesizing

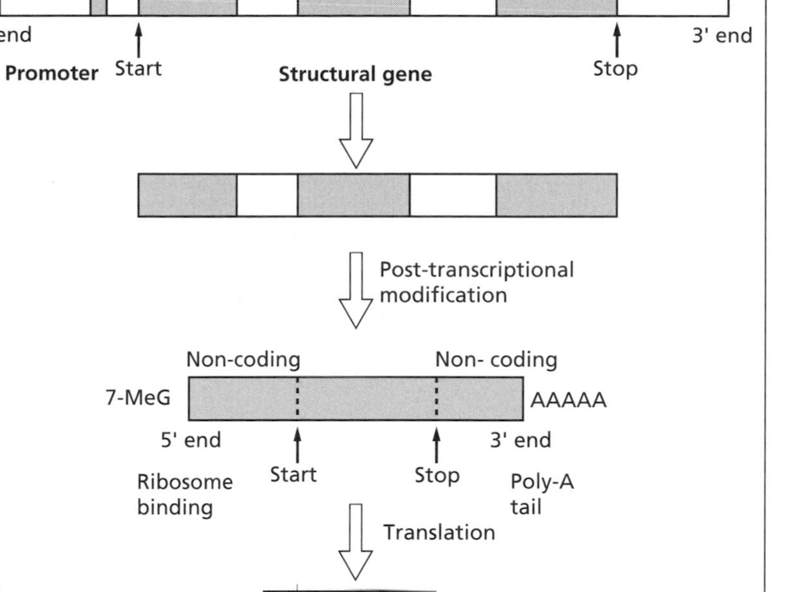

Figure 1.7 A schematic representation of the structure of a gene and of the events leading to synthesis of a peptide hormone. The gene consists of double-stranded (ds) deoxyribonucleic acid (DNA). At its 5′ end (the 'upstream' side) is the regulatory region known as the promoter, which includes the TATA box. This is followed by a series (variable in number and size) of exons and introns, which make up the structural gene. Ribonucleic acid (RNA) polymerase produces an RNA transcript of the exons and introns in the form of pre-messenger RNA (pre-mRNA). Removal of the RNA sequences derived from the introns is followed by splicing together of the exon-derived sequences. Further post-transcriptional changes include the addition of a 7-methyl guanosine (7-MeG) cap at the 5′ end and a poly A tail on the 3′ end. When the mature mRNA is bound to a ribosome, translation occurs, to give a peptide precursor that includes the signal peptide of the prehormone (or preprohormone). Post-translational processing (see Fig. 1.8) is needed before the hormone is ready for secretion.

cells, and is called rough endoplasmic reticulum (Fig. 1.6). The mature mRNA has a central region (Fig. 1.7), which is translated into protein, with 5′ and 3′ nontranslated regions on either side. The 5′ nontranslated region contains sequences that are important for the binding of ribosomes, made up of ribosomal RNA and protein, and factors that affect the efficiencies of translation. Translation of mRNA bound to a ribosome begins at the start signal, adenosine–thymidine–guanosine (ATG), which is the triplet base code for the amino acid methionine. Each triplet of bases on the mRNA represents a binding site for the specific transfer RNA (tRNA), and contains a triplet base sequence complementary to that of the mRNA. As each tRNA carrying its specific amino acid binds to the mRNA–ribosome complex, it is linked into the growing peptide chain. Peptide synthesis starts at the amino terminus and proceeds to the carboxy terminus, where translation of the mRNA ceases at a stop signal such as TGA.

Post-translational peptide modification

In general, mRNA codes for a peptide that is longer than the secreted form of the hormone. The precursor peptide, called a prohormone, carries a signal peptide extension at the amino terminus that is lipophilic. The endoplasmic reticulum has channel proteins that recognize the signal peptide sequence. These features enable the nascent peptide to cross the endoplasmic reticulum into the cisternal space, where the signal peptide is excised by a peptidase to leave the rest of the hormone in the cisternal space. Synthesis of a prohormone can be shown in cell-free translational systems that contain only mRNA, ribosomes and other cofactors, including tRNAs. Under these circumstances, the signal peptide remains attached to the rest of the hormone molecule, since there are no cisternal peptidases present. In the case of some hormones, apart from the prepeptide there may be another extension of the amino terminus, so that a 'preprohormone' is formed.

Other post-translational changes may be needed. As shown in Fig. 1.8a and c, disulphide bridges are formed in certain proteins within the cisternal space of the endoplasmic reticulum. The newly formed protein then travels through the endoplasmic reticulum, and certain carbohydrates may be added at this stage (Fig. 1.8d) if it is to be a glycoprotein. The protein or peptide hormone is

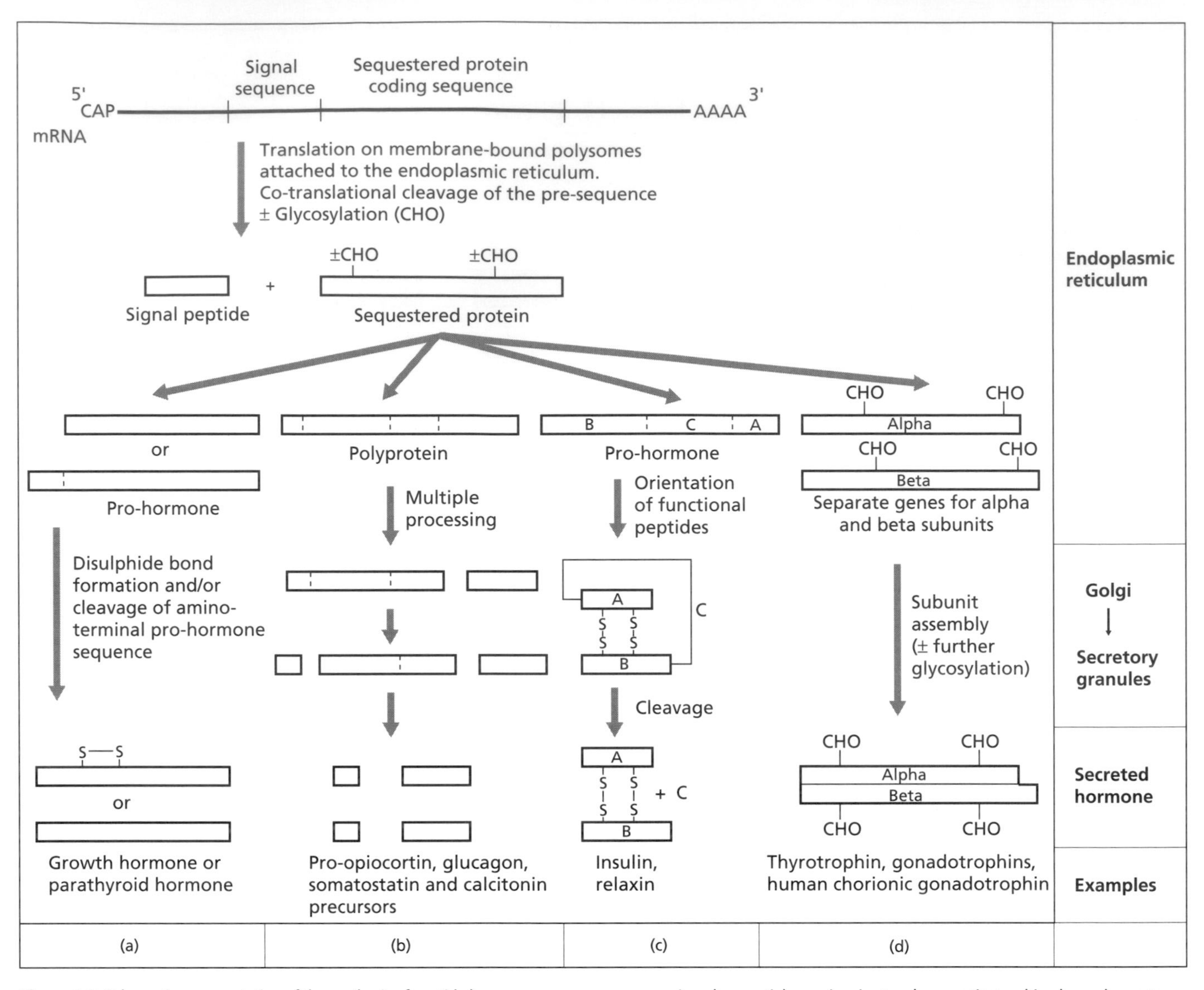

Figure 1.8 Schematic representation of the synthesis of peptide hormones, showing some post-translational changes. A signal peptide at the amino-terminal end facilitates movement of a prohormone across intracellular membranes of the endoplasmic reticulum. The signal peptide is removed, and the rest of the molecule is sequestered for further processing before it is secreted. Four types of post-translational modification are shown. (a) Where there is an amino-terminal extension in a prohormone, such as proparathyroid hormone, the extension is removed before secretion. Alternatively, as with growth hormone, the number of amino acids is not changed, but intrachain disulphide bonds are created before the hormone is secreted. (b) A polyprotein yields a number of peptides on specific hydrolysis by endopeptidases, and some of these peptides may be glycosylated. For example, pro-opiocortin (also called pro-opiomelanocortin) can give rise to adrenocorticotrophin plus melanocyte-stimulating hormone and β-endorphin; these peptides vary in length and have different biological activities. (c) Synthesis of highly active molecules such as insulin appears to proceed by folding of the peptide and formation of disulphide bonds. An active molecule is created by specific hydrolytic removal of a connecting (C) peptide, and so proinsulin gives rise to insulin plus C-peptide, which are secreted in equimolar proportions. (d) Synthesis of the larger protein hormones—such as thyrotrophin, the gonadotrophins, luteinizing hormone and follicle-stimulating hormone, as well as human chorionic gonadotrophin—proceeds from two separate peptides that come together to form the subunits of the protein. These four hormone molecules each have a very similar α-subunit and a hormone-specific β-subunit; both subunits are glycosylated.

transferred from the endoplasmic reticulum in vesicles to the Golgi complex, where further carbohydrate additions may occur, including the terminal sialic acid residues. The completed protein is then packaged into membrane-bound vesicles. For certain hormones, it has been shown that specific enzymes are packaged in an inactive form along with the prohormone. In this case, the enzyme is a specific endopeptidase, which is capable of cleaving the 'pro-' portion of the protein chain, as in the case of the C-peptide of insulin (Fig. 1.8c).

Storage

Protein or peptide hormone–secreting cells store the newly synthesized hormone in small vesicles or secretory granules. These may be observed under the electron microscope as electron-dense material scattered around the periphery of the cells, just inside the cell membrane. Movement of the vesicles from the Golgi apparatus to a position near the cell membrane is influenced by two types of filamentous structure, called microtubules and microfilaments, which are found in all eukaryotic cells. Microtubules are made up of polymerized protein molecules (tubulin), which form rods within the cell. Microfilaments consist of the 'muscle-like' protein actin, and are about 5 nm in diameter. Groups of these are arranged in bundles at strategic positions within the cell. Actin is associated with myosin subunits, and is probably involved in the movement and control of the positions of subcellular vesicles within the cell. It has been suggested that tubulin acts as the cytoskeleton, giving the cell some degree of rigidity, and that it provides a framework on which the other cytoskeletal elements, such as microfilaments, are able to control the movement of subcellular organelles within the cell.

Secretion

The cell requires some stimulus before the stored prohormone is activated and released. The term 'stimulus–secretion coupling' has been used to describe the latter process. The stimulation may be hormonal, and usually involves a change in permeability of the cell to Ca^{2+} ions. The divalent metal ions are required for interaction between the vesicle and plasma membranes and for the activation of enzymes, microfilaments and microtubules. Specific endopeptidases present together with the prohormone in the storage vesicle are activated during the secretory process, and produce the active form of the hormone for release from the cell.

The mode of secretion from the cell is called exocytosis (Fig. 1.6a). The membrane of an intracellular storage granule fuses with the plasma membrane of the cell; this parts near the point of fusion, and the content of the vesicle is secreted into the extracellular space surrounding the blood vessels. The membrane that originally surrounded the vesicle is quickly recycled within the cell. Large changes in the turnover of membrane phospholipids occur during this period of exocytotic activity.

Steroids

Synthesis

Cholesterol is the natural precursor of all steroid hormones. The biochemical pathway for steroid synthesis starts from acetate, via mevalonate, hydroxymethylglutaryl coenzyme A (CoA) and squalene, to cholesterol. All the steroid hormone–synthesizing cells of the body—i.e. the adrenal cortex, placenta, testis and ovary—contain intracellular fat droplets in the cytoplasm (Fig. 1.6b). These are composed principally of cholesterol esters, the storage form of the hormone precursor. Steroid-secreting cells, unlike protein-producing and peptide-producing cells, do not store hormone in a state ready for secretion, but synthesize hormone for secretion as required. Appendix 3 gives a description of the biosynthetic pathways for the major steroid hormones, together with a discussion of their key structural features.

TRANSPORT OF HORMONES IN THE BLOOD

Most peptide and protein hormones are hydrophilic, at least on the exterior surface, and they therefore generally circulate in the bloodstream with little or no association with serum proteins. The more hydrophobic a molecule, the less likely it is to circulate in the free state, and the more closely it associates with serum proteins for transport. Thus, there are specific transport proteins in the circulation that bind thyroxine and many of the steroid hormones. These include thyroxine-binding globulin, cortisol-binding globulin and sex hormone–binding globulin. The high specificity of these transport proteins is such that minor changes in the structure of hormones affect binding. Thus, aldosterone, for example, is only weakly bound to cortisol-binding globulin. Many hormones may also loosely associate with other circulating proteins, especially albumin.

Protein-bound hormone is in equilibrium with 'free' (or unbound) hormone. The free hormone can diffuse to tissues more readily, and so the physiological state usually corresponds more closely with the concentration of the free hormone. As a result of changes in the concentration of binding protein, the total and bound concentrations of hormone may alter quite markedly, while this is accompanied by only a small change in the free hormone concentration, with the result that the physiological status remains unaltered.

CONTROL OF THE ENDOCRINE SYSTEM

Hormones provide a mechanism by which the body can relay chemical signals throughout the hierarchy of different cell types perfused by the bloodstream. Homeostatic (self-regulating) control systems are features common to engineering and electronic design; the basic principles of such systems also apply to biological systems. Since the

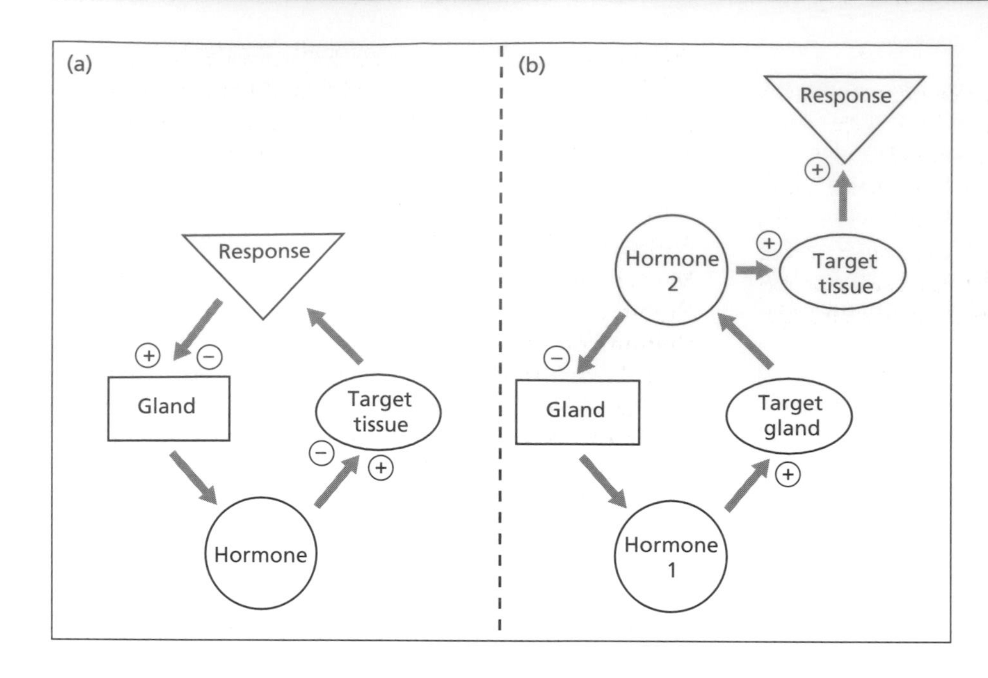

Figure 1.9 Two outline schemes for control of hormone synthesis, secretion and action. (a) The gland releases a hormone, which acts on target tissue to stimulate (+) or inhibit (−) a response. The response itself may either inhibit or stimulate the original gland to decrease or increase supply of the original hormone. (b) The gland produces a hormone (1), which acts on a second gland. The latter target is stimulated to produce a second hormone (2), which then acts on target tissues to induce a response. In addition, the second hormone is capable of controlling release of the first hormone by feedback inhibition (−).

primary role of the endocrine system is one of control, it is useful to consider the possible available mechanisms. In the following discussion, the hormone will be considered to be the signal, and the target cell will yield the response to it (Fig. 1.9).

Simple control

An elementary control system is one in which the signal itself is limited, either in magnitude (i.e. amplitude) or duration (i.e. frequency); thus, enough signal or hormone is produced at a time to induce only a transient response. Certain neural impulses are of this type. A refinement, which is introduced to discriminate a positive signal from background 'noise', is to ensure that the target cell cannot or does not respond below a certain threshold level of the signal. An example of this is the pulsatile release of gonadotrophin-releasing hormone from the hypothalamus.

Negative feedback

This is probably the commonest form of control in biological as well as other systems. In essence, the signal produces a response, which feeds back on the signal generator to decrease the level of signal. Examples are found in metabolic reaction sequences, where the product of a reaction sequence will feed back and inhibit its own production when the concentration builds up to a certain level (e.g. histidine synthesis). In order to regulate hormone release by this mechanism, the hormone must act on its target cell to produce, as a response, a substance that is capable of entering the bloodstream and acting on the releasing cell to inhibit or modulate production of the original stimulator. Thus, many of the hormones of the anterior pituitary—which are trophic or stimulating hormones and act on other endocrine glands such as the thyroid, adrenal cortex, or gonads to stimulate production of other hormones—are controlled by negative feedback; the resulting thyroid or steroid hormones then act on the pituitary to decrease the amount of the respective trophic hormone being released.

Positive feedback

In this system, the signal generator is stimulated by the response it induces. In engineering terms, this is an intrinsically unstable control system, but there are specific biological systems in which such a 'control' system can be of benefit. Control, used in the positive feedback situation, refers to a continued generation of the signal, as cessation of the stimulus only occurs when the system inducing the response cannot function any longer: in this case, the positive feedback has led to termination of the event. Examples of such a positive feedback system are relatively rare, but two situations involving the peptide hormone oxytocin are worth describing briefly. During childbirth, the stretch receptors in the distended vagina send neurological signals to the brain, where oxytocin release from the posterior pituitary is stimulated. This hormone is carried in the blood, and causes the uterus to contract; this activates the cervical receptors to stimulate more oxytocin release, and delivery terminates the positive feedback. In a similar manner, suckling causes stimulation of the nipple receptors, which results in increased oxytocin release, with a corresponding increase in the milk-ejection reflex; removal of the stimulus terminates the response, which is the release of oxytocin.

Inhibitory control

Certain hormones either have a very general action on a variety of target cells (e.g. GH), or do not produce a specific product that is released into the bloodstream (e.g. PRL, which stimulates milk synthesis in the breast). These hormones can be controlled by an inhibitory hormone, which prevents their release, and it is only when these inhibitory hormones or factors are suppressed (for example, by neurological or other factors) that release of the hormones is permitted.

Metabolic control

To some extent, this is an extension of negative feedback. Certain hormones have to be converted to an active form in order to act; for example, testosterone has to be converted to dihydrotestosterone in the testis and genitalia, and thyroxine has to be converted to triiodothyronine for expression of thyroid hormone action in almost all cell types. This control is probably regulated locally by the levels of the product or active hormone to which the precursor hormone is converted.

Endocrine disorders

In any complex regulatory system, it is likely that disordered function will have important consequences, and the endocrine system is no exception. Underproduction or overproduction of hormones can occur. For example, lack of GH in children causes dwarfism, while excess of the hormone leads to gigantism. The effects of overproduction of GH in adults (in whom the epiphyses have fused) are rather different, and lead to a condition called acromegaly. Many clinical disorders were recognized before the endocrine disturbance was understood, and it was only after further study that the underlying causes were revealed. For example, Addison described the effects of disease of the adrenal cortex when there is a lack of cortisol and aldosterone. Because of the decrease in circulating cortisol, there is compensatory overproduction of ACTH by the anterior pituitary. Apart from stimulating cortisol production, this pituitary hormone is cosecreted with melanocyte-stimulating hormone, which causes melanocytes in the skin to produce melatonin; this explains the pigmentation that is one of the features of Addison disease. Thus, attempted correction of a deficiency of one hormone by overproduction of another can have important consequences.

In other conditions, disordered synthesis—such as that of a steroid hormone—may occur when a particular enzyme is missing (arising from a genetic defect). The consequences of this can arise in part from the lack of that steroid and in part from an accumulation of other precursor steroids, which build up as a result of the enzyme deficiency. One of the commonest endocrine diseases is diabetes mellitus. This can be due to lack of secretion of insulin from the β-cells of the islets of Langerhans in the pancreas. The same clinical disease can, however, be caused not by lack of insulin secretion, but by resistance to its actions—i.e. a receptor disorder.

Endocrine rhythms

Most, if not all, organized bodily activities show periodic rhythmic or cyclic changes. Ultimate control of these rhythms probably arises from the nervous system, and some brain areas have been identified as centres for such regulation—e.g. the suprachiasmatic nucleus in the hypothalamus. Some rhythms controlled by these endogenous mechanisms appear to be independent of environmental change. Others are co-ordinated, and are said to be 'entrained' by external (exogenous) cues, such as the 24-hour light–dark cycle. These external cues are called 'Zeitgebers' —literally, time-givers.

Rhythms based on the 24-hour cycle are called 'circadian' (*circa* = about, *dies* = day). Those with a shorter period are termed 'ultradian', and those with a period longer than 24 hours are termed 'infradian'—e.g. the 28-day menstrual cycle in women, or seasonal reproductive periods in animals. Many hormone functions show a circadian rhythm. For example, cortisol secretion is maximal between 4 and 8 a.m., while GH and PRL are maximally secreted about 1 h after an individual has gone to sleep. Hormonal rhythmicity also changes during the life cycle of an individual: in puberty, gonadotrophins are secreted in relatively large amounts and the concentrations are maximal at night, whereas in sexually mature individuals they are secreted in a pulsatile fashion throughout the 24-hour period.

From a practical point of view, knowledge of the rhythmicity of hormone secretion is clearly very important. Sampling the blood concentration of a hormone for clinical or experimental reasons must take into account the variability of hormone levels throughout the day and night; otherwise, such measurements are not useful in providing diagnostic or other scientific information.

MEASUREMENT OF HORMONES IN THE CIRCULATION

Understanding endocrine control systems and the disturbance of normal regulation associated with endocrine diseases depends on the ability to measure levels of the appropriate hormones in the circulation. The methods for the determination of hormone concentrations, referred to as 'assays', usually depend on either the measurement of physiological responses induced by the hormone (bioassays) or the recognition of the hormone by antibodies that are raised to bind to specific antigenic sites on the hormone (immunoassays). The measurement of hormones in serum samples by immunoassay is now a matter of routine biochemical testing, and it is carried out on a large scale in clinical chemistry. Because of the favourable characteristics of antibody–antigen binding systems, immunoassays have been developed that are sufficiently sensitive, precise and hormonally specific to meet the analytical challenges presented by the endocrine systems. Bioassays are less suitable for the demands of routine clinical chemistry, and their use is generally restricted to more detailed research purposes. It is unlikely that they would be used for hormones with relatively simple structures, e.g. steroids or thyroid hormones, but they continue to play a role in measuring the potency of hormones with more complex structures—particularly the large protein and glycoprotein hormones produced by the anterior pituitary. Molecular structure also influences the choice of the design of immunoassays, as is detailed in Appendix 1.

CHAPTER 2

The Molecular Basis of Hormone Action

SUMMARY

This chapter outlines the major receptor-mediated pathways by which hormones regulate the functions of their target cells. Two superfamilies of receptors are described. The first are the receptors for water soluble hormones such as insulin, growth hormone, TSH, LH and FSH, for which the lipid barrier of the plasma membrane is impenetrable. Through necessity receptors for these hormones are located on the cell surface and are embedded in and bridge the plasma membrane.

The second receptor superfamily consists of the intracellular receptors that interact with the steroid and thyroid hormones which are lipid-soluble and can therefore pass into the cell. These receptors are located in either the cytosol or the nucleus of the target cell.

The cell surface receptors may be further subdivided into two distinct groups which differ in their intracellular signalling mechanisms. The first group, which includes receptors for insulin or growth hormone, act via phosphorylation cascades which are initiated by phosphorylation of tyrosine residues on key signalling proteins. The second group, such as those for TSH, LH or FSH are linked to G-proteins and signal either via the catalytic subunit phopholipase C or adenylate cyclase; this in turn generates intracellular phosphorylation cascades, governed largely by the phosphorylation of serine or threonine residues on key proteins, or via changes in intracellular calcium. These changes are mediated by the second messengers cAMP, diacylglycerol and IP_3.

The second receptor superfamily, the nuclear as opposed to the cell surface receptors, can be subdivided into two classes. Class I, typified by those responsive to cortisol, are, in their resting state, located in the cytosol, where they are complexed with inactivating heat-shock proteins (hsp). Binding of the steroid leads to dissociation of the hsp and relocation of the occupied receptor to the nucleus where it then acts as a transcription factor. Class II, exemplified by receptors for T_3 and calcitriol, are to be found bound to DNA in the target cells even in their resting state, and as with Class I, function as hormone-activated transcription factors.

The hormones which stimulate nuclear receptors may be enzymically modified by their target cells themselves, e.g. the deiodination of T4 to T3 by 5′-deiodinase. This provides an important mechanism for the local regulation of hormone action at the level of the target tissue. As always, defects in key components in these complex pathways, be they the receptors themselves or their intracellular mediators, can lead to illustrative endocrinopathies.

This chapter presents only the rudiments of the molecular grammar of the response systems. Given the large number of hormones and target tissues, through necessity the integrated system must be complex so that it may support the versatility of the *in vivo* situation. One complexity that is not addressed in this chapter is that of the cross-talk between the individual pathways. For the sake of clarity the individual pathways have been described as independent sytems. However, there is increasing evidence of interaction between the separate pathways. For example, MAP kinase has been reported to phosphorylate serine residues in the N-terminal domain of the oestrogen receptor and thereby enhance its transcriptional activation function, and STAT 5 has been shown to interact with glucocorticoid receptors.

INTRODUCTION

Hormones interact with their target cells via hormonally specific receptors. Some important characteristics of these hormone receptors are summarized in Table 2.1.

Clearly a receptor must be readily accessible to its hormone and thus the cellular location of a receptor reflects the chemical characteristics of its specific cognate hormone. For example, the water-soluble hormones such as the pituitary derived proteins and glycoproteins, are hydrophilic and cannot cross the lipid barrier presented by the cytoplasmic membrane. These therefore interact with receptors located on the cell surface. In contrast, lipid-soluble hormones such as the steroids and thyroid hormones, bind to intracellular receptors; these are located either in the cytosol or the nucleus. Each of these two major categories of receptor will be considered in turn. The diversity of the different receptor subdivisions is outlined in Fig. 2.1.

Table 2.1 Notable characteristics of hormone receptors

1 Hormones react with their receptors in a reversible manner. This can be described by the equation

$$H + R \rightleftharpoons HR$$

where the position of equilibrium lies well to the right, i.e. hormones have high affinities for their receptors. The reversible nature of this reaction and the saturability of the sytem can be demonstrated with a series of classical ligand binding experiments. Quantitative measurements of affinity constants and numbers of receptors per cell can be established by the application of the Law of Mass Action. Kd values range between pico- and nanomolar concentrations which is appropriate for hormones since they circulate at these low concentrations. See Appendix 2 for further discussion of the kinetics of hormone/receptor interactions.

2 Receptors exhibit high degrees of hormonal specificity.

3 The locations of receptors are appropriately tissue specific.

4 For some hormones, e.g. aldosterone, hormone specificity is crucially achieved by target tissue conversion.

5 Receptors for hormones fall into several discrete groups in terms of their structure and subcellular localization (Fig. 2.1). These reflect the biochemical characteristics of their cognate hormones.

6 Receptors on cell surfaces trigger a wide range of intracellular signal transduction pathways. These also fall into several catagories (Fig. 2.1).

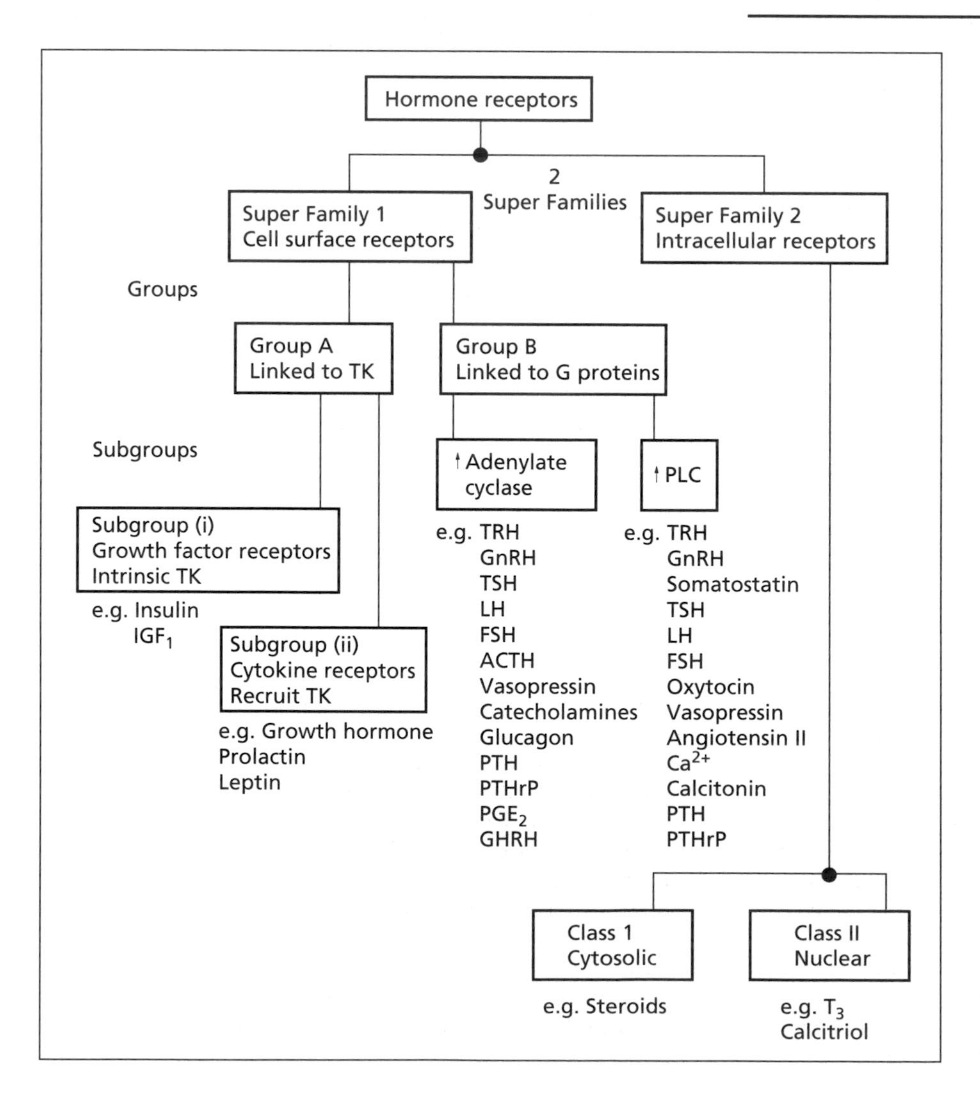

Figure 2.1 A composite diagram showing the different classes of hormone receptors. The details of each of these receptor classes will be discussed in the text. In addition to the classification shown here, receptors for some hormones can occur in more than one type. For example, different types of PTH receptors link to different G-proteins which then either couple to adenylate cyclase or phospholipase C (PLC). TK = Tyrosine kinase.

CELL SURFACE RECEPTORS FOR HORMONES

There are 2 superfamilies of cell surface receptors. The first is linked to tyrosine kinase and the second to G-proteins (Fig. 2.1). There is however, an underlying structural unity in all of these receptors. Each holoreceptor is comprised of three segments (Fig. 2.2).

1 An extracellular component, otherwise known as the ectodomain, which binds the hormone with a high affinity.

2 A membrane spanning region; this varies in structure from a simple linear hydrophobic region to a more serpentine structure which crosses the membrane seven times.

3 A cytosolic domain which initiates the intracellular signalling cascade. These intracellular pathways can themselves be complex, with several branch points and they will be discussed in detail later on. Protein phosphorylation of sequences of proteins plays an important role in signal transduction.

Protein phosphorylation

The amino acids serine, threonine and tyrosine each carry a polar hydroxyl group (Fig. 2.3). These amino acids can be phosphorylated when a phosphate group is transferred from ATP and substitutes for the polar hydroxyl group on the amino acid. This generates a covalently bound phosphate (Fig. 2.4a). The energy transfer during this reaction leads to an activating conformational change of the phosphorylated protein. In many signalling pathways, the activated phosphorylated protein is then itself able to act as a protein kinase and phosphorylate the next protein in the sequence. In this way a phosphorylation 'cascade' is generated which relays the intracellular signal along a pathway (Fig. 2.4b).

Serine or threonine vs. tyrosine phosphorylation

Protein phosphorylation acts as a key molecular switch. The polar hydroxyl groups of serine and threonine are far more abundantly phosphorylated than those of tyrosine. Thus phosphoserine and phosphothreonine residues

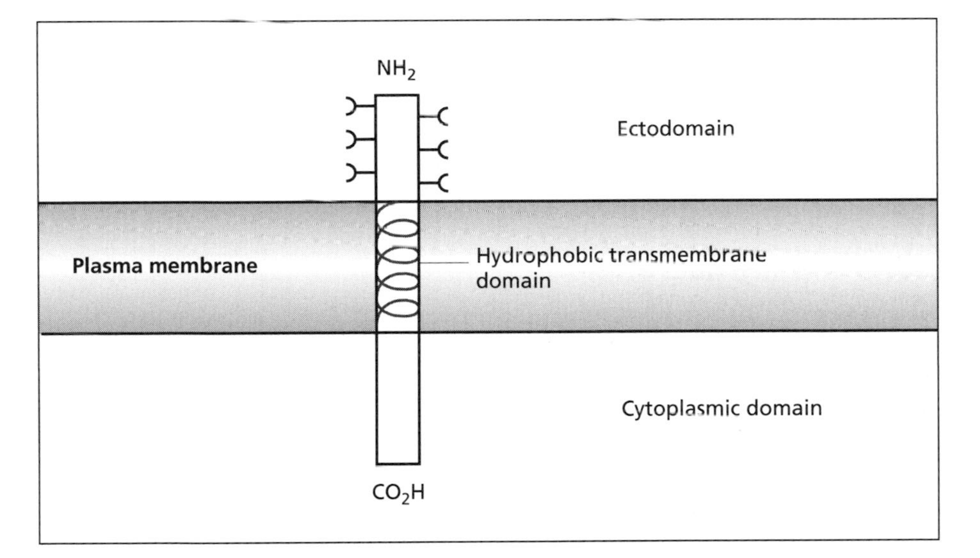

Figure 2.2 Schematic representation of a membrane-spanning cell-surface receptor. These receptors have 3 clearly identifiable domains: the ectodomain, which is bridged by a membrane-spanning component to the intracellular cytoplasmic domain. Each domain has characteristic structural features which reflect its location and function. The hormone binds with a high degree of specificity to a ligand binding pocket in the ectodomain. The N-terminal ectodomain is rich in glycosylation sites (—C), but the functional significance of the attached oligosaccharide moieties is not known. The ectodomain is comparatively rich in cysteine residues. These form internal S-S bonds and repeated loops are vital for the correct folding of this receptor region. The ectodomain of receptors for some hormones can also be identified as a separate entity in the circulation. For example, the free ectodomain for growth hormone forms a circulating binding protein. Moreover it has long been recognized that the ectodomain of the TSH receptor can be cleaved relatively easily. Fragments of the TSH receptor ectodomain in the circulation may be important for the so far unexplained induction of thyroid stimulating antibodies which are antireceptor autoantibodies which mimic TSH action. As might be expected, the membrane-spanning domain is rich in hydrophobic and noncharged amino acids. Approximately 25 of these are required to bridge the typical cytoplasmic membrane which is 100 Å across. To do this they form an α-helix. The structure of the transmembrane domain can however, be much more complex than is shown in this diagram (see Fig. 2.11). The C-terminal cytoplasmic domain either contains within its own structure, or links with, separate catalytic systems which initiate intracellular signals. Using recombinant technology, chimeric receptors have been formed by mixing and recombining segments of different receptors which fall within one of the receptor subdivisions (see Table 2.1). These demonstrate the functional independence of the 3 segments.

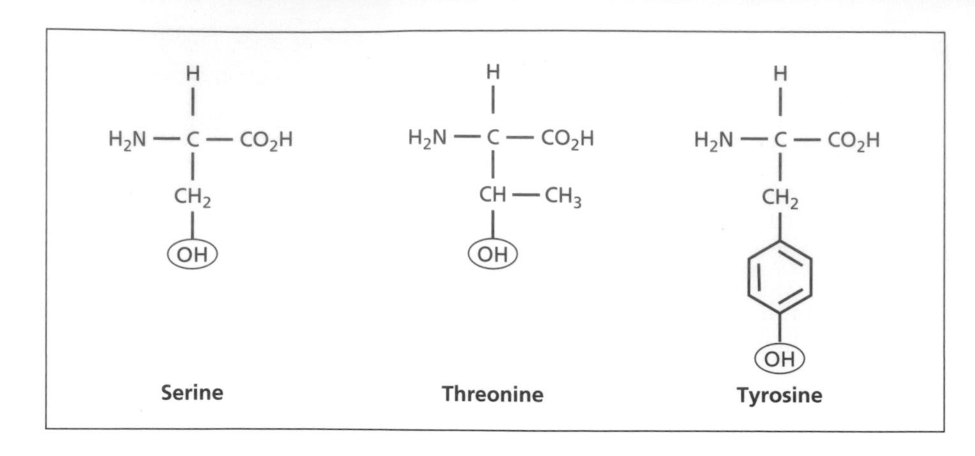

Figure 2.3 The structures of the amino acids serine, threonine and tyrosine which carry polar hydroxyl groups which can be phosphorylated. Tyrosine is distinguished from the others since it is the only amino acid with a phenolic group. Phosphorylation of the latter provides a particularly distinctive molecular switch in intracellular signalling pathways. Over 99% of all protein phosphorylations occur on serine and threonine residues.

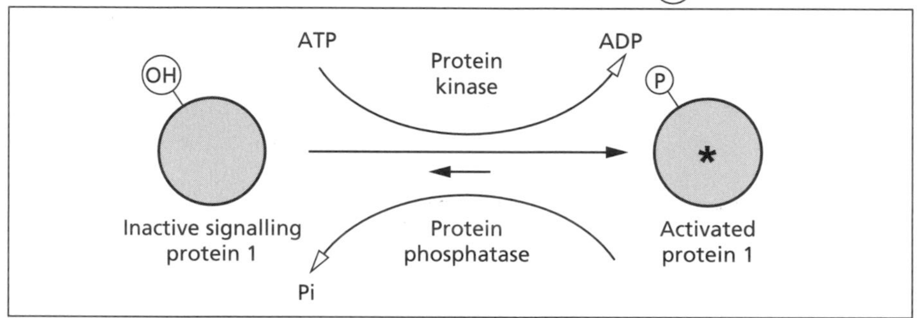

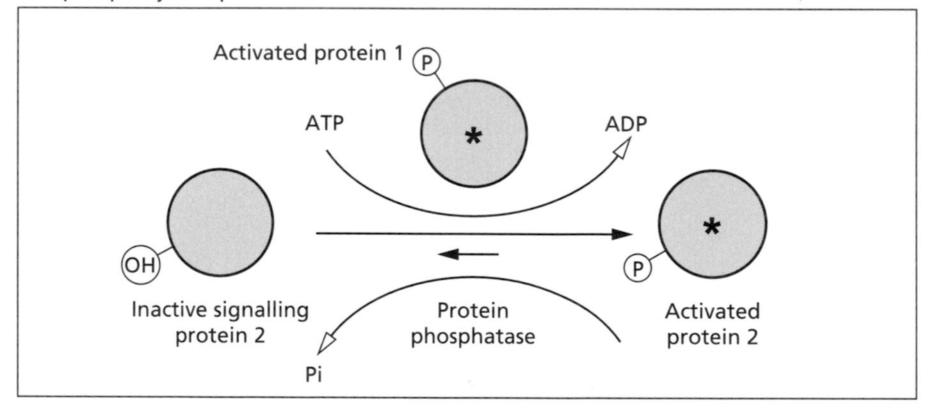

Figure 2.4 Protein phosphorylation and the generation of phosphorylation cascades. (a) Phosphorylation of Protein 1 induces an activating conformational change due to the energetically favourable phosphorylation Ⓟ of a hydroxyl group (OH). (b) The initiation of a phosphorylation cascade. Phosphorylated Protein 1 acts as a kinase and phosphorylates Protein 2. The forward and backward reactions are catalysed by protein kinases and phosphatases, respectively. There is a high degree of amino acid specificity so that serine/threonine kinases usually show essentially no cross-reactivity with tyrosine residues. Conversely the kinases and phosphatases that react with tyrosine residues do not usually react with serine or threonine residues. The enzymes which are specific for either serine/threonine or tyrosine residues are inhibited by different compounds: this is used in their identification, as are antibodies capable of distinguishing the phosphoamino acids. The catalytic domain of tyrosyl phosphatases bear no resemblance to those of serine/threonine phosphatases or of the alkaline or acid phosphatases. The symbol Ⓟ is an abbreviation for phosphate.

account for the major fraction of the 10% of the proteins which are phosphorylated at any given time in a mammalian cell. Indeed, until 1980, only phosphoserine and phosphothreonine had been identified as naturally occurring phosphoamino acids. Only about 0.1% of the phosphorylated proteins contain phosphotyrosine residues. However, the relatively long side chain of phosphotyrosine, together with the unusual negative electron density of its aromatic ring (Fig. 2.3), makes tyrosine phosphorylation a particularly distinctive molecular switch. As is discussed in more detail below, tyrosine phosphorylation plays a particularly prominent role in signal transmission for hormones such as insulin and growth hormone.

Phosphorylation of tyrosine not only activates the recipient protein but can also create important 'docking' sites for subsequent protein/protein interactions. This is due to complementary conserved protein modules, known as SH2 and SH3 domains, on the docking proteins. These are approximately 100 amino acids long and contain a crucially positioned arginine (Arg-175) which facilitates binding to phosphotyrosine but not phosphoserine or phosphothreonine residues. The relatively long side chain of phosphotyrosine provides the appropriate length to dock into the grooves of the SH2/SH3 domains or the catalytic clefts of tyrosine phosphatases.

SH2/SH3 domains, with their highly distinctive molecular topologies, can be found in a diverse array of cytoplasmic signalling proteins. As detailed later, they are important for the docking of inactive, soluble tyrosine kinases to receptors which are anchored in the plasma membrane but which have been activated by hormone binding. These domains also play a more 'passive' role where they appear to link signalling proteins within a phosphorylation cascade. An appropriate analogy for this would be the use of 'adaptor' plugs or even transformers when connecting electrical equipment.

Cell surface receptors and intracellular signalling

There are two major groups of cell surface receptors linked to intracellular signals (Fig. 2.1). The first relies upon tyrosine kinase for the initiation of the downstream signals. The second major group is linked to G-proteins. These generate intracellular messages which activate pathways which preferentially utilize serine/threonine kinases.

Tyrosine kinase linked cell surface receptors

These have a relatively simple transmembrane segment and either (i) have intrinsic tyrosine kinase activity located in the cytosolic domain or (ii) recruit tyrosine kinases subsequent to receptor activation by the binding of the hormone (Fig. 2.1).

Receptors with integrated tyrosine kinase activity

The most prominent member of this subgroup from an endocrine perspective is the receptor for insulin. However, these receptors typically bind ligands such as epidermal growth factor (EGF) or fibroblast growth factor (FGF) which stimulate cell growth and proliferation and are therefore frequently referred to as 'growth factor receptors'. The receptor for insulin-like growth factor 1 (IGF 1) is also a member of this subgroup.

The fundamental structure of these receptors is as depicted in Fig. 2.2. For ligands such as EGF and FGF, receptor occupancy is followed by dimerization of two adjacent monomeric receptors. Such dimerization of ligand-coupled receptors is a well recognized phenomenon. This then leads to activation of the tyrosine kinase which is integrated into the structure of the cytosolic domain. In contrast, both the receptor for insulin and IGF 1 pre-exist in their unoccupied state as preformed dimers (Fig. 2.5). However again, occupancy of the ligand-binding pocket formed by the two alpha subunits, by one molecule of insulin or IGF 1, results in activation of the tyrosine kinase integrated into the structure of the cytosolic domain.

Signalling pathways activated by insulin. The earliest response to insulin binding to its receptor is autophospho-

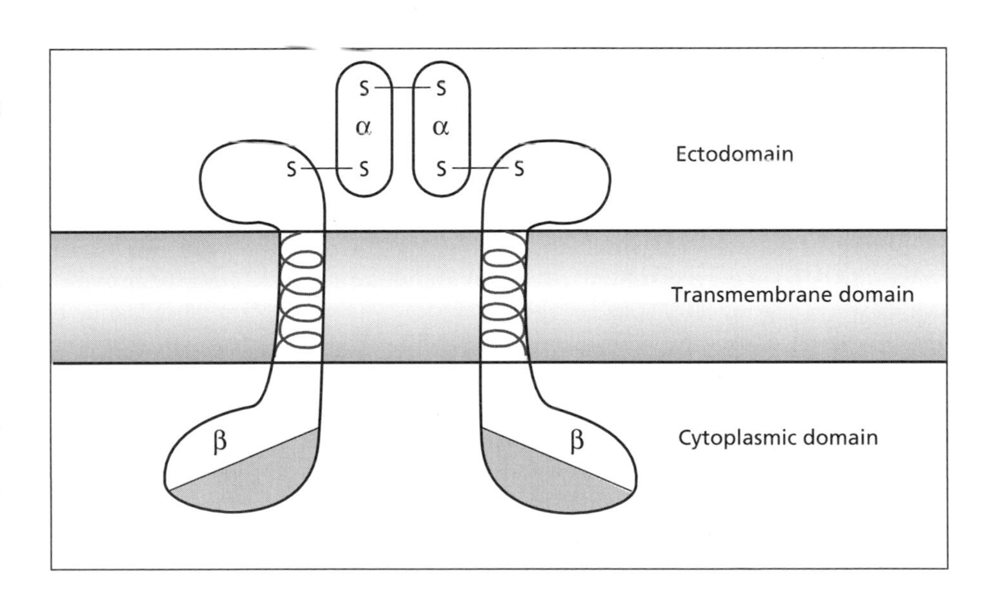

Figure 2.5 Outline structure of the insulin receptor. The receptor is a heterotetrameric structure comprised of 2α and 2β subunits as shown. Both subunits are derived from a single amino acid chain precursor. The molecular weight of the holoreceptor is ~400 kDa. One molecule of insulin binds to the ectodomain. The N-terminus of the first third of the β-subunit (193 amino acids) lies on the extracellular side of the membrane. The transmembrane domain consists of 23 hydrophobic amino acids organized in an α-helix whilst the cytoplasmic domain (402 amino acids) accounts for approximately two-thirds of the β-subunit. The integrated tyrosine kinase domain is indicated by the hatched area of the cytoplasmic domain. The structure of the receptor for IGF-I, but not IGF-II, is similar to that of the insulin receptor. There is homology between both the insulin and IGF-I receptors and the structure of IgG. The number of insulin receptors on insulin target cells is very variable (100–200 000) with adipocytes and hepatocytes expressing the highest numbers.

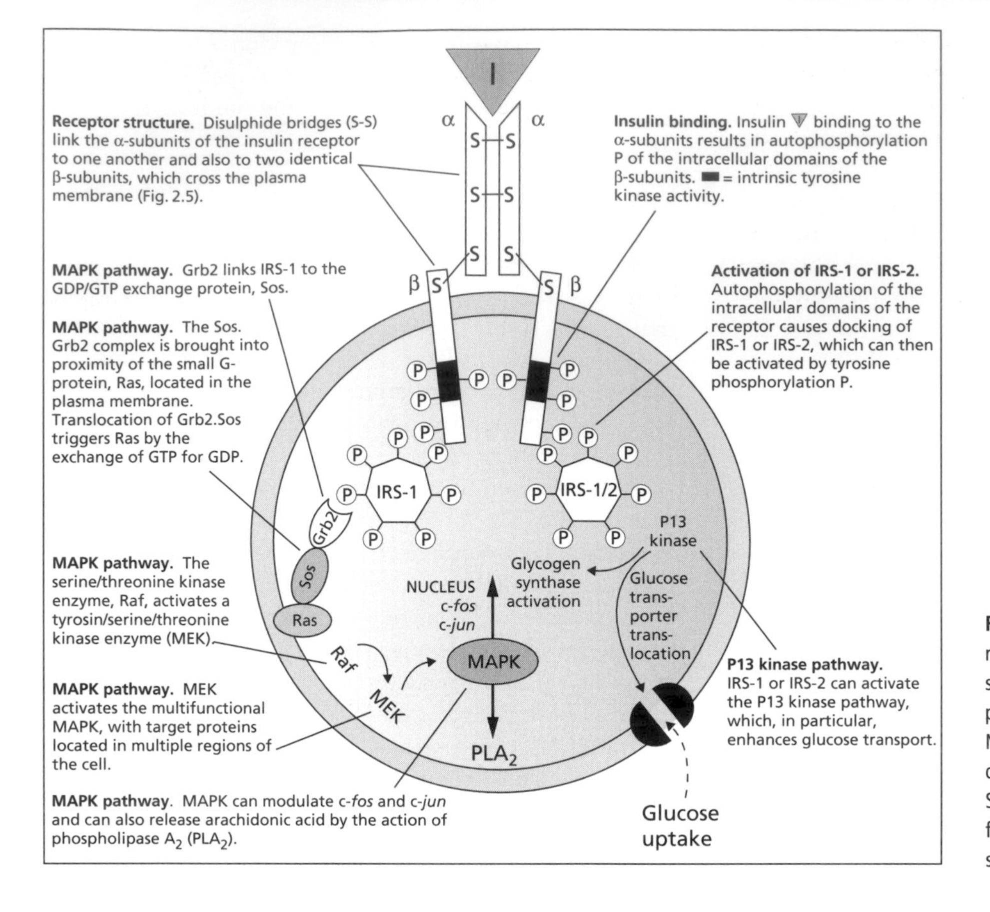

Figure 2.6 The insulin receptor: an example of a receptor with intrinsic tyrosine kinase activity, showing the major intracellular signalling pathways which may be activated by insulin. Note: there is also a well-recognized pathway, not dependant on IRS-1, for stimulation of Grb2, via Shc (src homology collagen-like protein), which, for the sake of clarity of representation, is not shown.

rylation of the cytosolic domain of the β-subunits themselves (Fig. 2.6). This initiates a complex series of response cascades that involve over 50 enzymes. The receptor's tyrosine kinase next phosphorylates a key substrate, namely Insulin Receptor Substrate 1 or 2 (IRS 1 or 2). This phosphorylation is thought to be essential for almost all subsequent biological actions of insulin. IRS-1 is a 131-kDa protein which itself has 21 potential tyrosine phosphorylation sites, at least 8 of which are phosphorylated by the activated insulin receptors.

Multiple phosphorylation of IRS-1 leads to the docking of several proteins with SH-2 domains, and the activation of divergent intracellular signalling pathways. For example, docking of the p85 subunit of phosphatidylinositol-3-kinase (PI 3-kinase) leads to regulation of glucose transporter translocation. There is a superfamily of glucose transporters (GLUT 1–4 and SGLT 1). In the prime organs of insulin action, such as adipose tissue and skeletal or cardiac muscle, the predominant isoform is GLUT 4. This is a 520-amino acid protein which spans the membrane 12 times and catalyses glucose uptake into the cell. Insulin binding to its receptor leads to translocation of GLUT 4 from intracellular vesicles to the cell membrane. After removal of bound insulin, the transporter returns to the intracellular pool. A branch point in this pathway leads to increased glycogen synthase activity with consequent enhancement in glycogen synthesis together with increased gene expression for hexokinase-2 in these tissues. Reduced glycogen synthase and hexokinase-2 has been observed in muscle biopsies from noninsulin-dependent diabetes melitus (NIDDM) patients. In addition reduction in levels of IRS-1 and the p85 subunit of PI 3-kinase have been reported for these subjects.

The mitogenic effects of insulin are signalled via an alternative pathway which diverges from phosphorylated IRS-1. Instead of binding to the SH2 domains of PI 3-kinase it docks with the SH2/SH3 domains of the growth factor receptor-bound protein 2 (Grb 2 protein). This adaptor protein links tyrosine phosphorylated receptors or cytoplasmic tyrosine kinases to regulators of small G-protein activity (Fig. 2.6). In this particular pathway, Grb 2 links IRS-1 to the GDP/GTP exchange protein, Sos (Son of sevenless protein). In turn, this brings the Sos.Grb2 complex into the proximity of the small G-protein, Ras, located as depicted in the plasma membrane (Fig. 2.6). This triggers Ras by the exchange of GTP for GDP.

Ras activation stimulates a downstream cascade in which serine/threonine kinases, such as Raf, play an important role, with the latter activating a tyrosine/serine/threonine kinase (MEK) which subsequently activates a multifunctional serine/threonine kinase which is of central importance. This was originally named microtubule-associated protein kinase. However in recognition of its broader role, it is now more commonly referred to as mitogen-activated protein kinase (MAP kinase). This kinase has target proteins located in multiple regions of the cell that are coupled to both cytoplasmic and nuclear responses. The latter lead to stimulation of gene expression, protein synthesis and cell growth.

Defects in the insulin receptor/signalling pathways and consequent insulin resistance syndromes. Over 50 different mutations in the insulin receptor itself have been reported. There are three associated congenital syndromes of severe insulin resistance which are, in ascending order of clinical severity, Type A insulin resistance, Rabson–Mendenhall syndrome and Leprachaunism/Donahues syndrome. As would be expected, all patients have impaired glucose metabolism together with raised insulin concentrations. Whereas patients with Type A insulin resistance are usually not diagnosed until puberty, at the other end of the spectrum, namely Leprachaunism, there is severe intrauterine growth retardation and the patients rarely survive beyond the first year of life. This extreme form of insulin resistance is considered to arise because of the absence of any functional insulin receptors. In contrast, Rabson–Mendenhall syndrome is probably the result of mutations which result in a severely defective, but not totally inactive, insulin receptor. Some patients with Type A Insulin Resistance have mutations clustering in the tyrosine kinase domain of the receptor. The majority of Type A patients have normal insulin receptors. These patients may harbour as yet unidentified mutations in any of the other critical insulin signalling molecules indicated in Fig. 2.6.

Receptors which recruit tyrosine kinase activity

The best known endocrine members in this second subgroup of receptors are those for growth hormone (GH), prolactin (PRL) and leptin. These hormones, together with cytokines such as the interleukins and erythropoietin share a common major structural feature in that they have 4 long alpha—helices arranged in an antiparallel fashion. As a consequence, this subgroup is commonly referred to as the cytokine/haemopoietic receptors. There are at least 20 members, all of which share the basic receptor structure shown in Fig. 2.2. The ectodomain which binds the ligand is about 200 amino acids long and is the region of major homology. It has several conserved features and a characteristic ligand-binding pocket formed from two barrel-like modules. The cytoplasmic regions are variable in length and exhibit only limited similarities. However one motif, which is found close to the membrane and is known as Box 1 is relatively highly conserved. This appears to be particularly important for the stimulation of mitogenic activity in the target cells.

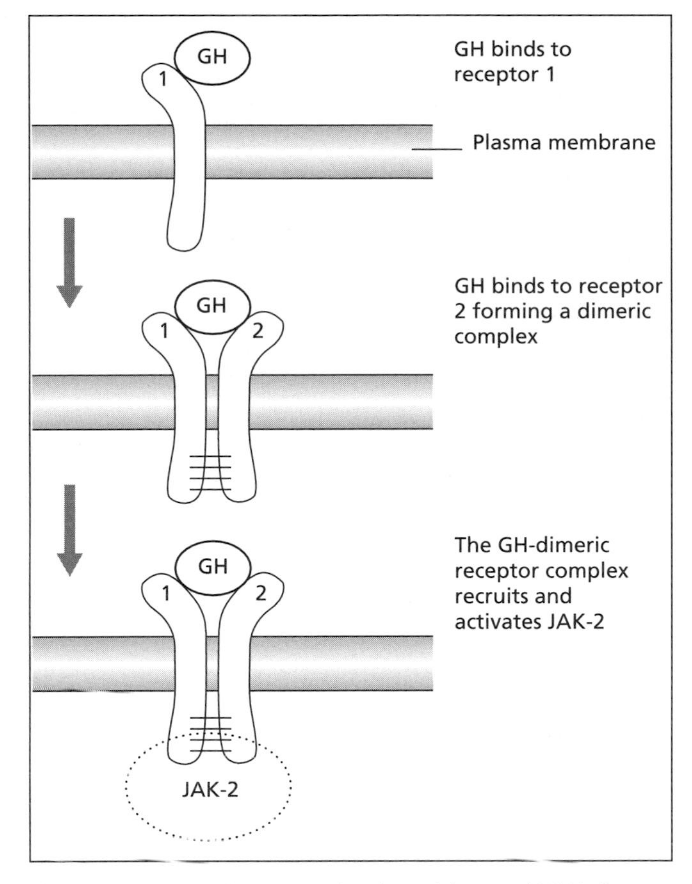

Figure 2.7 Diagrammatic representation of growth hormone (GH) binding to its cell-surface receptors and, via the formation of receptor dimers, subsequently recruiting Janus Associated Kinase 2 (JAK-2). The two receptors depicted (1 and 2) have identical structures.

GH and PRL signalling pathways. The co-crystal structure of human GH with its receptor was analysed in 1992 and shown to be a ternary complex consisting of a single molecule of the hormone and two receptors. Parallel studies using mutational analysis of residues in the hormone revealed that each molecule of GH had two different sites, each of which can bind to the receptor. Moreover the formation of the signal-transducing complex is sequential. Thus after GH has bound to one molecule of receptor, this is followed by association of this complex with a second receptor molecule (Fig. 2.7). The dimerization of the cytoplasmic region in the ternary complex is particularly important for signal transduction. Such receptor homodimerization has also been reported for PRL and erythropoietin. However further studies with cytokines generally, have shown that this homodimerization model in fact only

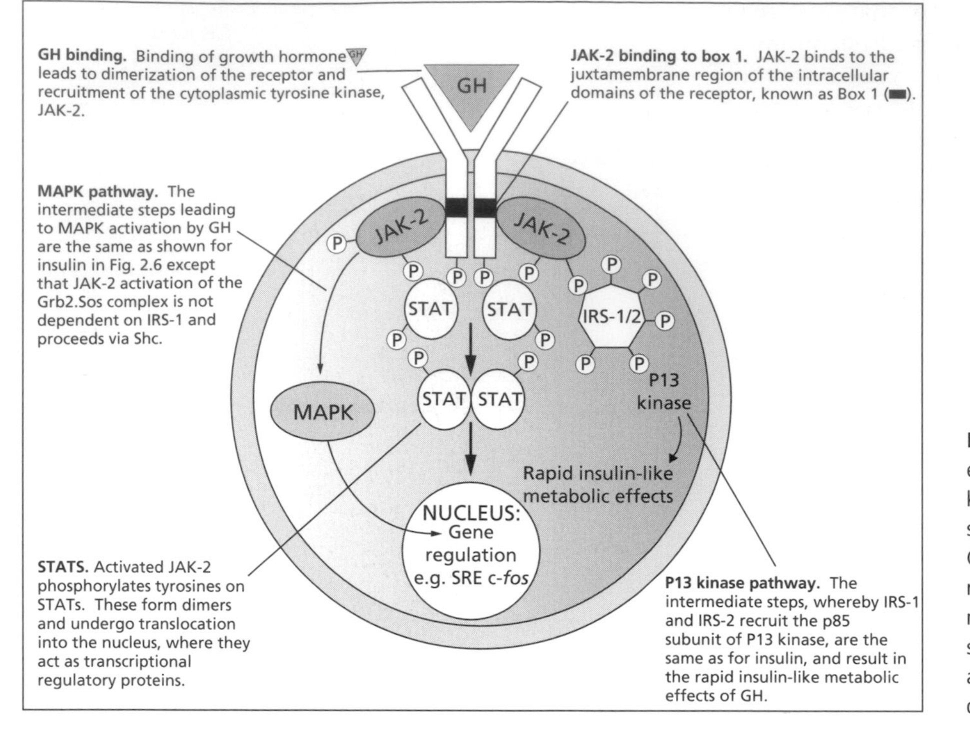

Figure 2.8 The growth hormone receptor: an example of a receptor which recruits tyrosine kinase activity, showing the major intracellular signalling pathways which may be activated by GH. SRE's (specific response elements) are MAPK-responsive upstream regulating sequences, which mediate the induction of early response genes, such as *c-fos*. These events contribute to the ability of GH to promote cell growth and differentiation.

applies to a minority of cytokine receptors. The majority form heterodimers and oligomers with diverse cytoplasmic proteins.

(i) *Tyrosine kinase recruitment.* Although cytokine receptors themselves contain no identifiable enzymatic motifs which could function as tyrosine kinases, cytokines such as interleukins 2 and 3 together with GH and PRL rapidly induce tyrosine phosphorylation of proteins, including regions of the cytoplasmic domain itself. Within a few minutes of exposure of the target cells to the extracellular stimulators, tyrosine phosphorylation can be detected. Indeed, using cross-linking and immunoprecipitation techniques, it was deduced that tyrosine kinase was not only stimulated by GH occupancy of its receptor but that the kinase activity was also closely associated with the receptor. This kinase, which was recruited by dimerized receptors, was identified as Janus Associated Kinase-2 (JAK-2) (Fig. 2.8).

(ii) *Janus Associated Kinases.* When first identified the JAK family of kinases were 'orphan kinases' since their regulators and functions were not then known; accordingly they were first named JAK for 'just another kinase'. However the 4 members of the family (JAK1–3 and Tyk-2) were eventually shown to contain as a distinctive structural feature, two tandem kinase domains, which were located at their carboxy terminals. Because of this they were renamed Janus Associated Kinase, after the Roman deity Janus who had two faces.

These cytosolic kinases are 120–135 kDa proteins which are 40% identical. Kinase activity is due to a JH1 domain at the C-terminus, and there is a second JH2 domain which, whilst being similar to known kinases, lacks a motif for ATP-binding: this may regulate JH1 activity. They are devoid of SH2/SH3 domains and the details of the mechanism by which they are recruited by the occupied cytokine receptors have yet to be established. GH and PRL receptors both recruit JAK-2 as does erythropoietin (Fig. 2.8) although there is some evidence that JAK-2 is constitutively associated with the PRL receptor. For GH and PRL receptors, a proline-rich docking site in the cytoplasmic domain, named Box 1, is key for JAK-2 association and subsequent activation. It is probable that the close association of the cytoplasmic domains of the dimerized receptors brings together the two JAK-2 molecules and that this allows cross-phosphorylation of each catalytic domain.

(iii) *STATs.* The major JAK substrates are, apart from themselves and the cytokine receptors, the so-called STAT proteins. These are latent transcription factor proteins, which contain 700–800 residues and share 30–40% identity. A crucial tyrosine residue is located in the carboxy terminal in a homologous position in all STAT proteins (residue 694), and phosphorylation of this is essential for STAT-activation. STAT proteins have dual functions: (i) *s*ignal *t*ransduction in the cytoplasm, followed by (ii) *a*ctivation of *t*ranscription in the nucleus. The family members of STAT proteins have been named in the order of their identification. Both GH and PRL, together with erythropoietin, induce tyrosine phosphorylation of STAT proteins 1, 3, 5a and 5b but STAT 5 is probably the major axis of the JAK-STAT cascade. STAT phosphorylation is also an early response and can be detected within minutes of exposure of the target cells to these hormones.

SH2 domains on STAT proteins allow them to dock onto crucially positioned phosphotyrosines on the cytokine receptors (Fig. 2.8). The STAT proteins are themselves then phosphorylated by the JAK proteins which have been recruited by the ligand occupied receptors. Phosphorylated STAT proteins then dissociate from the occupied receptor/kinase complex and form dimers, to give homo- or heterodimers in the cytosol. Dimerization appears to be essential for their final translocation to the nucleus. Here they activate immediate early response genes which regulate proliferation, or more specific genes which determine the differentiation status of the target cell.

(iv) *Alternative pathways*. GH and PRL do not activate their target cells exclusively via the JAK/STAT pathway. As shown in Fig. 2.8, occupancy can also lead to stimulation of the MAPK and PI 3-kinase pathways. This overlapping of signalling pathways for GH and insulin may account for the acute insulin-like effects of GH.

Defects in the GH receptor/signalling pathways and consequent GH resistance syndromes. Resistance to GH was first reported by Laron in 1966. Since then, severe resistance to GH, characterized by grossly impaired growth despite normal or elevated GH levels in serum, has been termed Laron syndrome (Fig. 2.9). Molecular genetic investigations have shown that this disorder is mainly associated with mutations in the gene for the GH receptor. These can result in defective hormone binding to the ectodomain or reduced efficiency of dimerization of the receptor after hormone occupancy. It is an autosomal recessive disorder and it is now appreciated that there is a range of phenotypic presentations.

As might be expected (see Chapter 3), exceptionally low levels of circulating IGF-1 and its principal carrier protein, insulin-like growth factor binding protein 3, are also observed in Laron syndrome. Thus the patients themselves form an *in vivo* bioassay for GH suggesting that either the GH, which was present at a high concentration in the circulation, was bioinactive, or that the receptor/signalling pathway was nonresponsive. The finding that the administration of exogenous fully bioactive GH to Laron syndrome patients failed to elevate IGF-1 levels supported the latter hypothesis. This was confirmed after the cloning of the gene for the GH receptor and the subsequent identification of multiple mutation sites in the gene in Laron patients.

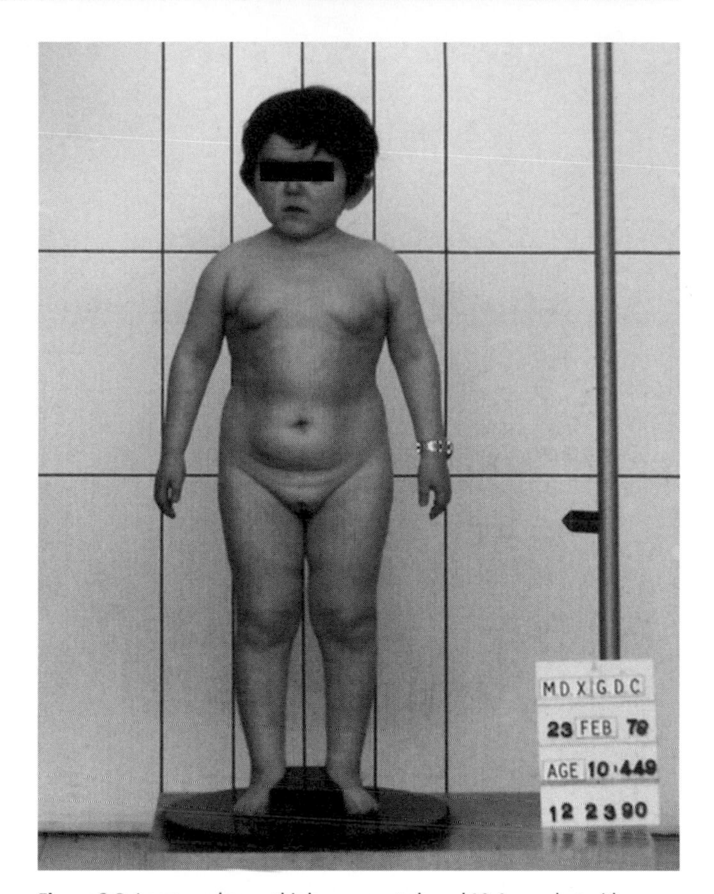

Figure 2.9 Laron syndrome: this boy presented aged 10.4 years but with a height of only 95 cm, which is equivalent to that of a 3-year-old. Note the prominent forehead, depressed nasal bridge, under-development of the mandible, truncle obesity and a very small penis. These features could have been a manifestation of severe growth hormone (GH) deficiency but the concentration in a basal serum sample was elevated (15.6 mU GH/L). However the additional finding that the serum IGF-1 concentration was undetectable, despite the elevated GH, was consistent with a diagnosis of Laron syndrome which is due to nonfunctioning receptors for GH.

The gene for the GH receptor contains 10 exons. Relatively early on, in 1989, large deletions were detected in exons 3, 5 and 6 in two Laron syndrome patients. Since exons 2–7 encode the signal peptide and the ectodomain of the GH receptor, and thus affect receptor binding, it was predictable that such large gene deletions at these loci would result in GH-resistance.

The majority of defects reported subsequent to this early study have identified point mutations, i.e. the alteration of a single nucleotide in the DNA to another. Nonsense, missense, splice and frameshift mutations have now been reported in exons 4 and 7, which will again affect the extracellular domain of the receptor for GH.

As previously mentioned (Fig. 2.2), the ectodomain of the GH receptor can be identified in the circulation where

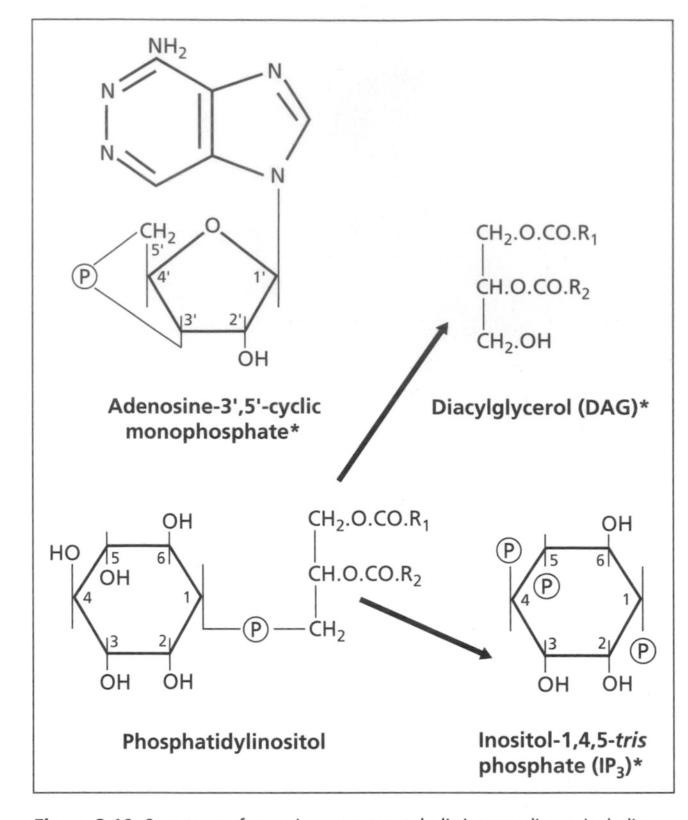

Figure 2.10 Structures of some important metabolic intermediates, including 'second messengers' (which are marked by an asterisk,*), involved in the mechanism of hormone action. The symbol Ⓟ is the abbreviation for phosphate, PO^{-}_{4}. Numbers close to the angles of the carbohydrate rings show the chemical numbering convention used to identify substituents attached at these positions. R_1 and R_2 represent fatty acid chains, e.g. $(CH_2)_kCH_3$, where k is variable and there may be 12 or more carbon atoms in the chain. In addition, there are usually one or two unsaturated bonds such as CH ═ CH also present.

it forms a GH-binding protein (GHBP). Normal levels of GHBP together with suspected Laron syndrome, would suggest that the defect was occurring post-receptor binding. It is significant therefore that patients with normal GHBP levels typically exhibit a milder phenotype: in fact 20–25% of Laron patients now fall into this category. For example, a missense mutation in the ectodomain which is not part of the GH binding site has been shown to result in defective receptor dimerization despite unimpaired GH binding. Moreover mutations in exons 8–10 occur, which affect the transmembrane or cytosolic domains giving rise to inefficient or absent interactions with JAK-2 and consequently impaired intracellular signalling. On the other hand, Laron patients are recognized who have no apparent mutation in the gene coding for GH receptors. It is possible that their defect could be attributed to mutations in genes regulating downstream signalling. Furthermore, a partial deletion in the gene coding for IGF-1, which would render the GH-IGF 1 axis ineffective, has been associated with a condition exhibiting severe intrauterine growth retardation followed by postnatal growth failure, sensorineural deafness, GH resistance and mild mental retardation.

Table 2.2 Examples of G-protein coupled receptors

Hormone	Dominant G-protein α-subunit(s)
Thyrotrophin-releasing hormone	$G_q\alpha$
Corticotrophin-releasing hormone	$G_s\alpha$
Gonadotrophin-releasing hormone	$G_q\alpha$
Somatostatin	$G_i\alpha/G_q\alpha$
Thyroid-stimulating hormone	$G_s\alpha/G_q\alpha$
Luteinizing hormone/human chorionic gonadotrophin	$G_s\alpha/G_q\alpha$
Follicle-stimulating hormone	$G_s\alpha/G_q\alpha$
Adrenocorticotrophic hormone	$G_s\alpha$
Oxytocin	$G_q\alpha$
Vasopressin	$G_s\alpha/G_q\alpha$
Catecholamines (β-adrenergic)	$G_s\alpha$
Angiotensin II	$G_i\alpha/G_q\alpha$
Glucagon	$G_s\alpha$
Calcium	$G_q\alpha/G_i\alpha$
Calcitonin	$G_s\alpha/G_i\alpha/G_q\alpha$
Parathyroid hormone (PTH)/ PTH-related peptide (PTHrp)	$G_s\alpha/G_q\alpha$
Prostaglandin E_2	$G_s\alpha$

Note: for somatostatin, vasopressin, angiotensin II, calcitonin and PTH/PTHrp, different receptor subtypes determine α-subunit specificity, and there may be differential tissue distributions of these receptor subtypes. This phenomenon provides opportunities to develop selective therapeutic antagonists.

G-protein coupled receptors (GPCRs)

Receptor Structure

The second major group of cell surface receptors are those which couple with G(guanine)-proteins associated with the inner surface of the cell membrane (Fig. 2.1). This leads to the generation of intracellular second messengers such as cyclic adenosine monophosphate (cAMP) and inositol 1,4,5-tris phosphate (IP_3) (Fig. 2.10). This is the largest of the cell surface receptor groups with over 140 members. Some are listed on Fig. 2.1 and in Table 2.2. Other extracellular receptors, including glutamate, thrombin, odourants and those responsible for the visual transduction of light also act via GPCRs. Although the fundamental design of these receptors is as depicted in Fig. 2.2, the most striking structural difference from the tyrosine kinase linked receptor group discussed under Section A, lies in the transmembrane region. This takes the form of an elaborate

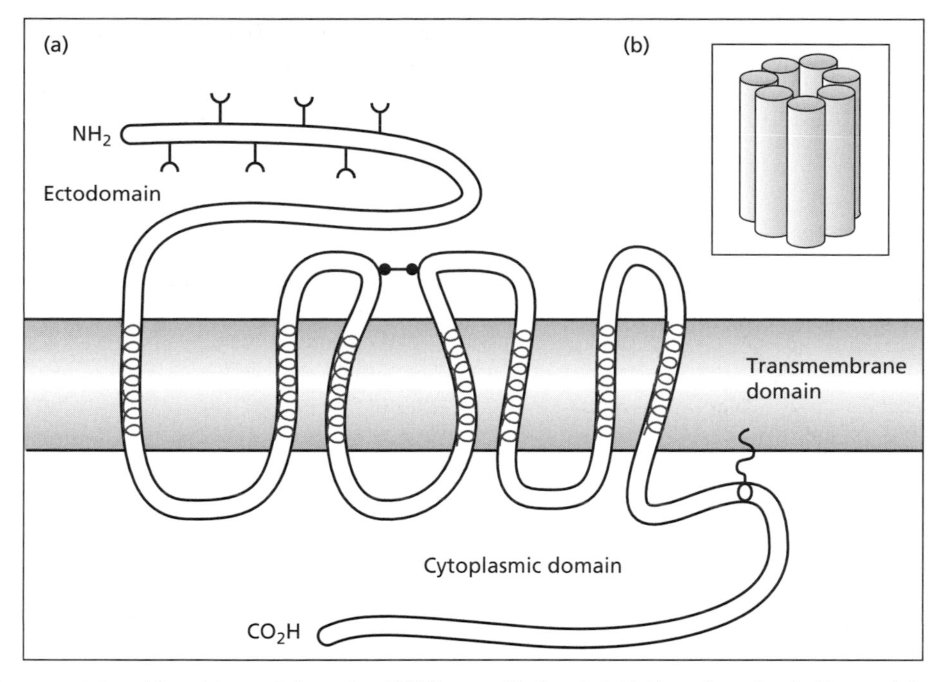

Figure 2.11 A schematic representation of G-protein coupled receptors (GPCR) showing the 7 transmembrane domains. (a) The structure is an elaborate variation of the 3 segment design depicted in Fig. 2.2. The size of the N-terminal ectodomain is generally in proportion to the size of the cognate ligand, except that the Ca^{2+} receptor has an unexpectedly large ectodomain. In the ectodomain, which obviously plays a key role in ligand binding, homology is lower than among the transmembrane and cyotoplasmic domains. For example, for the TSH, LH/hCG and FSH receptors, homology in the ectodomain is only 35–45%, but is far higher in the midregions. The ectodomain can be heavily glycosylated; this may contribute to as much as 40% of its mass. The ligand binding site is highly conformational with several discontinuous elements contributing to the binding. The transmembrane domain has a characteristic heptahelical structure, most of which is embedded in the plasma membrane and provides a hydrophobic core. An intraloop disulphide bridge between the second and third extracellular loops may be formed by conserved cysteine residues, as shown. The cytoplasmic domain links the receptor to the signal-transducing G-proteins. For the β-adrenergic receptor it has been shown that specific regions in the third intracellular loop together with sections of the C-terminal tail are critical for G-protein coupling. (b) Showing the rearrangement of the 7 transmembrane α-helices to form a hydrophobic pore.

serpentine membrane-spanning structure, which crosses the lipid bilayer of the plasma membrane 7 times (Fig. 2.11a). The conserved hydrophobic transmembrane helices which make up this domain can be arranged to create a hydrophobic pore (Fig. 2.11b).

The size of the GPCR ranges from that for gonadotrophin releasing hormone, with only 337 amino acid residues to the largest, which is the calcium sensing receptor which has 1085 residues. The latter has an extended ectodomain (613 amino acids) which appears to bind Ca^{2+} with a low affinity compared to the classical hormone receptors. This would be consistent with the higher concentration of Ca^{2+} relative to that of hormones.

Coupling to plasma membrane G-proteins. G-proteins are key participants in cell activation by GPCR. The linking G-proteins are the larger members of a superfamily of regulatory proteins which function as molecular switches by binding and then hydrolysing GTP to GDP. The Ras protein (Fig. 2.6) was an example of the smaller membrane-associated G-proteins.

Hormone occupancy of a GPCR results in conformational changes in the receptor which are transmitted across the plasma membrane and so alter the extent and/or nature of receptor interaction with G-proteins. This is brought about by contacts between the intracellular loops and the C-terminal tail of the receptor and specific regions of the G-protein complex. This results in GTP exchange for GDP on the G-protein. The activated proteins then undergo major structural modifications and ultimately modulate the catalytic activity of adenylate cyclase or phospholipase C (PLC) within the membrane structure (Fig. 2.12).

The G-protein hetero-trimeric complex in action

In their resting state, the G-proteins exist as heterotrimeric complexes with α, β and γ subunits. The oligomer has a molecular weight of about 90 000 with the α, β and γ subunits each contributing approximately 45 000, 35 000 and 5000, respectively. In practice the β and γ subunits associate with such a high affinity that the functional units are $G\alpha$ and $G\beta/\gamma$ (Fig. 2.13). In the absence of a hormone-

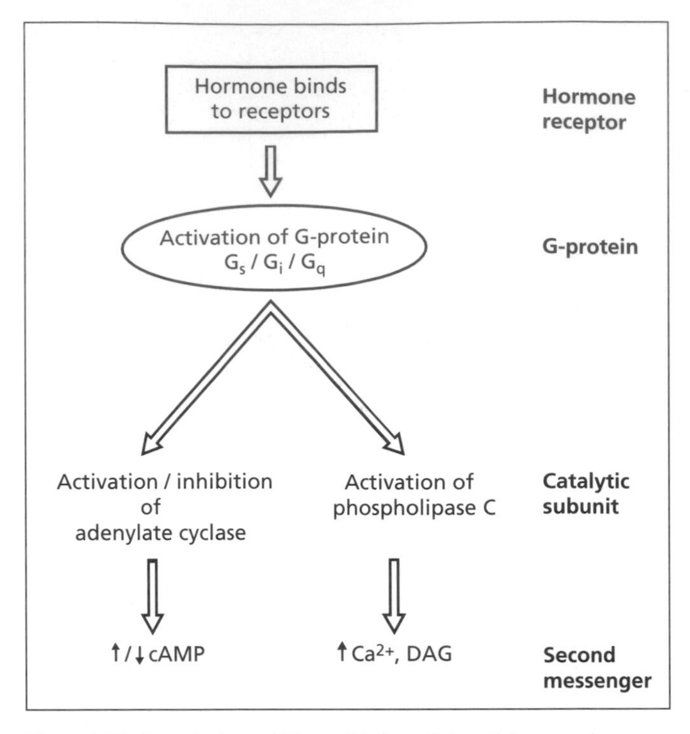

Figure 2.12 General scheme of the modulation of intracellular second messengers by hormonal activation of G-protein–linked cell-surface receptors. Note that, for a given hormone or extracellular modulator, the two alternative pathways are not mutually exclusive, and they may in fact interact.

occupied and activated receptor these complexes form a 'G-protein pool' within the membrane.

After association of the G-protein complex with the occupied receptor, conformational changes in the α-subunit lead to an increased rate of dissociation of GDP which is replaced by GTP. This guanine nucleotide exchange in turn causes the α-subunit to dissociate from the heterotrimeric complex. The liberated α-subunit, together with its activating GTP then binds to a downstream catalytic unit which is either adenylate cyclase or PLC (Fig. 2.12).

G Subunits. Although there are now known to be over 20 isoforms of the Gα subunit, these may be grouped into 4 major subfamilies which have great functional significance. These are $G_s\alpha$ and $G_i\alpha$, which activate or inhibit adenylate cyclase, respectively, $G_q\alpha$ which activates PLC and $G_o\alpha$ which activates ion channels (Fig. 2.12). A given

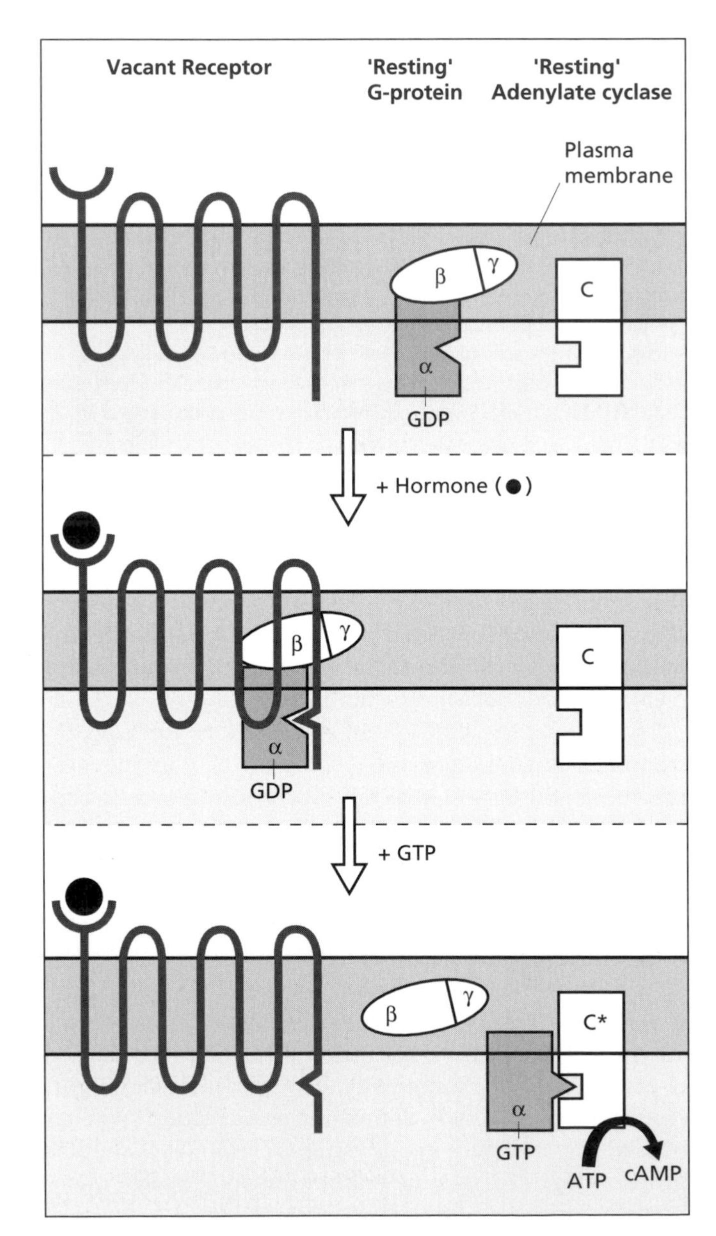

Figure 2.13 (right) A diagrammatic representation of G-protein-modulated activation of a membrane-bound enzyme, such as adenylate cyclase. A hormone, such as adrenaline, binds to the extracellular region of the receptor. The third intracellular loop and the C terminus of the receptor then associates with a G-protein, which has three subunits named α, β, and γ. This leads to displacement of guanosine diphosphate (GDP) by guanosine triphosphate (GTP) and dissociation of the activated G-protein from the hormone–receptor complex. This results in release of the α-subunit from the heterotrimer, and the GTP-activated α-subunit of the G-protein subsequently diffuses in the lipid bilayer and binds to the catalytic subunit. This induces a conformational change, which activates C to C*, and the generation of many molecules of cyclic adenosine 5′-monophosphate (cAMP). As explained in the text, the entire system is reversible. Because of the interactions between the G-protein and the nucleotides, it is sometimes referred to as a nucleotide regulatory complex, when the abbreviation 'N-complex' is then used. It is important to note that variants of the basic model shown in this figure have been proposed. Also, there is a plant-derived diterpene, known as forskolin, which directly activates the catalytic subunit, and acts independently of G-proteins. This action has been important in establishing the independence of the catalytic subunit for adenylate cyclase. As might be predicted from the model shown, forskolin is a ubiquitous stimulator of adenylate cyclase activity.

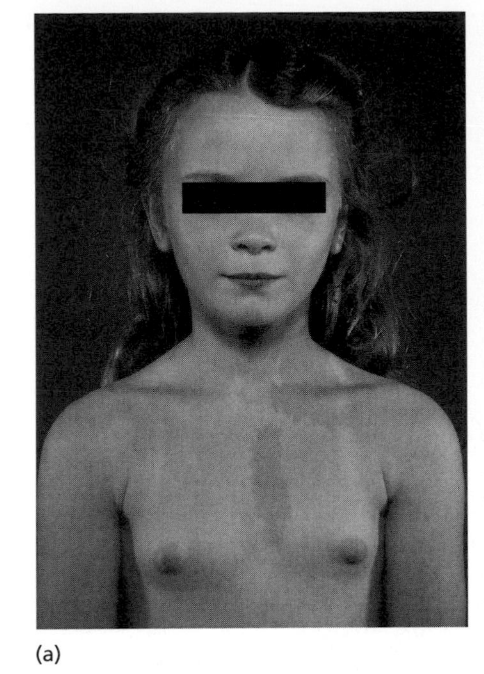

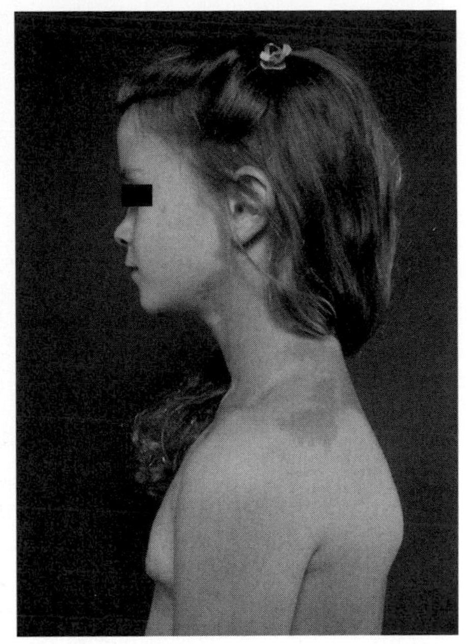

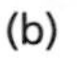

Figure 2.14 McCune–Albright syndrome: at 6 years of age, this girl presented with breast development (Fig. 2.14a) and vaginal bleeding. However, gonadotrophin concentrations were undetectable. Skin pigmentation was also noticeable (Fig. 2.14a & b). The latter was due to a gain in $G_s\alpha$ function, which would normally be stimulated by MSH, in the skin. Similarly, the early breast development was because of an analogous gain in $G_s\alpha$ function, and consequent constitutive activation, in the ovary. In some cases, but not this particular one, gain of $G_s\alpha$ function can also be seen in bones, causing the condition known as fibrous dysplasia, the adrenals and the thyroid resulting in Cushing syndrome and thyrotoxicosis, respectively.

(a) (b)

receptor may interact with one or more of these family members as listed in Table 2.2. Of those listed, more than half can be seen to interact with more than one Gα subunit and thus moderate contrasting and sometimes apparently conflicting intracellular second messenger systems. This receptor promiscuity can be attributed to, amongst other things, different receptor subtypes. In the case of calcitonin these are differentially expressed at different stages of the cell cycle. On the other hand, the particular Gα subunit selected for coupling may depend upon the concentration of the hormone. For example, TSH, calcitonin and LH/hCG receptors activate adenylate cyclase at low concentrations, whilst with higher concentrations, $G_q\alpha$ is recruited to activate PLC.

Structural studies, using chimeric Gα subunits and mutagens, or deletion of residues in the C-terminus of the Gα subunit, emphasize the importance of this region in determining which Gα subunit is recruited by an activated receptor. In fact both the C-and N-termini of Gα subunits lie in close proximity to each other and face the plasma membrane, with its embedded Gβ/γ heterodimer, the receptor and the catalytic subunits. Anchorage to the membrane is provided by lipid modification of the C- and N-termini of Gα amongst other structural features.

Selection is of course a two-way process, and complementary structural features on the cytoplasmic domain of the receptor also determine which Gα subunit is coupled. The third intracellular loop and C-terminal tail are crucial for the coupling of $G_s\alpha$ subunits to the β-adrenergic receptor or $G_q\alpha$ to the angiotensin II receptors. Moreover, progressive truncations of the C-terminal tail of PTH receptors results in a decrease in Gα subunit selectivity. As might also be anticipated, using polypeptides corresponding to specific regions of the cytoplasmic domain of receptors, direct, receptorless activation of Gα has been obtained. Conversely, polypeptides have been synthesized which will block receptor/Gα subunit coupling and thus selectively inhibit endogenous signal transduction pathways.

Gα subunits can also function as a GTPase which cleaves a phosphate from the GTP, resulting in GαGDP. This endows the G-proteins with a mechanism for switching off their activation of the catalytic subunit. Hydrolysis of the GTP bound to Gα due to its intrinsic GTPase activity liberates the Gα subunit from the catalytic subunit and allows reassociation of GαGDP with the Gβ/γ. This newly reformed heterotrimer then returns to the G-protein pool in the membrane. In this way an individual G-protein complex is recycled, so that it can respond to another receptor.

G-protein and GPCR aberrations. There are several examples of endocrinopathies which occur due to activating or inactivating mutations of G-proteins or receptors coupled to them. Pseudohypoparathyroidism (Fig. 7.9) and Albright's Hereditory Osteodystrophy are associated with a loss of $G_s\alpha$ function whereas McCune–Albright Syndrome (Fig. 2.14) and some cases of acromegaly are linked to a gain in $G_s\alpha$ function and constitutive activation. The complex constellation of abnormalities can be explained in the terms of trophic hormones that raise intracellular cAMP and drive the function and proliferation of different endocrine organs. On the other hand nephrogenic diabetes insipidus can be the result of a

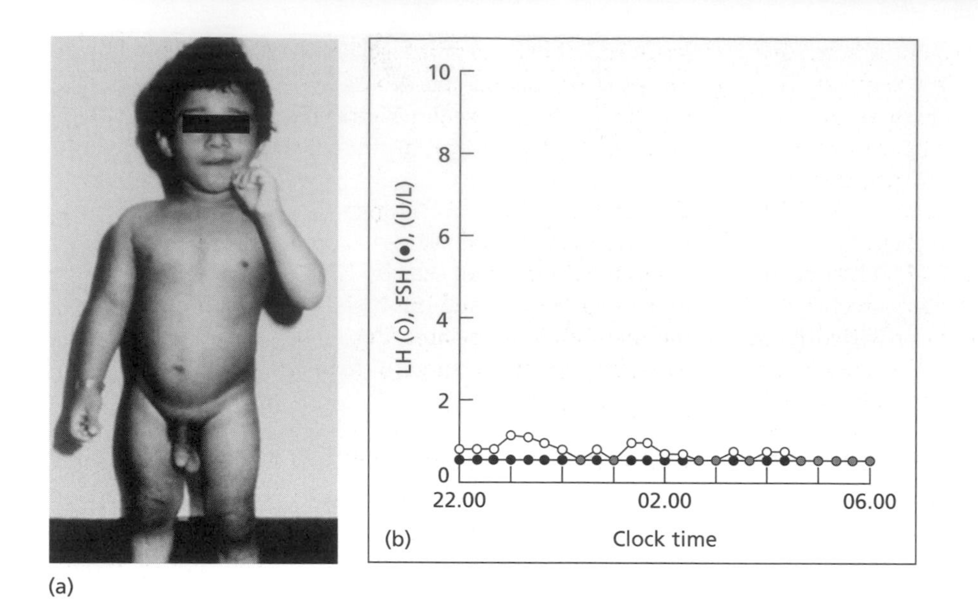

Figure 2.15 Familial male precocious puberty: this 2-year-old came from Pakistan with signs of precocious puberty. He was the size of a 4-year-old. His overnight gonadotrophin profile revealed undetectable concentrations of LH and FSH indicating that the testosterone was arising from antonomous function of the Leydig cells.

mutation in the GPCR itself. Germline mutations on *Xq2.8*, coding for the V2 receptor lead to a loss of receptor function so that circulating vasopressin, despite being very high, cannot increase urine concentration. Conversely familial male precocious puberty, or testotoxicosis (Fig. 2.15), which is an autonomous form of endocrine hyperfunction, occurs as a result of germline activating missense mutations in the gene for the LH receptor. Thus whereas GPCRs normally occur in a constrained, inhibited form, activating mutations presumably relieve crucial helix–helix interactions which are normally relieved only by hormone occupancy. Activating mutations in the transmembrane domain of the TSH receptor have been reported in toxic thyroid adenomas and a mutation in $G_s\alpha$ has been associated with autonomous thyroid nodules. In addition resistance to TSH has been attributed to mutations in the ectodomain of the TSH receptor.

Intracellular second messengers

cAMP. $G_s\alpha$ activates membrane bound adenylate cyclase which catalyses the conversion of ATP to the potent second messenger cAMP (Figs 2.12 and 2.13). This cyclic nucleotide in turn activates a cAMP dependent protein kinase (PKA) which modulates multiple aspects of cell function.

There are least 10 isoforms of adenylate cyclase. Each has 2 sets of 6 membrane-spanning domains together with 2 cytoplasmic domains. They differ in particular in their interaction with negative regulators such as $G_i\alpha$ and $G\beta/\gamma$.

cAMP reacts with a repressive regulatory subunit on PKA, which then dissociates from the holoenzyme and unmasks a catalytic site which phosphorylates serine and threonine residues (Fig. 2.16). Thus $G_s\alpha$ subunits, via cAMP and PKAs regulate major metabolic pathways,

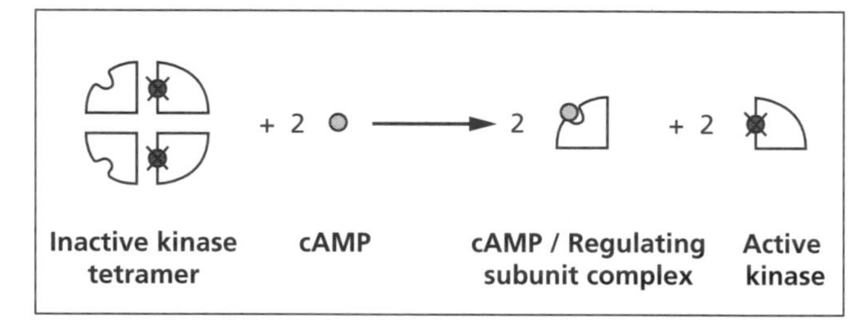

Figure 2.16 The activation of cyclic adenosine 5′-monophosphate (cAMP)-dependent protein kinase. Cyclic AMP binds to the regulatory subunits, and this frees activated kinase subunits.

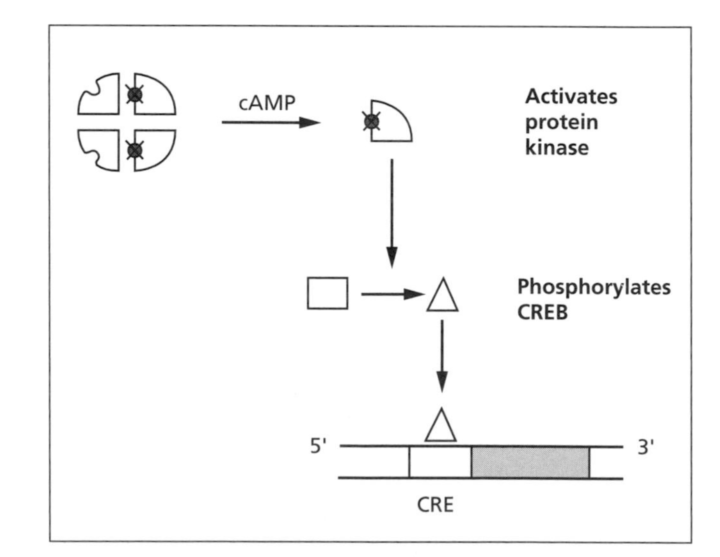

Figure 2.17 Cyclic adenosine 5′-monophosphate (cAMP) can activate the transcription of specific genes—for example, that for the peptide hormone somatostatin, via the cyclic AMP-response element-binding protein (CREB). The latter binds to the cAMP response element (CRE) and switches on transcription of the cAMP-inducible gene ▭. Thus CRE is the ultimate target for control of transcription by cAMP.

including those for lipolysis, glycogenolysis and steroidogenesis (Table 2.2). PKA phosphorylates a transcription factor called CREB (*c*AMP *r*esponse *e*lement *b*inding protein). This is then translocated to the nucleus where it binds to a short palindromic sequence in the promotor regions of cAMP-regulated genes referred to as CRE (*c*AMP *r*esponse *e*nhancer element) and thereby has a direct effect on gene transcription (Fig. 2.17). This mechanism mediates the induction of genes for somatostatin.

The major signal terminating system is provided by a large family of phosphodiesterases (PDEs) which can be activated by a variety of systems, including direct PKA phosphorylation. PDEs rapidly hydrolyse cAMP to the inactive 5′AMP and thereby close a feedback loop. In addition, cAMP activated PKA, PKC and other more recently identified receptor kinases (GRKs) may phosphorylate serine and threonine residues in the intracellular loop and the C-terminal tail of GPCR which leads to receptor desensitization. An increase in a particular GRK, directed at the β-adrenergic receptor, has been reported in patients suffering from chronic heart failure.

Diacylglycerol and Ca^{2+}. More than 20 different extracellular regulators, including TRH, GnRH and oxytocin, stimulate their target cells by GPCR which recruit G proteins with the $G_q\alpha$ subunit (Table 2.2). The latter activates the membrane associated PLC. This enzyme, which has 3 major isoforms (β, γ and α) catalyses the reaction

$$PIP_2 \rightarrow DAG + IP_3$$

where PIP_2 is phosphatidylinositol 4,5—bisphosphate and DAG is diacylglycerol (Fig. 2.10). PIP_2 is a minor membrane phospholipid, accounting for less than 1% of the total phopholipids in the plasma membrane. DAG and

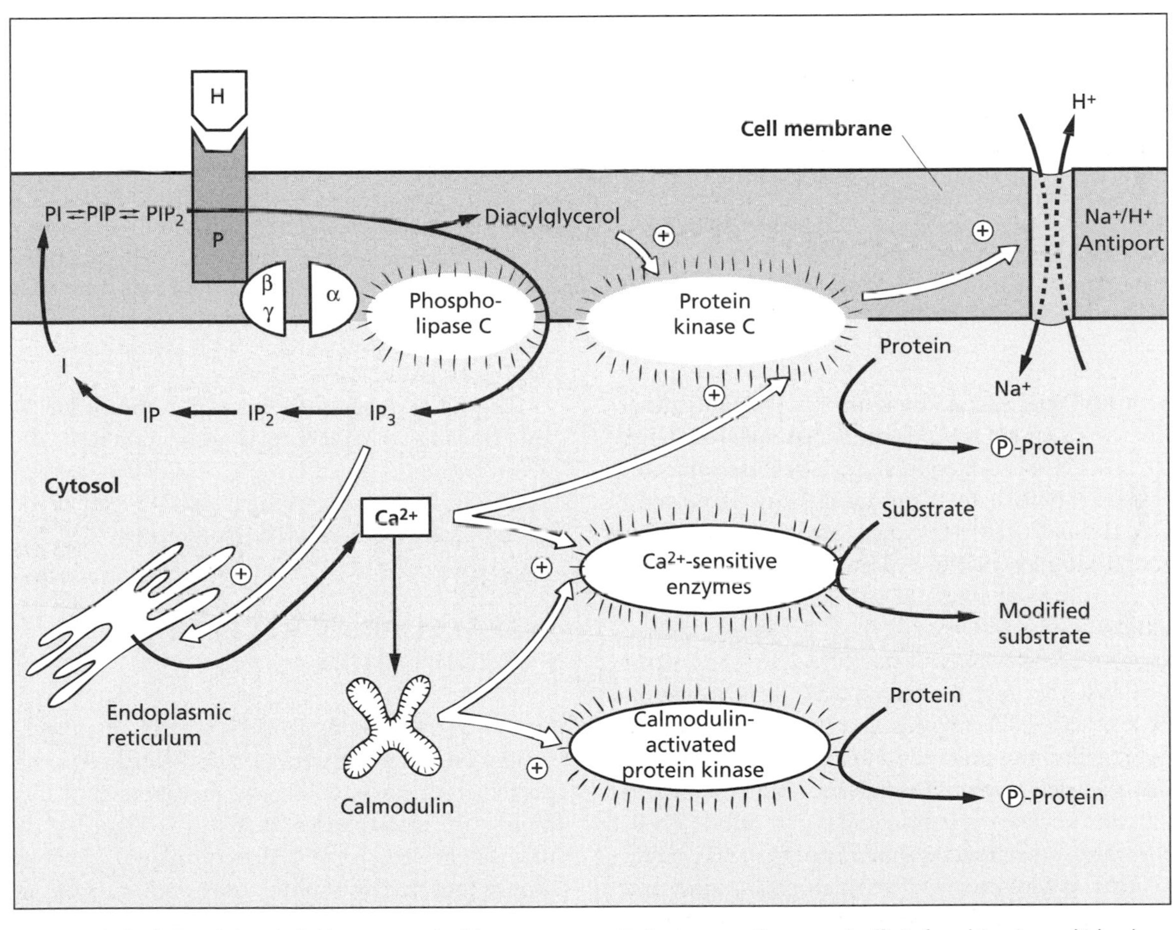

Figure 2.18 Hormonal stimulation of phospholipid turnover and calcium metabolism within the cell. Metabolism of phosphatidylinositol (see Fig 2.10) is shown in an abbreviated form on the left of this figure, with the phospholipids (PI, PIP, PIP_2) present in the membrane and the inositol phosphates (IP, IP_2, IP_3) in the cell cytoplasm. Hormone action stimulates phospholipase C, which then hydrolyses phosphatidylbisphosphate (PIP_2) to yield diacylglycerol (DAG) and inositoltrisphosphate (IP_3). IP_3 mobilizes calcium from the intracellular stores, particularly the endoplasmic reticulum, while DAG activates protein kinase C. It also increases the enzyme's affinity for calcium ions, which enhances activation. The effects of the hormone action on these enzyme systems are to stimulate the phosphorylation of proteins and enzymes, and hence alter intracellular metabolism. The sodium/hydrogen ion (Na^+/H^+) antiport is also stimulated by action of some growth factors to decrease the intracellular H^+ concentration and hence raise the intracellular pH; this can affect a variety of enzymes and intracellular reactions.

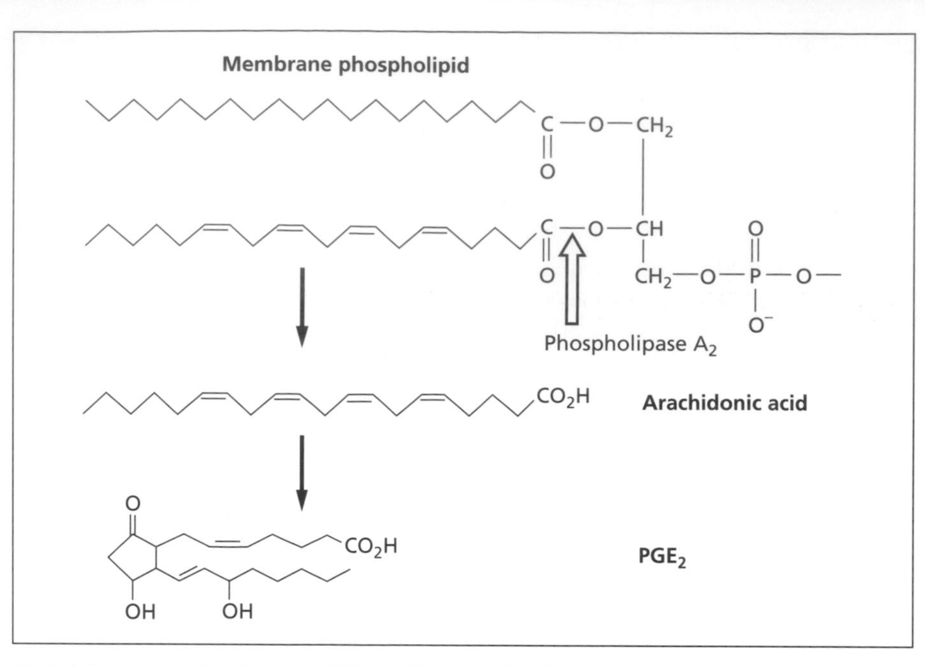

Figure 2.19 Calcium-ion-activated phospholipase A_2 releases arachidonic acid from the 2 position of specific glycerophospholipids. Arachidonic acid is the most abundant unsaturated fatty acid in tissue phospholipids. It is the rate limiting precursor of important chemically related signalling molecules, the eicosanoids. The conversion occurs via cyclooxygenase and lipoxygenase pathways. The eicosanoids include thromboxanes, leucotrienes, lipoxins and prostaglandins. Control of their production is exerted mainly by varying the activity of phospholipase A_2. A pathway for prostaglandin E_2 is outlined above. There are at least 16 different prostaglandins, which are all structurally related, 20-carbon, fatty-acid derivatives. They are released from many different cell types and influence both the adjacent cells and also the cell that has produced them. They have only short half-lines in the circulation of 3–10 minutes and are inactivated by a single passage through the systemic circulation. This autocrine action may amplify or prolong the response to the original stimulus, thereby causing synergy. Prostaglandins stimulate a wide variety of bioactivities, including inflammation responses and contraction of uterine smooth-muscle cells. Aspirin inhibits the production of prostaglandins at sites of inflammation.

IP_3 act as intracellular second messengers. DAG, together with a cofactor, phosphatidylserine, activates the cell membrane associated PKC, whilst IP_3 is released into the cytosol whence it binds to calcium-mobilizing IP_3 receptor channels in the endoplasmic reticulum (Fig. 2.18). This causes a rapid 10-fold rise in cytosolic free Ca^{2+}, from a resting concentration of about 0.1 μM.

Ca^{2+} activates several Ca^{2+}-sensitive enzymes, including the protein kinase calmodulin (Fig. 2.18), and some isoforms of PKC. In fact the name PKC was coined to reflect this Ca^{2+}-dependency. It also activates phospholipase A_2, which liberates arachidonate from phospholipids and thereby generates potent local tissue activators which are collectively known as eicosanoids (Fig. 2.19). These include thromboxanes, leucotrienes, lipoxins and prostaglandins. The latter are well recognized para- and autocrine mediators which may amplify or prolong the responses to the original hormonal stimulus. Ca^{2+} ions also activate cytosolic guanylate cyclase, an enzyme that cataylses the formation of another cyclic nucleotide, cyclic guanosine monophosphate (cGMP). The effects of atrial natriuretic peptide (Chapter 4) are mediated by receptors linked to guanylate cyclase.

Through necessity, the rise in intracellular free Ca^{2+} is only transient and calcium mobilization is de-activated by several systems. For example, PLC-β can increase the rate of GTP hydrolysis from the $G_q\alpha$/GTP activated complex, by acting as a GTPase-activating protein (GAP).

INTRACELLULAR RECEPTORS FOR HORMONES

Steroid and thyroid hormones are not, in molecular terms, similar chemical structures, but nevertheless they bind to protein receptors which are members of a large superfamily of intracellular receptors (Fig. 2.1) which are themselves structurally closely related. Since these hormones are hydrophobic, they can diffuse across the plasma-membrane of their target cells and so gain access to these intracellular receptors which are found in either the cytosol or the cell nucleus. These receptors function as hormone-regulated transcription factors (Fig. 2.20), controlling the expression of specific target genes by interaction with regions close to the gene promotors. Compared with the hormones which act via the rapidly

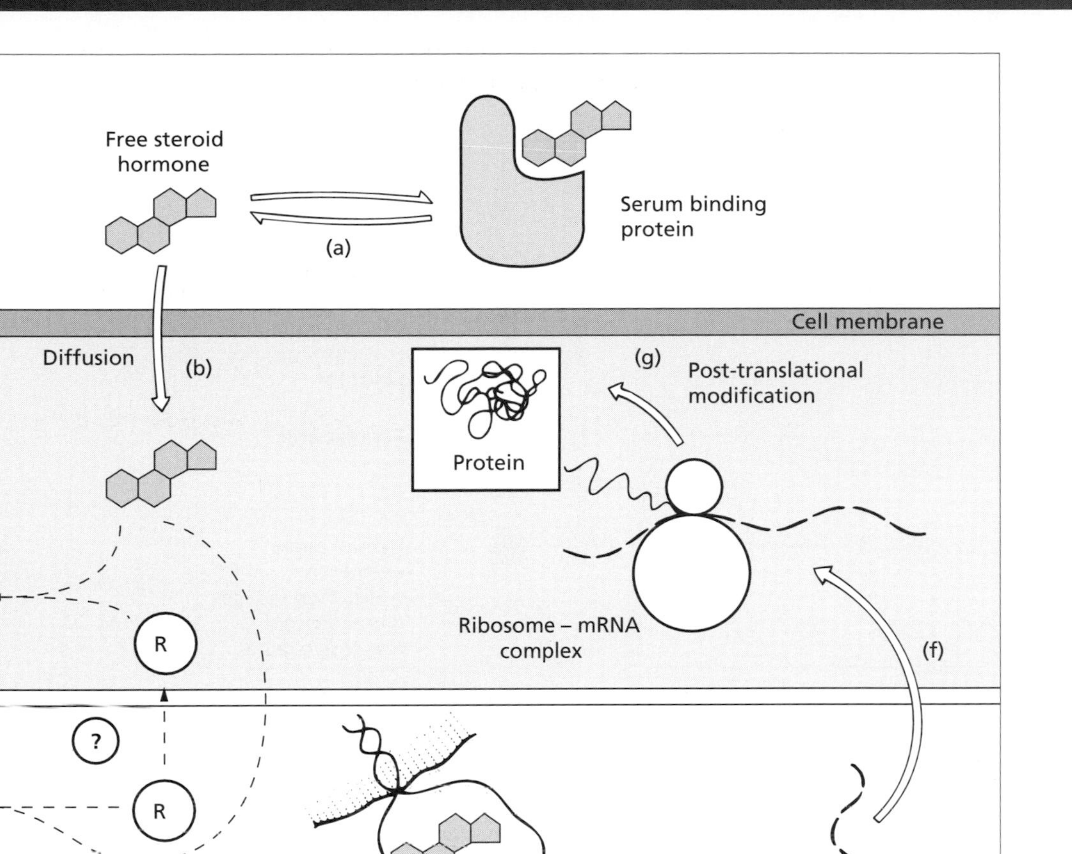

Figure 2.20 Outline of the mechanism of steroid hormone action. Free steroid is in equilibrium with that bound to serum binding-proteins (a), and it diffuses across the target-cell membrane (b). Binding to the steroid hormone-receptor protein ® may occur in the cell cytoplasm or in the cell nucleus. The hormone–receptor complex (c) interacts with chromatin, which is attached to the nuclear-matrix structures. The hormone–receptor complex binds to a receptor site on the regulatory region of one deoxyribonucleic acid (DNA) strand associated with a particular gene (d). This region is known as the hormone-response element (HRE). This interaction influences the promoter region, which then permits DNA-dependent ribonucleic acid (RNA) polymerase to start transcription of the triplet base code by separation of the two strands of DNA to yield a specific messenger RNA (e). Post-transcriptional modification and splicing of the exon sequences follows, and messenger RNA passes out of the nucleus (f). Peptides and proteins are formed by translation of the message on ribosomes attached to the endoplasmic reticulum. Finally, modification of the protein occurs to give the final gene product (g).

responsive cell-surface receptor/second messenger systems discussed above, the ultimate biological responses to steroid and thyroid hormones are sluggish. This is because they generate their responses via promotion of RNA and protein synthesis. There is therefore a characteristic lag period between the time of exposure of the target cell to the hormone and the onset of an *in vivo* biological response.

The superfamily of receptors for steroid and thyroid hormones

There are more than 150 members of this superfamily of receptor proteins. The majority are at present 'orphan' receptors, since no cognate ligand has been identified for them, but the most important, from an endocrine perspective, are listed in Fig. 2.21. Each consists of a single

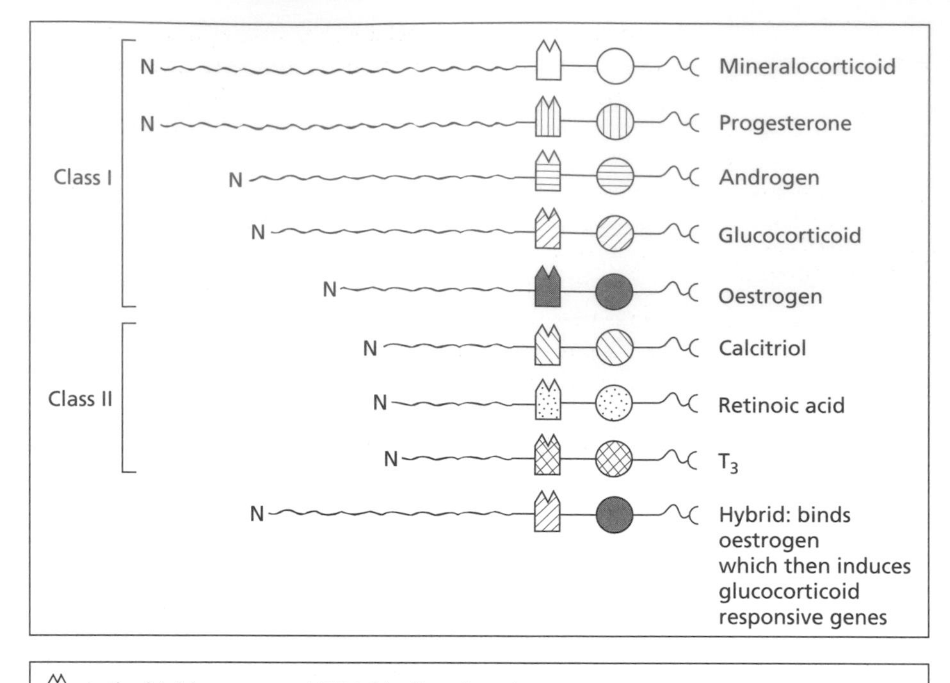

Figure 2.21 The steroid—thyroid hormone receptor superfamily. Diagrammatic representation showing the relative sizes of these evolutionarily related proteins, which range in size from 395 to 984 amino acids.

polypeptide chain. Within this structure, 3 distinctive major modules can be identified. These are as follows.

1 A hormone-specific binding domain, which at the C-terminus contains a region (AF2) responsible for hormone dependent transcriptional activation; the ligand binding site itself is a hydrophobic pocket.

2 A highly conserved DNA-binding domain.

3 An N-terminal domain which is hypervariable both in length and composition. For some receptors, the latter appears to exert a transcriptional-activation function, due to a region referred to as AF1; this activation is not hormone dependent, i.e. it is constitutive. The modules in a given holoreceptor function independently, as can be demonstrated by the construction of hybrid or chimeric receptors in domain-exchange experiments (Fig. 2.21).

The molecular weights of these receptors range from 46 kDa for the T_3 receptor to 100 kDa for the receptors for progesterone and mineralocorticoids. Notable regions of homology between the receptors, which can be as high as 60–90%, occur, indicating that they are related evolutionarily. It is speculated that the oncogene *v-erb A* or *c-erb A* may be their common ancestor. The nuclei of cells which express these receptors can be immunostained with antisera which are highly receptor specific. The superfamily is usually subdivided into 2 classes (Figs 2.1 and 2.21) on the basis of both their mode of action when activating transcription and the forms which they assume when they are unoccupied. All steroids act via Class 1 receptors, whereas calcitriol, retinoic acid and T_3 utilize Class II.

The DNA-binding domain

This domain is characterized by the presence of 2 'zinc fingers'. These are 2 polypeptide loops, each of which is 10–20 amino acids long. A single zinc ion co-ordinates 2 cysteine and 2 histidine residues in each loop and this stabilizes the structure. The 2 fingers are separated by approximately 12 amino acids. These distinctive fingers are obligatory for interlocking of the receptor with the target acceptor DNA and form the principal interface when this takes place.

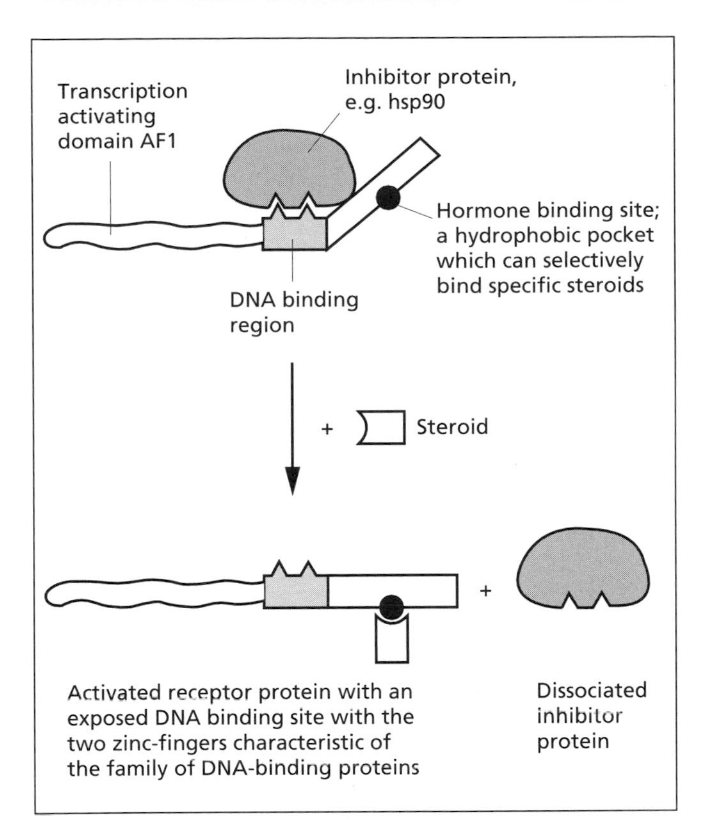

Figure 2.22 Diagrammatic representation using a linear representation of the mechanism of activation of a steroid hormone receptor protein. Note: (1) hsp90 is a heat-shock (or stress) protein with a molecular weight of 90 kDa. It is highly conserved in evolution. Its production by many different cell types increases with heat. (2) Although receptors for steroid and thyroid hormones have similar structures, those for thyroid hormones are not held in an inactive state by an inhibitor protein such as hsp90. In contrast, receptors for thyroid hormones, as well as those for calcitriol and retinoic acid, are bound to deoxyribonucleic acid (DNA) in the 'resting state'. They are activated by occupancy of the receptor by the appropriate ligand. Receptors for steroid hormones are referred to as class I receptors and those for thyroid hormones as class II receptors (Figs 2.1 and 2.21).

For Class I steroid receptors, when in their resting state, the zinc fingers are masked by the association of the receptor with a dimerized heat-shock protein such as hsp 70, hsp 90 or others (Fig. 2.22). These high molecular weight complexes are partitioned between the cytosol and the nucleus with a steroid-specific distribution. For example, whilst 90% of the resting glucocorticoid receptors are cytosolic, those for the androgens are predominantly nuclear. Clearly, when the receptors are associated with the hsp dimers, which obscures their zinc fingers, they cannot bind to nuclear DNA. Occupancy of the hormone binding site by a given steroid however, leads to dissociation of the hsp dimer. This reveals the zinc fingers and translocation to the nucleus then takes place if required. The receptors themselves then dimerize and bind with 4 zinc fingers to a short region of DNA. The latter is referred to as the hormone response element (HRE) or, in the case of the T_3 receptor, the thyroid hormone response element (TRE). Each zinc finger is thought to recognize a specific sequence of about 5 nucleotide pairs in the HRE. X-ray crystallographic analysis and protein nuclear magnetic resonance spectroscopy have been used to reveal the molecular details of zinc finger proteins interacting with the major groove of DNA.

Targeting of the hormone/receptor complex to the HRE acceptor is directed by remarkably few amino acids in the DNA binding domain. These occur in a region called the P Box which is located at the base of the first zinc finger. For example, alteration of just 2 amino acids in the zinc finger of the glucocorticoid receptor leads to less stringent targeting so that the receptor can then bind to and activate oestrogen-responsive genes as well. Thus with this receptor design, 2 sites on the receptor confer hormonal specificity: the hormone binding site itself and also the DNA binding domain.

As explained in the legend to Fig. 2.22, receptors for thyroid hormones are located excusively in the nucleus. In their resting state they are already bound to the DNA, and are activated by occupancy of the hormone binding domain by thyroid hormones. This model also applies to receptors for calcitriol and retinoic acid and these receptors are therefore grouped into a subclass, Class II, within the superfamily (Figs 2.1 and 2.21). T_3 receptors, which are constitutively nuclear, may inhibit or 'silence' basal gene transcription in the absence of the ligand. They may do this by recruiting a corepressor protein which inhibits basal promotor activity, but which dissociates from the receptor in the presence of T_3.

Transcriptional-activation

As outlined above, receptor dimerization is required before the ligand-occupied nuclear receptors can bind to their HRE. For Class I steroid receptors, homodimers are formed which then bind to palindromically arranged hexanucleotide half-sites (Fig. 2.23). In contrast, with a Class II receptor, such as that for T_3, the receptor is usually bound to the acceptor DNA as a heterodimer with an unoccupied retinoid X receptor, although homodimeric interactions have also been reported.

The dimers are bound to the HRE which is upstream from the target gene and its promotor region. DNA-dependent RNA polymerase action is controlled by the promotor region, and this in turn is subject to enhancing, or occasionally supressive influence by the dimerized hormone complex, bound to the HRE. Specific coactivator,

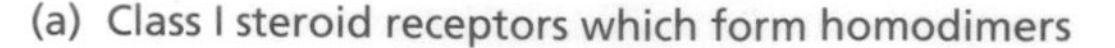
(a) Class I steroid receptors which form homodimers

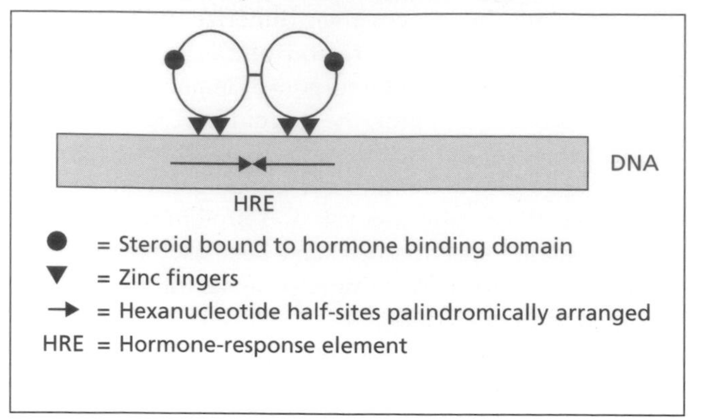

(b) Class II receptors e.g. for T_3, which form heterodimers

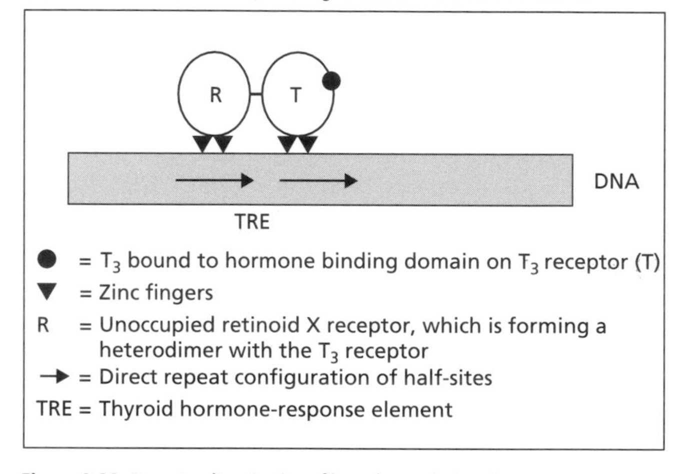

Figure 2.23 Receptor dimerization of ligand-occupied nuclear receptors. (a) Class I steroid receptors which form homodimers. (b) Class II receptors, e.g. for T_3, which form heterodimers.

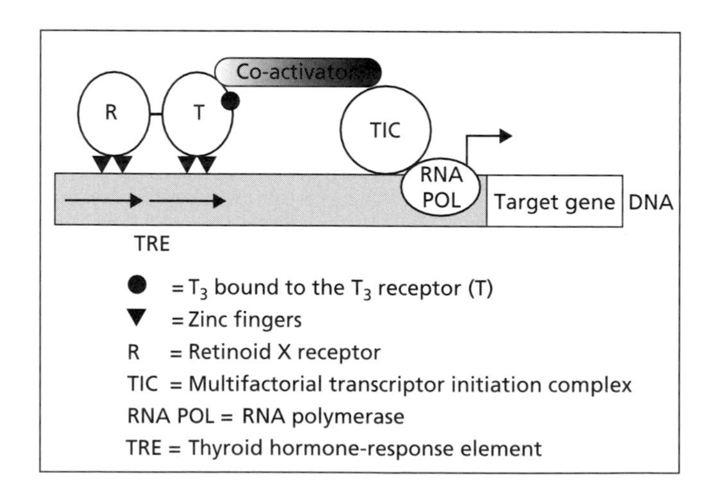

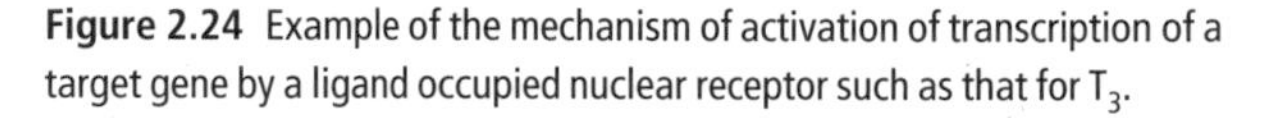
Figure 2.24 Example of the mechanism of activation of transcription of a target gene by a ligand occupied nuclear receptor such as that for T_3.

or even corepressor proteins are recruited by the ligand occupied dimerized receptors as shown in Fig. 2.24. These enhance or repress the function of the transcription-initiation complex which is assembled from a number of additional transcription factors together with RNA polymerase.

The mRNA produced by transcription is further processed by splicing together the exon sequences (Fig. 1.7). Final expression of steroid hormone action is manifested by the synthesis of specific proteins within the cell (Fig. 2.20). However, in a given cell, only a small number of the genes present will be regulated directly and only a limited number of proteins will be produced in the first instance. In some steroid-responsive cells, however, this early primary response is followed by a secondary response. The delayed response is due to proteins of the primary response inducing multiple sites of RNA synthesis themselves. In this way a co-ordinated and amplified response is obtained.

Defective nuclear receptors

Since the isolation of the cDNA for nuclear receptors, extensive work has been undertaken to identify mutations in their genes which might then be associated with specific endocrinopathies. Table 2.3 attempts to summarize the progress which has been made, linking in many cases hormone resistance syndromes, which are characterized by reduction in target organ responsiveness to the circulating hormone, to identified clinical defects.

Mutations have been identified which lead to reduced ligand binding to the hormone-binding domain, impaired receptor dimerization and also a decrease in binding of the occupied receptor/dimer to the HRE.

Pit-1: another endocrine transcription factor

Apart from the transcription factors such as CREB (Fig. 2.17) and the nuclear hormone receptors discussed above (Fig. 2.21), another transcription factor has been identified in the pituitary which regulates the expression of genes coding for growth hormone, prolactin and the β-subunit of TSH. This is known as Pit-1 and is a homeobox protein that is a member of the POU family of transcription factors, which are important for mammalian development. Pit-1-binding elements are found in the promotor regions of the target genes for growth hormone, prolactin and TSH-β. This could explain the paradoxical lack of hormonal specificity, whereby TRH simultaneously stimulates the secretion of both prolactin and TSH. Growth hormone is not normally secreted in response to TRH except in acromegalics; this may be explained by the finding that transcription of the gene for growth hormone requires relatively high levels of Pit-1. Patients with point

Table 2.3 Examples of underlying molecular defects and associated clinical effects of mutated nuclear receptors.

Receptor	Clinical Effects	Molecular defects reported to date
Androgens (AR)	Partial or complete androgen insensitivity syndromes	↓Receptor number ↓Androgen binding ↓AR dimerization
	Breast cancer Prostate cancer	↓AR dimerization AR responds to progesterone
Glucocorticoid (GR)	Generalized inherited glucocorticoid resistance	↓Hormone binding ↓GR number ↓DNA binding
Oestrogen (ER)	Usually lethal Oestrogen resistance	↓Hormone binding ↓DNA binding
T_3 (TR)	Resistance to thyroid hormone	TRβ gene defects ↓T_3 binding
Calcitriol (VDR)	Calcitriol-resistant rickets	↓VDR dimerization

mutations in Pit-1 have been identified and they show reduced or absent growth hormone, prolactin and TSH levels, which do not respond to provocation. This can be associated with short stature and, as a consequence of late diagnosed hypothyroidism, severe learning disability.

Target cell conversion of circulating hormones destined for nuclear receptors

There are several examples in which the target cell for hormones which act via nuclear receptors, express a tissue specific enzyme which locally converts a circulating hormone to a more potent metabolite. This then acts on the receptors with an increased affinity. For example, tissue-specific 5′ deiodinases convert thyroxine to T_3 (Fig. 5.3), 5α–reductase metabolizes testosterone to dihydrotestosterone (Fig. 6.6) and 1α–hydroxylase in the mitochondria of cells in the renal tubule converts 25-OH vitamin D to calcitriol (Fig. 7.13).

Conversely, in aldosterone-responsive cells of the kidney, an 11β-hydroxysteroid dehydrogenase (11β-HSD) converts and thereby deactivates cortisol to its 11-keto-metabolite, cortisone (Fig. 2.25). This is important since cortisol, but not cortisone, binds to the mineralocorticoid receptor. Since cortisol is present in the circulation at concentrations which are 2–3 orders of magnitude higher than those of aldosterone, if not deactivated in this way it would cause inappropriate over activation of the mineralocorticoid receptor. Because of the action of this 11β-HSD, the surprisingly 'promiscuous' mineralocorticoid receptor is therefore 'protected' from over stimulation by cortisol. Deficiency or impaired function of this enzyme leads to the hypertension and hypokalaemia characteristic of the Apparent Mineralocorticoid Excess (AME) syndrome.

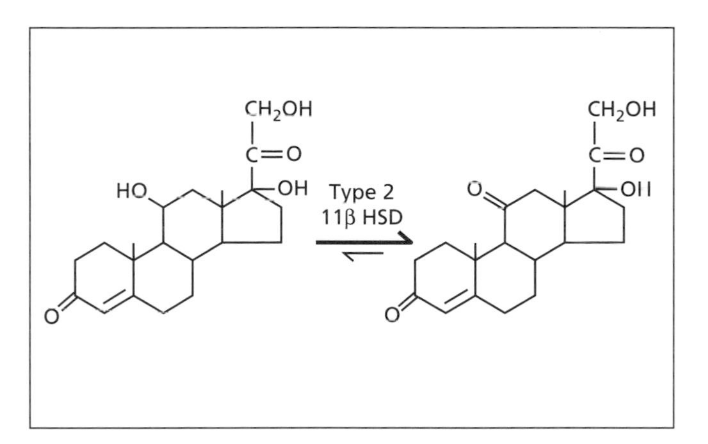

Figure 2.25 The crucial conversion of cortisol to cortisone affected by 11β hydroxysteroid dehydrogenase (11βHSD). Unlike cortisol, cortisone no longer binds to the mineralocorticoid receptor and this provides a mechanism for attaining aldosterone specificity for its nonselective receptor. There are at least 2 types of 11βHSD. Type 2 drives the reaction from left to right, whereas Type 1 favours the reverse reaction.

CHAPTER 3

The Hypothalamopituitary Axis

SUMMARY

The hypothalamopituitary axis plays a central role in the endocrine system. It organizes the appropriate hormonal responses to stimuli from higher centres, which arise from changes in the external environment. These range from alteration in the supply of nutrients and ambient temperature to challenges that result in physical or psychological stress. Secretion of most of the hormones from the anterior pituitary is stimulated by peptide-releasing hormones, which are secreted from the hypothalamus directly into the adenohypophyseal portal vasculature. The delivery of these releasing hormones, which have short half-lives, is dependent on an intact pituitary stalk.

Most of the hormones from the anterior pituitary are also regulated by negative-feedback inhibition: the pituitary hormones in the circulation interact with their target tissues, which are stimulated to secrete further hormones that feed back to inhibit release of the pituitary hormones. For example, cortisol inhibits adrenocorticotrophin, gonadal hormones inhibit luteinizing hormone and follicle-stimulating hormone secretion, and the thyroid hormones control thyrotrophin release. Where the target tissue does not produce a circulating hormone, such as in the case of growth hormone or prolactin (PRL), pituitary secretion is controlled by inhibitors. Prolactin is under inhibitory control of dopamine, but both releasing and inhibiting hormones from the hypothalamus (as well as inhibition by glucose) control growth hormone release.

In contrast to the anterior pituitary, the two neurohypophyseal hormones, oxytocin and vasopressin, are synthesized in the supraoptic and paraventricular nuclei in the hypothalamus. They are transported to the terminals of the nerve fibres, which are located in the posterior pituitary, in the form of storage granules. Oxytocin is released in response to peripheral stimuli of the cervical stretch receptors and suckling at the breast. Vasopressin (antidiuretic hormone) release is stimulated by changes in the activity of the hypothalamic osmoreceptors.

INTRODUCTION

The existence of the pituitary gland has been known for at least 2000 years. According to Aristotle, the pituitary was the organ through which one of the four essential humours of the body, the phlegm or pituita, passed from the brain into the body. In the nineteenth century, Rathke studied the development of the pituitary (hypophysis), and showed that it consisted of two parts—the anterior pituitary (or adenohypophysis) and the posterior pituitary (or neurohypophysis). Pierre Marie described the association between acromegaly (a condition characterized by the increased growth of the extremities) and pituitary tumours, and in 1909 Cushing was the first to remove part of the pituitary of an acromegalic patient and notice an improvement in the condition. Evans and Long showed that injections of crude extracts of the anterior pituitary in animals caused increased growth and even gigantism. These studies led, eventually, to the isolation of growth hormone (GH).

Other functions of the pituitary were discovered; it affects lactation (through prolactin, PRL) and regulates the function of the thyroid (through thyrotrophin, thyroid-stimulating hormone, TSH), the adrenals (through adrenocorticotrophin, adrenocorticotrophin hormone, ACTH) and the gonads (through luteinizing and follicle-stimulating hormones, LH and FSH). In recognition of the importance of the hormones that are secreted by the anterior pituitary, it was suggested that the pituitary could be considered as the 'conductor of the endocrine orchestra', although this view has now to be modified, since the pituitary is itself regulated by the nervous system through the hypothalamus.

The posterior part of the pituitary, the neurohypophysis, secretes two hormones, vasopressin and oxytocin; these are released from neurones whose cell bodies are in the hypothalamus. The anterior pituitary does not have neuronal connections with the hypothalamus, even though it is under hypothalamic control: this control occurs through a system of portal veins, the blood flowing downwards from the hypothalamus to the pituitary. From these observations, Harris developed the concept of the control of the adenohypophysis by humoral factors produced in the hypothalamus. This led to the award of the Nobel prize to Schally and Guillemin, who independently isolated and established the structures of some of these so-called 'releasing hormones'.

MORPHOLOGY OF THE MAMMALIAN HYPOTHALAMOHYPOPHYSEAL SYSTEM

Development

The hypothalamohypophyseal system is derived from two ectodermal components. One of these is Rathke's pouch, a dorsal outgrowth of the buccal cavity developing just in front of the buccal membrane. Rathke's pouch detaches itself and develops into the anterior pituitary. The second ectodermal component, the infundibulum, develops as a downgrowth from the neuroectoderm forming the floor of the third ventricle immediately caudal to the future optic chiasma. This develops into the pituitary stalk and the posterior pituitary. The remainder of this ventral neuroectoderm forms the median eminence, while the hypothalamic nuclei differentiate in its lateral walls and form the sides of the third ventricle.

Anatomy

In the adult, the pituitary lies in a bony cavity, the sella turcica or pituitary fossa, in the sphenoid bone (Fig. 3.1). The human adult pituitary weighs about 0.5 g, but this can double during puberty or pregnancy. The anterior pituitary accounts for about three-quarters of its weight. The pituitary is connected to the hypothalamus by a stalk (Fig. 3.2), which carries axons to the neurohypophysis, as well as blood vessels. The pituitary gland is closely related to a number of other important structures. Superiorly, there is the optic chiasm; anteriorly and below is the sphenoid air sinus, which provides a useful passage for neurosurgical operations on the gland through the nose; laterally are the cavernous venous sinuses, through which the third, fourth and sixth cranial nerves run.

Blood flows from the primary capillary plexus in the median eminence down the portal veins to the sinusoidal vessels in the anterior pituitary (Fig. 3.2). Anatomical and physiological studies strongly suggest that there may be a reverse flow of hypothalamic and pituitary peptides along the pituitary stalk and back to the brain; this may account for their presence in the spinal fluid. Venous blood from the pituitary stalk and the pituitary gland drains by a number of veins into the adjacent cavernous sinuses.

Hypothalamic nuclei

There are two groups of nuclei in the hypothalamus with neuroendocrine functions. One is composed of the paired supraoptic and paraventricular nuclei in the anterior hypothalamus and the other group is referred to collectively as the hypothalamic–hypophyseotropic nuclei (Fig. 3.2). Posterior pituitary function is dependent on the former group, and the anterior pituitary on the latter.

The supraoptic and paraventricular nuclei. The posterior pituitary (or neurohypophysis) consists of nerve fibres whose terminals abut on capillaries. These fibres arise from the neurones of the paired supraoptic and paraventricular nuclei in the anterior part of the hypothalamus. The neurones are large and characterized by the presence of cytoplasmic secretory droplets 120–200 nm in diameter. They are the cells of origin of vasopressin and oxytocin, which are stored in, and secreted from, the posterior pituitary.

The newly synthesized hormones are packaged in granules with a larger protein, neurophysin. The granules are

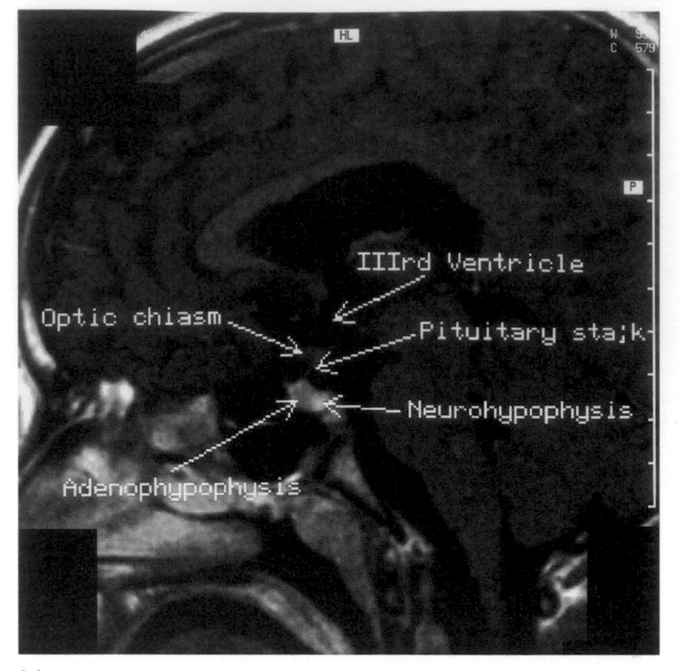

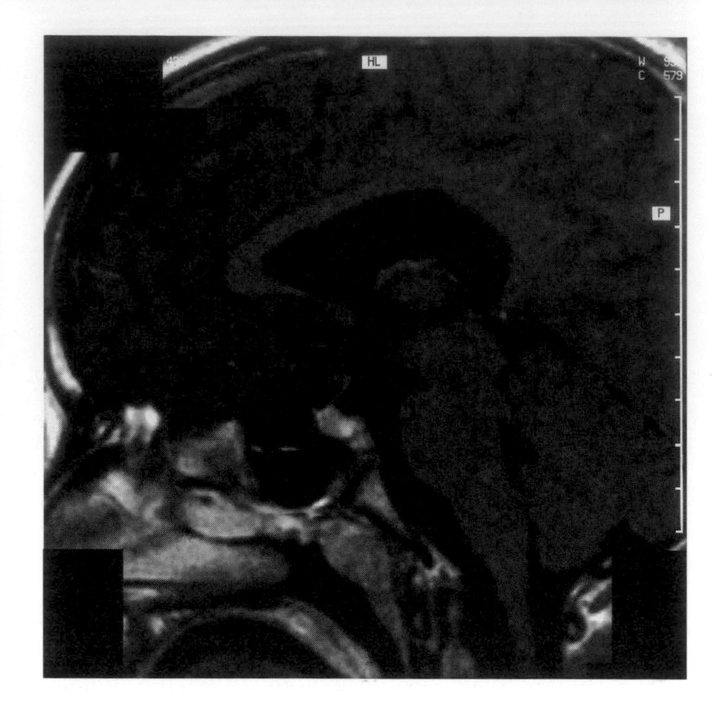

(a)

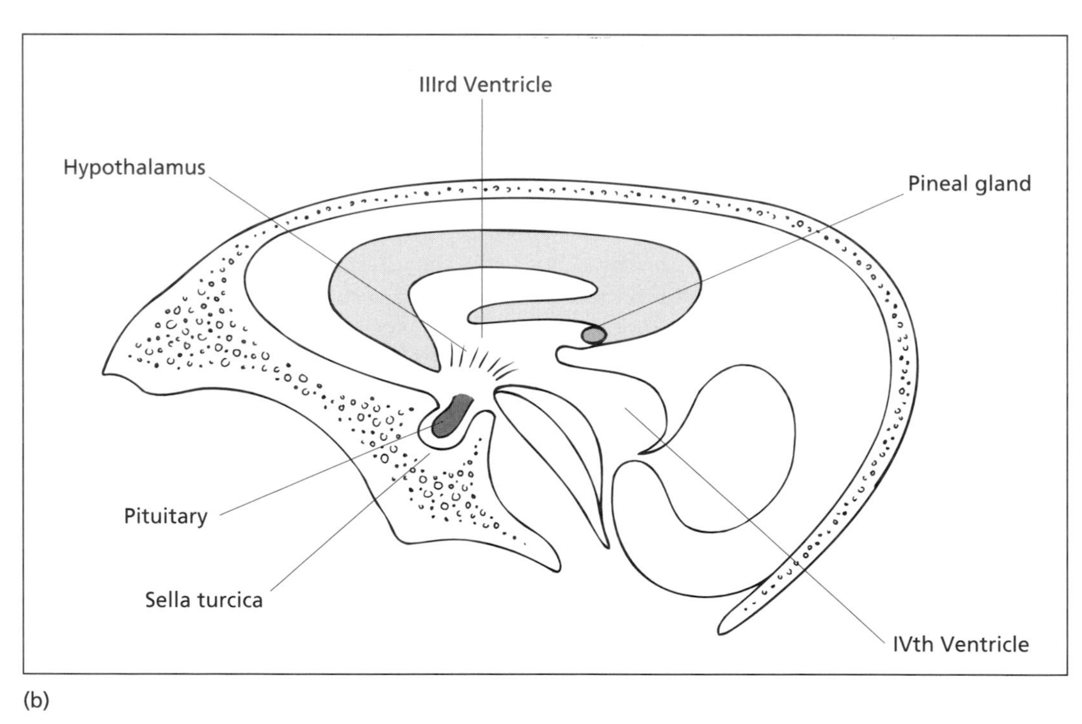

(b)

Figure 3.1 (a) A magnetic resonance imaging (MRI) scan to show the anatomy of the hypothalamopituitary axis. (b) Location of the pituitary gland in the sella turcica.

transported down their fibres to the terminals of the axons at a rate of 8 mm/h. When the neurones are stimulated, the granules are released by exocytosis and their contents diffuse into the adjacent, fenestrated, capillaries. Stimulation of release of these two hormones by dehydration or suckling leads to the disappearance of stainable neurosecretory material from the neurones. Immunocytochemical studies show that neuronal perikarya staining for either vasopressin or oxytocin is scattered through both the supraoptic and the paraventricular nuclei. In addition to the nerve fibres projecting down to the posterior pituitary, some vasopressin-positive fibres have been shown to

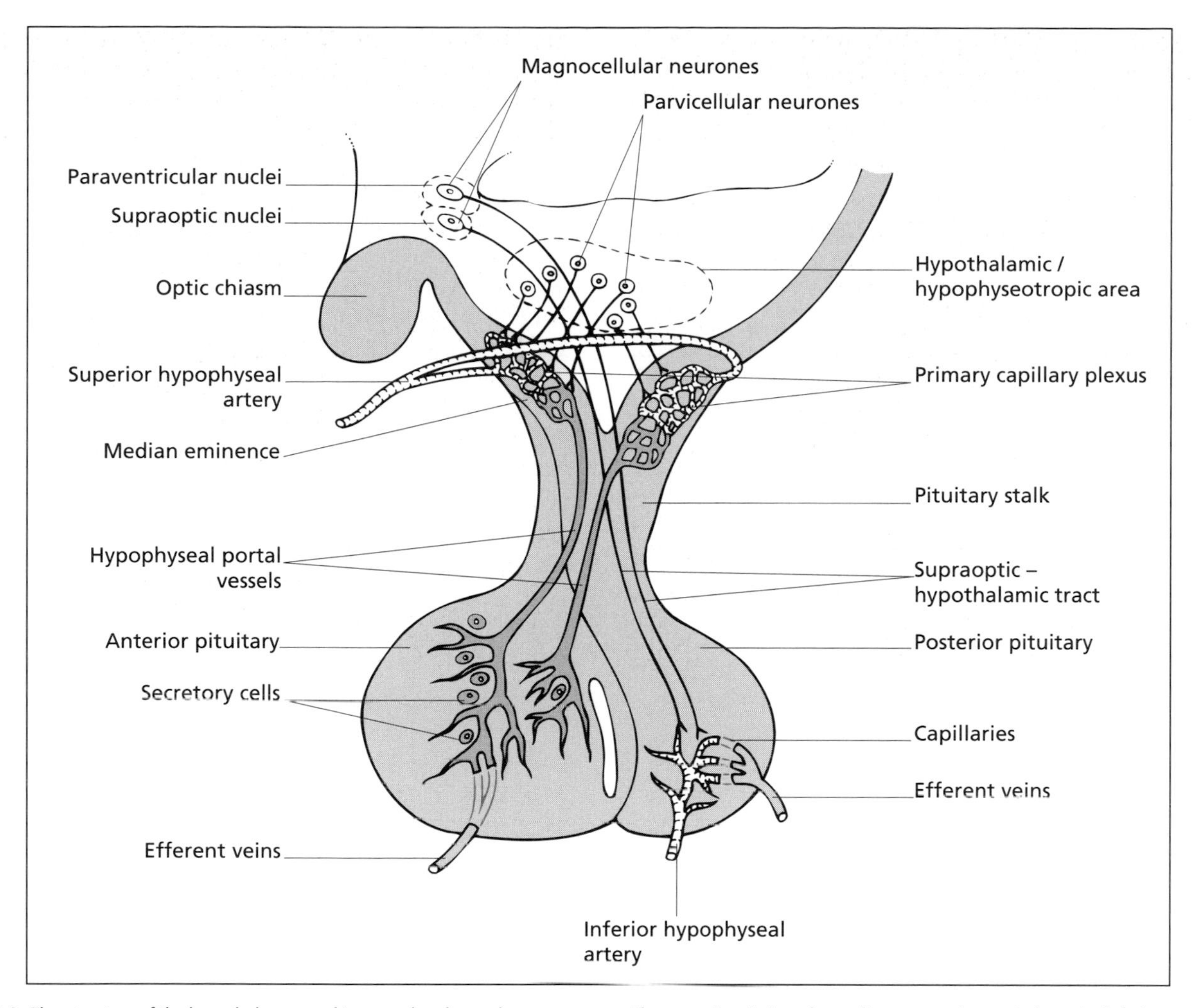

Figure 3.2 The structure of the hypothalamus and its neural and vascular connections with the pituitary. The blood supply to the median eminence consists of the superior hypophyseal artery, whose branches form the primary capillary plexus in the median eminence and the upper part of the pituitary stalk. From the plexus arise the hypophyseal portal vessels, which terminate in the anterior pituitary to form a secondary plexus of sinusoidal capillaries and supply its secretory cells. Efferent veins drain the anterior pituitary into dural sinuses. The posterior pituitary has a direct systemic supply from the inferior hypophyseal artery. Note that the axons from the parvicellular neurones of the hypothalamic–hypophyseotrophic area (shown in white) terminate close to the primary capillary plexus. The axons of the magnocellular neurones of the supraoptic and paraventricular nuclei run down the pituitary stalk as the supraoptic–hypothalamic tract, and terminate close to the capillaries supplying the posterior pituitary. The optic chiasm is also shown.

terminate in the external layer of the median eminence. This is important clinically, because it means that a patient who loses the posterior pituitary can recover vasopressin function.

Hypothalamic–hypophyseotropic nuclei. These are found in the lateral wall of the third ventricle (Fig. 3.1); there is functional overlap between morphologically distinguishable nuclei in the hypothalamic–hypophyseotropic area (Fig. 3.2). The neurones in this region are smaller, and neurosecretory droplets cannot be demonstrated in them; they terminate in the external layer of the median eminence, in close proximity to the capillaries of its primary plexus. These nerve terminals contain small dense-cored vesicles, 80–120 nm in diameter, which can be demonstrated by immunohistochemical techniques to be the storage form of the releasing hormones that control the anterior pituitary. The discharge of these releasing hormones involves exocytosis and they diffuse into the adjacent capillaries of the primary plexus. The boundaries of the hypothalamic nuclei from which these neurones arise outline the hypophyseotropic area, although these are less easily defined than the supraoptic and paraventricular nuclei.

Innervation of neurosecretory neurones. The hypothalamus receives nerve fibres directly or indirectly from virtually all areas of the brain, and so its activity must, in part, be regulated by higher centres. This complex neural input reflects the role of the hypothalamus as a regulatory centre for many vital functions. Hypothalamic peptidergic neurones are capable by themselves of sustaining a certain degree of autonomous function, as indicated by experiments in which the hypothalamopituitary complex has been surgically disconnected from the rest of the brain. In such experiments, the basal secretions of GH, FSH and LH are largely unchanged, and release of ACTH in response to insulin-induced hypoglycaemia or stress is unaffected. However, superimposed on this autonomy are inputs to these neurones both from within the hypothalamus and from other parts of the brain, such as the septum, hippocampus, anterior thalamus, amygdala, pyriform cortex and midbrain.

Pathways that release norepinephrine, epinephrine, dopamine, serotonin and acetylcholine are of major importance in the control of the neurosecretory cells of the hypothalamus. Monoaminergic nerve terminals have been demonstrated synapsing on hypothalamic peptidergic neurones and on their axons in the median eminence near the perivascular space adjacent to the primary capillary plexus. Peptide neurotransmitters or neuromodulators—for example, opioid peptides, substance P and bombesin—are likely to be involved in the modulation of hypothalamic releasing hormone secretion; some of these opioid peptides have been shown to exert effects on the secretion of pituitary hormones.

Anterior pituitary: cytology

The secretory cells of the anterior pituitary are arranged in clumps or in branching cords of cells separated by the sinusoidal capillaries arising from the hypophyseal portal vessels. They are held together in a reticular fibre framework (Fig. 3.2). Using light-microscope techniques, the cells of the anterior pituitary are classified as chromophobes (poorly stained) and chromophils (well stained), which are further subdivided into those that stain with acid dyes (acidophils) and those that stain with basic dyes (basophils).

Electron microscopy has revealed that the cells of the anterior pituitary possess all the characteristics of protein-secreting cells (see Fig. 1.6). Hormones are released by exocytosis of the secretory storage granules and diffuse through the perivascular space to the blood vessels. The chromophobe cells are sparsely granulated, while the chromophils are richly granulated.

Using immunocytochemical stains for particular hormones, acidophils can be divided into two subgroups, the somatotrophs, which secrete GH, and the mammotrophs, which produce PRL. The basophils can be divided by similar criteria into three populations of cells, the thyrotrophs producing TSH, the gonadotrophs producing LH and FSH and the corticotrophs producing ACTH. It is now generally agreed that most chromophobes are quiescent forms of the several kinds of chromophils. In addition, there are some undifferentiated cells and, in some species (but not in humans), there are melanotrophs, which produce melanocyte-stimulating hormone (MSH).

HYPOTHALAMIC HORMONES THAT CONTROL THE ANTERIOR PITUITARY

Discovery

A number of hypothalamic hormones that are secreted into the hypophyseal portal vessels and subsequently regulate anterior pituitary function have been isolated and characterized (Table 3.1). Since they are produced from several groups of peptidergic neurones, which function as endocrine cells, they are referred to as neurohormones. Their existence had been predicted by Harris, who proposed the 'portal-vessel chemotransmitter hypothesis', based on the evidence summarized in Table 3.2.

Initially, crude extracts prepared from the hypothalamus and median eminence were used to demonstrate the existence of 'factors' that could stimulate or inhibit the secretion of specific hormones from the anterior pituitary. Chemical identification of each factor and attribution of its major functions followed, and each factor was ultimately established as a regulatory hormone. Synthetic forms of each of these hypothalamic hormones are now available for use, both therapeutically and for the biochemical testing of the integrity of pituitary function.

Mechanism of action

Hypothalamic hormones have short half-lives in circulation, and act rapidly on their specific anterior pituitary target cells. Their effects may be detected *in vivo* by measuring changes in the circulating concentrations of the relevant pituitary hormone—for example, by immunoassay of TSH in response to thyrotrophin-releasing hormone (TRH). *In vitro* systems can also be used. In these, pituitary glands, isolated pituitary cells, or cells from immortalized pituitary cell lines are either superfused or manipulated as cell cultures. The responses to added hypothalamic hormones, in terms of both intracellular signals and the release of the pituitary hormones, can then be monitored.

The hypothalamic hormones modulate the immediate secretion of the hormones from secretory granules, which accounts for their rapid actions *in vivo*. They bind to

Table 3.1 Hypothalamic hormones.

Name	Structure* and discovery date	Major functions
Thyrotrophin-releasing hormone (TRH)†	Tripeptide (1969)	Stimulates release of TSH and PRL; minor stimulation of FSH release
Gonadotrophin-releasing hormone (GnRH)	Decapeptide (1971)	Stimulates release of LH and FSH
Growth hormone-releasing hormone (GHRH)	Peptide: 44 aa (1982)	Stimulates release of GH
Growth hormone release-inhibiting hormone or somatostatin (SMS)	Peptide: 14 aa (1973)	Inhibits release of GH; also gastrin, VIP, glucagon, insulin, TSH and PRL
Corticotrophin-releasing hormone (CRH)	Peptide: 41 aa (1981)	Stimulates release of ACTH
Dopamine	Monoamine	Inhibits release of PRL

* Human.
† Abbreviation in common usage.
aa, amino acids; ACTH, adrenocorticotrophin hormone (adrenocorticotrophin); FSH, follicle-stimulating hormone; GH, growth hormone; LH, luteinizing hormone; PRL, prolactin; TSH, thyroid-stimulating hormone (thyrotrophin); VIP, vasoactive intestinal peptide.

Table 3.2 Key evidence in support of the portal-vessel chemotransmitter hypothesis.

Anatomical
- Blood flows to the anterior pituitary from the primary capillary plexus located in the median eminence
- In contrast to the posterior pituitary, there is little secretomotor innervation of the anterior pituitary

Experimental
- Lesions in the hypothalamus and median eminence produce atrophy of specific endocrine glands
- Electrical stimulation of localized regions in the anterior hypothalamus evokes secretion of specific anterior pituitary hormones
- Transection of the pituitary stalk, with the insertion of an impermeable barrier to prevent regeneration of the portal vessels, results in failure of gonadal, thyroid and adrenal function, and stunts growth
- Transplantation of the anterior pituitary into a well-vascularized region remote from its original site, e.g. under the renal capsule, fails to restore target organ function in hypophysectomized animals; however, replacement under the median eminence, so that the anterior pituitary becomes revascularized by the portal vessels, reverses the decline

specific receptors on the plasma membrane of their target cells. Feedback regulation may in part be due to changes in the numbers of these receptors. For example, increased thyroid hormones will cause a reduction in the number of TRH receptors.

Post-receptor intracellular signalling involves both phosphatidylinositol metabolism and the adenylate cyclase system (see Figs 2.10 and 2.12), and generally increases in intracellular calcium are associated with stimulation of pituitary hormone release. TRH and gonadotrophin-releasing hormone (GnRH) appear to activate both systems, with increases in inositol 1,4,5-triphosphate (IP_3), diacylglycerol (DAG) and cyclic adenosine 5′-monophosphate (cAMP) playing important roles as intracellular signals (see Figs 2.1, 2.12 and 2.18). However, the stimulatory action of corticotrophin-releasing hormone (CRH) and growth hormone-releasing hormone (GHRH) appear to be mediated primarily through the activation of adenylate cyclase.

The mechanism of action of inhibitory hormones is not well understood. Both somatostatin and dopamine inhibit adenylate cyclase via the inhibitory G-protein (G_i) nucleotide regulatory complex (Chapter 2). However, since they can also inhibit secretion induced by cAMP analogues, they probably do not act exclusively by reduction in intracellular cAMP.

Physiology of the control of anterior pituitary function

Regulation of the release of hormones by the anterior pituitary is a complex process. Our current understanding is summarized in Fig. 3.3. The release of the hypothalamic hormones is central to the system. They can be either stimulators or inhibitors of the secretion of specific hormones from the anterior pituitary (Table 3.1).

Since the release of the hypothalamic hormones is generally pulsatile and they have short half-lives, their actions on the pituitary are of limited duration. In several cases, these actions are also limited by a number of different negative-feedback systems, as illustrated in Fig. 3.3.

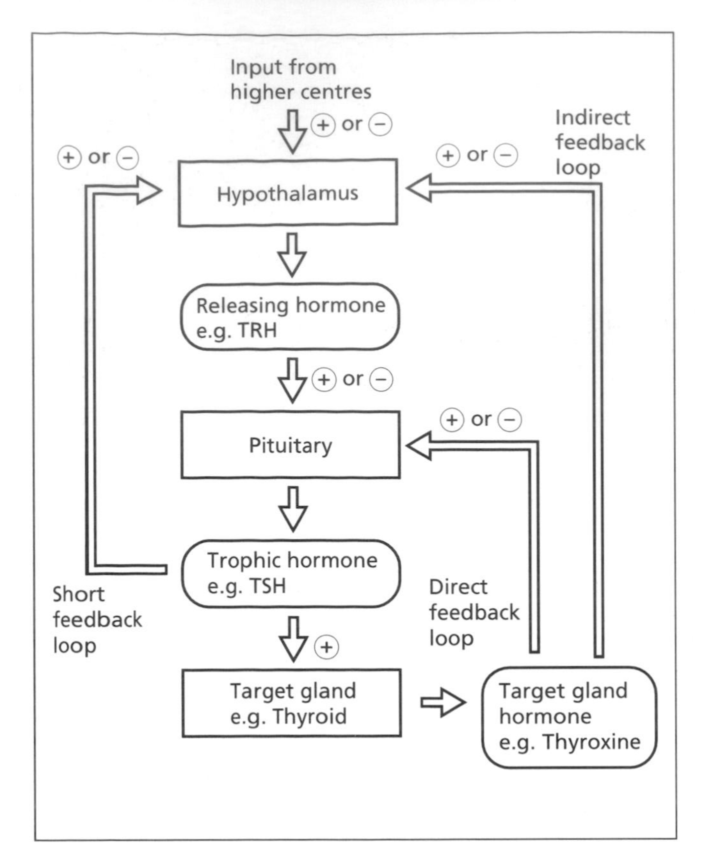

Figure 3.3 A schematic representation of the interactions between higher centres, the hypothalamus, the pituitary and peripheral endocrine glands, showing feedback regulation. The controlling factors can be stimulatory (+) or inhibitory (−).

For example, TRH stimulates TSH release from pituitary thyrotrophs, but this release is subject to negative feedback by thyroid hormones produced by the thyroid gland. Such feedback is described as a closed-loop system, and it may occur as either a direct or an indirect feedback loop (Fig. 3.3). In addition, open-loop neural transients from higher centres, such as acetylcholine and the monoamines discussed previously, modulate the system. Several endocrine responses to environmental changes, such as psychological stress, exercise and temperature changes, are mediated in this way.

Regulatory influences of this type may be especially important in controlling the secretion of GH and PRL. These are two hormones that affect a variety of target cells throughout the body, rather than having a distinct target gland capable of secreting a hormone that can inhibit the release of the pituitary hormone. Both of these hormones are under the control of two hypothalamic hormones, one of which is stimulatory, while the other plays an important role as a pituitary inhibitor. In addition to direct stimulation or inhibition, there is also interplay between the different endocrine units, so that other hormones may modify pituitary responses to hypothalamic hormones. For example, GH production from somatotrophs is dependent on an adequate supply of thyroid hormones.

Positive feedback loops also exist, and explain, for example, the mechanism whereby sustained high levels of oestradiol produced by the ovary induce a sudden rise in the secretion of LH in the middle of the menstrual cycle (see Chapter 6). Clearly, such positive-feedback loops are potentially unstable unless there are other regulatory factors.

The pulsatility of the release of hypothalamic hormones can be crucial to their action on the anterior pituitary. The frequency of the pulses and their amplitude form an additional important regulatory system. For example, in the treatment of the infertile female with GnRH, it is essential that the neurohormone is administered in discrete pulses with a well-defined frequency.

Several anterior pituitary hormones exhibit a circadian rhythm. With a hormone such as GH, this characteristic may be quite marked. The regulatory processes responsible for circadian rhythms in humans are at present poorly understood, but it is probable that the pineal gland (Fig. 3.1) plays a role. In all mammals, this gland appears to act as a neuroendocrine transducer that responds to changes in environmental light stimuli. Neural connections between the retina and pineal are responsible for a light-regulated daily cycle of the secretion of melatonin from the pineal gland. This is due to neural control of the enzyme *N*-acetyltransferase, which is rate-limiting for the conversion of 5-hydroxytryptamine to melatonin.

In mammals, melatonin secretion increases when light is reduced. Thus, in the winter months, the concentration of melatonin rises, which regulates the timing of the reproductive cycles of seasonal breeders such as hamsters. It is responsible for the gonadal regression that occurs in the winter. These actions may be associated with changes in the pulsatility of GnRH secretion and/or sensitivity to steroid negative feedback. No direct influences have yet been demonstrated in humans, but it is well recognized that melatonin rises at night and that the increase declines with age—which could be a trigger for the onset of puberty.

ANTERIOR PITUITARY HORMONES

The six major hormones produced by the anterior pituitary are listed in Table 3.3, where their structures are contrasted. GH and PRL (together with human placental lactogen) form a family of polypeptide hormones with considerable sequence homology. The glycoproteins TSH, LH and FSH form another family with structural similarities.

Table 3.3 Hormones of the anterior pituitary.

Name and common abbreviation	Amino acids*	Mol. wt*	Dominant second messenger system
Single-chain proteins			
Adrenocorticotrophin (ACTH)	39	4 500	cAMP
Growth hormone (GH)	191	22 000	STAT
Prolactin (PRL)	199	22 000	STAT
Glycoproteins with two subunits			
Luteinizing hormone (LH)	204	30 000	cAMP
Follicle-stimulating hormone (FSH)	204	30 000	cAMP
Thyroid-stimulating hormone (TSH)	204	30 000	cAMP

* Human.
cAMP, cyclic adenosine 5′-monophosphate.
STAT, signal transduces and activator of transcription.

Growth hormone (somatotrophin)

As its name implies, this hormone stimulates growth. In terms of weight, it is the most abundant hormone of the anterior pituitary, accounting for up to 10% of its dry weight.

Structure and synthesis

The major form of human GH (hGH) is a protein with 191 amino acids, two disulphide bridges and a molecular weight of 22 kDa. The somatotrophs of the human pituitary typically contain about 10 mg of the hormone. Slight variants of the basic structure exist, so that there is considerable microheterogeneity of the GH molecule in both pituitary extracts and plasma. The major variant is a shorter form, with a molecular weight of only 20 kDa. This contributes only about 10% of the hGH in the pituitary and even less to the circulating hormone. It may have a subtly different spectrum of bioactivities compared with the dominant 22 kDa form. In addition, there is a well-recognized tendency for these molecules to polymerize, particularly GH from nonprimate species. Both dimers (big GH) and oligomeric forms (big–big GH) have been observed in the circulation.

The structure of GH is species-specific, and hGH differs markedly from the nonprimate GHs. This is thought to reflect a dramatic increase in the rate of evolution of the GH/PRL gene family with the onset of the evolution of the primates. One practical consequence of this is that it is obligatory to use GH of human origin in the treatment of children with GH deficiencies. Until 1985, the only source of hGH was that extracted from human pituitaries. Unfortunately, some batches of the extracted hGH were contaminated with a protein particle (a prion) causing dementia and death (Creutzfeldt–Jakob disease). This problem stimulated the development of recombinant forms of hGH, based on the recent advances in genetic engineering techniques. Recombinant forms of both 22 kDa and 20 kDa GH with the same amino acid sequence and disulphide bonds as the native molecules can now be provided in unlimited quantities. In addition, mutants can be prepared that have deliberate changes made to the basic structure, and these are used in experiments aimed at mapping the sites on the GH molecule that determine its biological activities. They may lead to the construction of analogues with advantages for clinical use, such as a longer half-life in the circulation, or to the construction of antagonists.

Effects of growth hormone

GH has a wide spectrum of biological activities, which are summarized in Table 3.4 and Fig. 3.4. Its most spectacular effect—namely, the promotion of growth of bone, soft tissue and viscera—is due to both a direct action to stimulate fibroblast differentiation and an indirect action to promote clonal expansion of the newly differentiated cells mediated by insulin-like growth factors (IGF-I and IGF-II). Its metabolic effects are thought to be primarily the result of direct actions of GH on its target cells.

Direct effects. The best recognized are described in Table 3.4, although direct effects have also been reported in other tissues such as the hypothalamus, heart and diaphragm. These direct actions generally antagonize those of insulin, giving rise to the diabetogenic properties of GH, and synergize with cortisol.

Indirect effects. GH increases the production of IGFs from the liver and other tissues, which then mediate the growth-related effects attributed to GH (Table 3.4 and Fig. 3.4). GH stimulation of the local production of IGF-I and subsequent autocrine or paracrine regulation of cellular activity (see Fig. 1.2) can be very important, leading, for example, to the clonal expansion of chondrocytes. The indirect effects mediated by hepatic production of IGFs were discovered by the failure to reproduce *in vitro* some of the effects of GH seen *in vivo*. Initially, the putative mediators were variously named sulphation factor or somatomedins, but eventually the structures of two distinct mediators were identified, and because of the similarity of their structures to that of proinsulin they were renamed insulin-like growth factors (IGF-I and IGF-II). They have a molecular weight of about 7500 Da.

As might be expected, in contrast to the direct effects of GH, the indirect effects of GH via IGF-I and IGF-II are often insulin-like, and they can be antagonized by cortisol. They have insulin-like activities on fat cells, and stimulate

Table 3.4 Major biological effects of human growth hormone (hGH).

Direct	
Reduced glucose transport and metabolism	Reduction in insulin receptors, e.g. in the liver
Increased lipolysis	Localized decrease in adipose tissue: free fatty acids released, which then provide an energy source for muscles
Increased amino acid transport	Into muscle, liver and adipose cells
Increased protein synthesis	Increases in both transcription and translation, for example in the liver, leading to mitosis
Increased IGF production	From liver and other cells such as the pituitary and fibroblasts, where it acts locally
Increased fibroblast differentiation	Chondrocyte, osteoblast and adipocyte formation
Indirect	
Promotion of growth and endocrine effects	Via IGFs: bone, soft tissue, gonads and viscera; clonal expansion of chondrocytes

IGF, insulin-like growth factor.

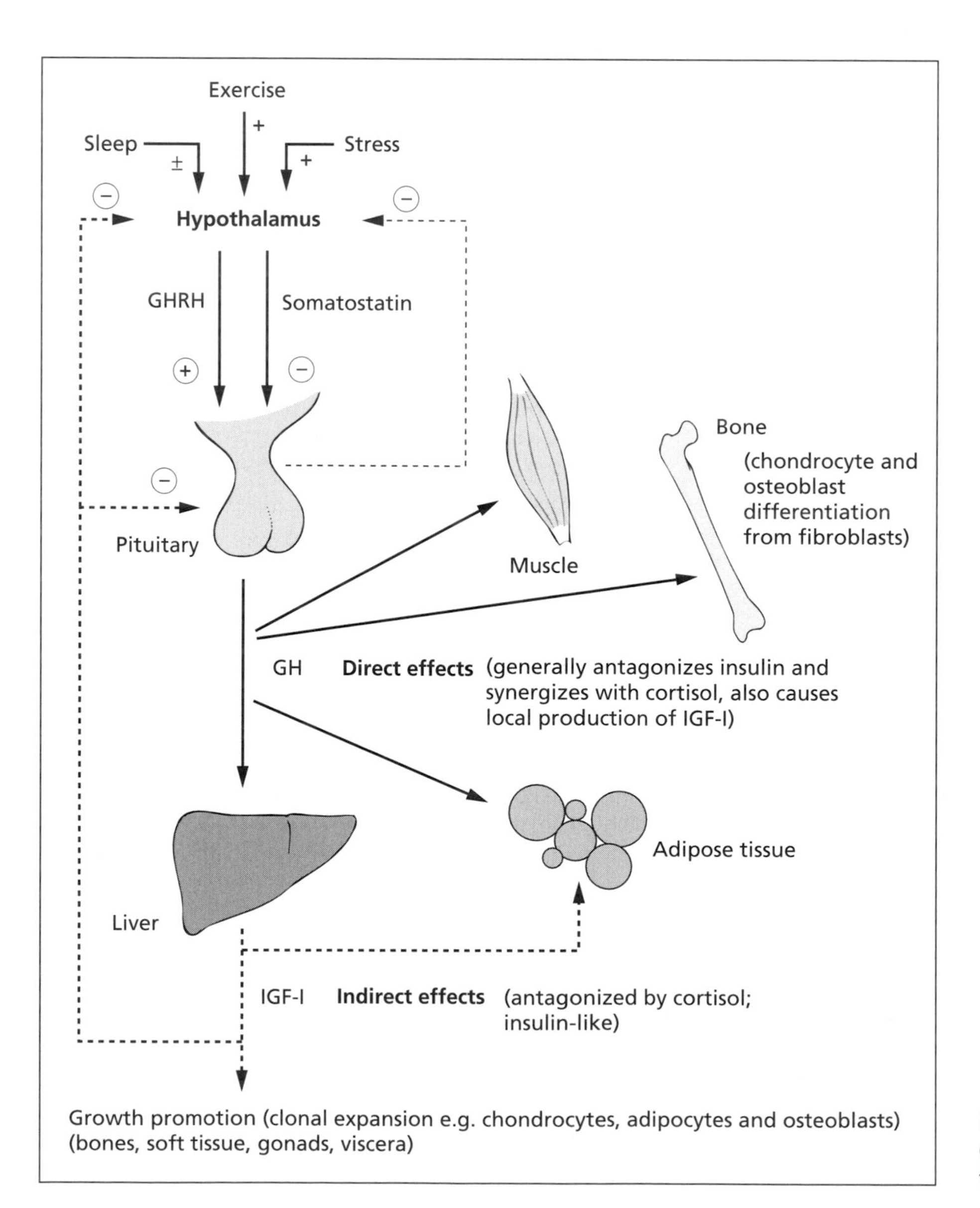

Figure 3.4 Summary of the regulation and effects of growth hormone. Glucagon and free fatty acids increase somatostatin release.

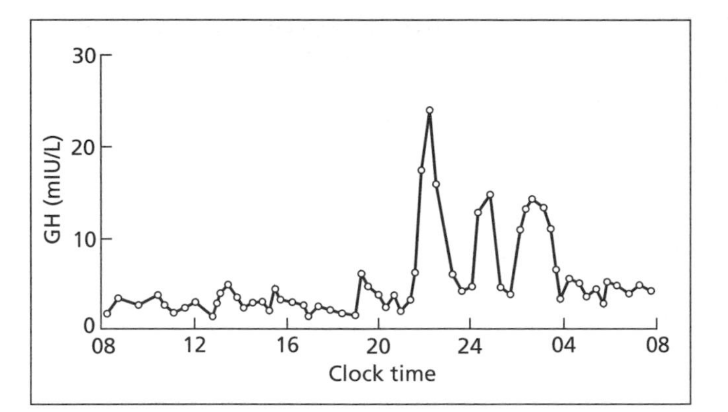

Figure 3.5 Diagram showing the pronounced fluctuation in the levels of growth hormone (GH) in the circulation of a normal 7-year-old child throughout a 24-h period. Irregular pulses occur, which are usually at their greatest magnitude during sleep. This pulsatility makes it inappropriate to rely on single measurements of the hormone for diagnostic purposes. It may, as a consequence, be necessary to sample at repeated intervals, e.g. 20 min, over a complete 24-h period, or to carry out a dynamic test such as one of those described in Fig. 3.6.

sulphate incorporation into cartilage, glycosaminoglycan and deoxyribonucleic acid (DNA) synthesis in cartilage, and collagen formation. In addition to these *in vitro* effects, administration of IGF-I stimulates increases in body weight, epiphyseal cartilage width and cartilage synthesis in hypophysectomized rats. Recombinant preparations of the IGFs are now available, and are being tested for potential therapeutic use.

Six different binding proteins for IGFs have been identified in serum. These binding proteins (IGFBPs) can be secreted locally by the target cells, together with specific proteases, which may in turn further regulate the bioavailability of IGFs. Serum proteases cause a striking reduction in IGFBP-3 in late pregnancy, but the physiological significance of this is not known. However, such observations form strong evidence for a complex controlling system that regulates the local delivery and actions of the growth factors. The concentrations of IGF in the serum appear to be relatively constant over extended periods, and so they do not reflect the wide fluctuations of GH, which occur on an hourly basis (Fig. 3.5). They are markedly influenced by the nutritional status of an individual.

The growth-promoting effects of GH via IGF-I are particularly important to growing animals, but both GH and IGF-I appear to be relatively unimportant to the fetus and neonate. IGF-II may be more important at this time. GH output increases with size to maintain the concentration of GH pulses needed to sustain growth during childhood. There is a marked rise in concentration at puberty. IGF-I levels reflect the rates at which children grow. GH and IGF-I promote growth of long bones at the epiphyseal plates, where there are actively proliferating cartilage cells. This effect ceases once the epiphyses of the long bones have fused at the end of puberty, and GH concentrations decline with advancing age.

Mechanism of action of GH and IGFs

GH receptors have been detected in all of the known target tissues, and they appear at the age of about 7 months. Recent cloning and complementary DNA (cDNA) sequencing shows that the receptor single-chain glycoproteins (molecular weight 130 kDa) span the plasma membrane (see Figs 2.2 and 2.7). Part of the extracellular region is homologous with the serum-binding protein for GH. One molecule of GH binds to two receptors, and the subsequent receptor dimerization within the plasma membrane is an important step in the activation of the target cell (see Fig. 2.8). This is then followed by the recruitment of a membrane-based tyrosine kinase (Janus-associated kinase 2, JAK 2). The number of receptors in a target tissue such as the liver can be changed both by peripheral factors, such as sex hormones, and also by GH itself, which induces 'down-regulation'.

The receptors for IGF-I are similar to those for insulin. These consist of a dimer of two glycoprotein subunits $(AB)_2$ (molecular weight 450 kDa), which span the membrane and have integral cytoplasmic tyrosine protein kinase domains (see Fig. 2.5). In contrast, the receptor for IGF-II is a single-chain structure that spans the membrane only once. Intriguingly, cloning has shown that it has 80% sequence homology with the mannose 6-phosphate receptor that transfers lysosomal enzymes from the Golgi apparatus to lysosomes. At present, there is little evidence that the IGF-II receptor itself activates intracellular signalling pathways. It may serve as a local 'capture' agent for IGF-II, which then subsequently acts on IGF-I receptors. IGF-II has only 10% of the affinity of IGF-I for the IGF-I receptor.

Growth hormone regulation

The major regulation systems are summarized in Fig. 3.4. The dynamic control of GH secretion from the pituitary is mediated by the interplay between GHRH and somatostatin. A feedback role for IGF-I at the pituitary and hypothalamus, together with a short-loop feedback by GH itself on the hypothalamus, has been proposed.

Release of GHRH and somatostatin is under the control of the central nervous system, so that stresses (e.g. exercise, excitement, cold, anaesthesia, surgery, haemorrhage) can all produce a rapid increase in the concentration of GH in serum. The most significant and consistent changes are associated with sleep, and bursts of secretion occur every 1–2 h during deep sleep (Fig. 3.5). The association with sleep is close—so that, if the onset of sleep is delayed,

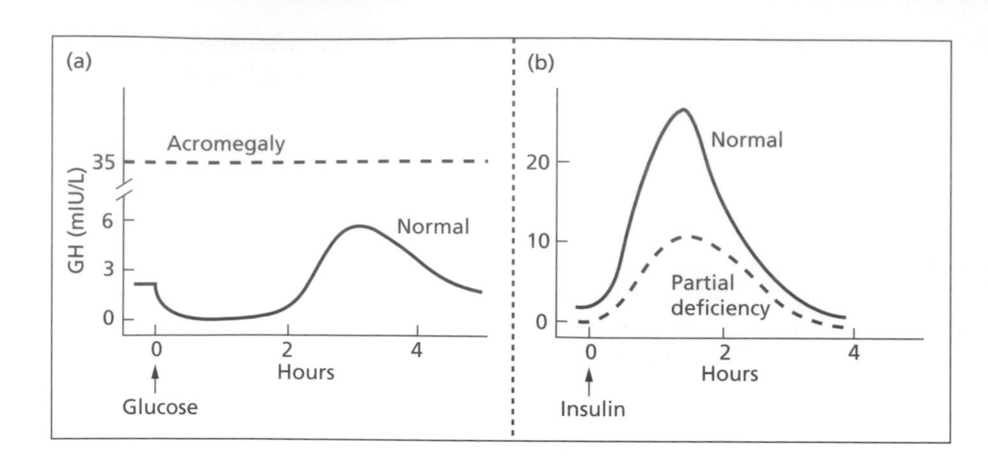

Figure 3.6 Dynamic tests of the regulation of the release of growth hormone (GH). (a) Oral administration of glucose normally suppresses GH release, although subsequently there is enhancement as blood sugar falls. In contrast, in acromegalic subjects, release of GH is not suppressed by administration of glucose, and so the excessive secretion of growth hormone continues. In these patients, there is sometimes a paradoxical rise in GH secretion. (b) Injection of insulin, by reducing blood sugar, increases the release of GH in normal subjects. This response is lacking in patients with complete hypopituitarism, but in those with partial deficiency there may be a reduced response.

the release of GH is also delayed. The highest levels of GH occur during sleep stages 3 or 4.

Since GH affects carbohydrate, protein and fat metabolism, it might be expected that metabolic products also influence its secretion—and this is indeed the case. Thus, an oral glucose load rapidly suppresses the secretion of GH (Fig. 3.6), and hypoglycaemia induced by insulin injection triggers release, which may be used as a test of GH secretion. Infusions of certain amino acids, particularly arginine, can also stimulate GH release, while elevated free fatty acid concentrations suppress it.

The secretion of GH is also modulated by other hormones. Glucocorticoids suppress secretion, while oestrogens sensitize the pituitary to the action of GHRH, so that basal and stimulated GH concentrations are slightly higher in women and rise early in the process of puberty in girls, but later in boys. Norepinephrine, dopamine and serotonin are also implicated in modifying GH secretion. As discussed in Chapter 5, thyroid hormone occupancy of nuclear receptors in somatotrophs results in transcriptional activation of genes responsible for GH production. As a consequence, GH secretion is compromised in hypothyroid children, who then suffer from stunted growth.

The basal concentration of GH in plasma is below 1 mIU/L, but it fluctuates rapidly, with peaks resulting from the pulsatile release of the hormone (see Fig. 3.5); bursts of hormone secretion are most frequent in adolescents, and account for the greatly increased total daily secretion in this age group. When secretion stops, the hormone disappears quite rapidly from the circulation, with a half-life of about 15 min. The presence of a GH-binding protein in serum increases this half-life, but the physiological significance of this protein is unknown.

Although the detailed mechanism that sets up the episodic nature of GH secretion is unknown, it appears to be the net result of the interplay between the two neurohormones, GHRH and somatostatin. GH peaks are virtually simultaneous with peaks of GHRH when somatostatin levels are low, and fall when somatostatin concentrations rise.

Assay

GH is measured for routine clinical purposes by immunoassay. Bioassays (see Appendix 1) are used to assess new GH preparations, such as pituitary extracts and recombinant products. They are also of obvious use when investigating the modified forms of GH that have been produced by recombinant technology in an endeavour to map the biologically active sites on the GH molecule. The most commonly used *in vivo* bioassay is the tibial assay, in which the GH-induced increase in width of the proximal epiphysis of the tibia is measured in hypophysectomized rats.

As would be expected from the diverse bioactivities of GH, it is possible to design an array of *in vitro* bioassays for GH. Two commonly used *in vitro* bioassays rely on the responses of immortalized cell lines, namely the Nb2 rat lymphoma cells and the 3T3-F442A mouse fibroblast cells, both of which respond to GH. These represent two classes of GH bioactivity. The Nb2 cells are exceptionally sensitive to both PRL and hGH, but will not respond to nonprimate GH. The response is usually a measure of the hormonally induced increase in activated cell proliferation. This class of GH bioactivity is referred to as lactogenic bioactivity. In contrast, the 3T3-F442A cells respond to both primate and nonprimate GH but not PRL. The response is a measure of the increase in transformation of the cells from a fibroblast form to adipocytes (Table 3.4). Since this is observed with GH only, this class of bioactivity of GH is referred to as its somatogenic bioactivity. Lactogenic bioactivity is thought to occur via receptors for PRL, whereas somatogenic bioactivity is mediated by receptors that are specific for GH (see Figs 2.1, 2.7 and 2.8). In addition, cell lines that express the human somatogenic receptor have now been engineered, and can be used to determine somatogenic bioactivity.

Prolactin

Structure

The structure of human PRL is very similar to that of GH, and for a long time it was believed that the human pituitary, unlike the pituitary of many animals, did not contain PRL. However, once PRL had been identified, a typical pituitary was found to contain 100 μg, i.e. 1% of the content of hGH by weight. Human PRL consists of 199 amino acids (Table 3.3), and is thus slightly longer than hGH. It has three disulphide bonds, in contrast to the two for hGH, and a molecular weight of approximately 22 kDa. PRL shows a similar tendency to that of GH to form oligomers in solution.

Effects of prolactin

The most obvious and perhaps main action of PRL is to stimulate lactation in the postpartum period (Fig. 3.7). It acts on the prepared breast to stimulate growth and support the secretion of milk. The mammary gland is rudimentary in young girls, but in the adolescent, oestrogen, GH and adrenal steroids act together to stimulate the growth of the duct system. Alveolar growth is stimulated by oestrogen, progesterone, adrenal steroids and PRL. Insulin and thyroid hormones are also necessary for mammary gland development, which is largely inhibited in

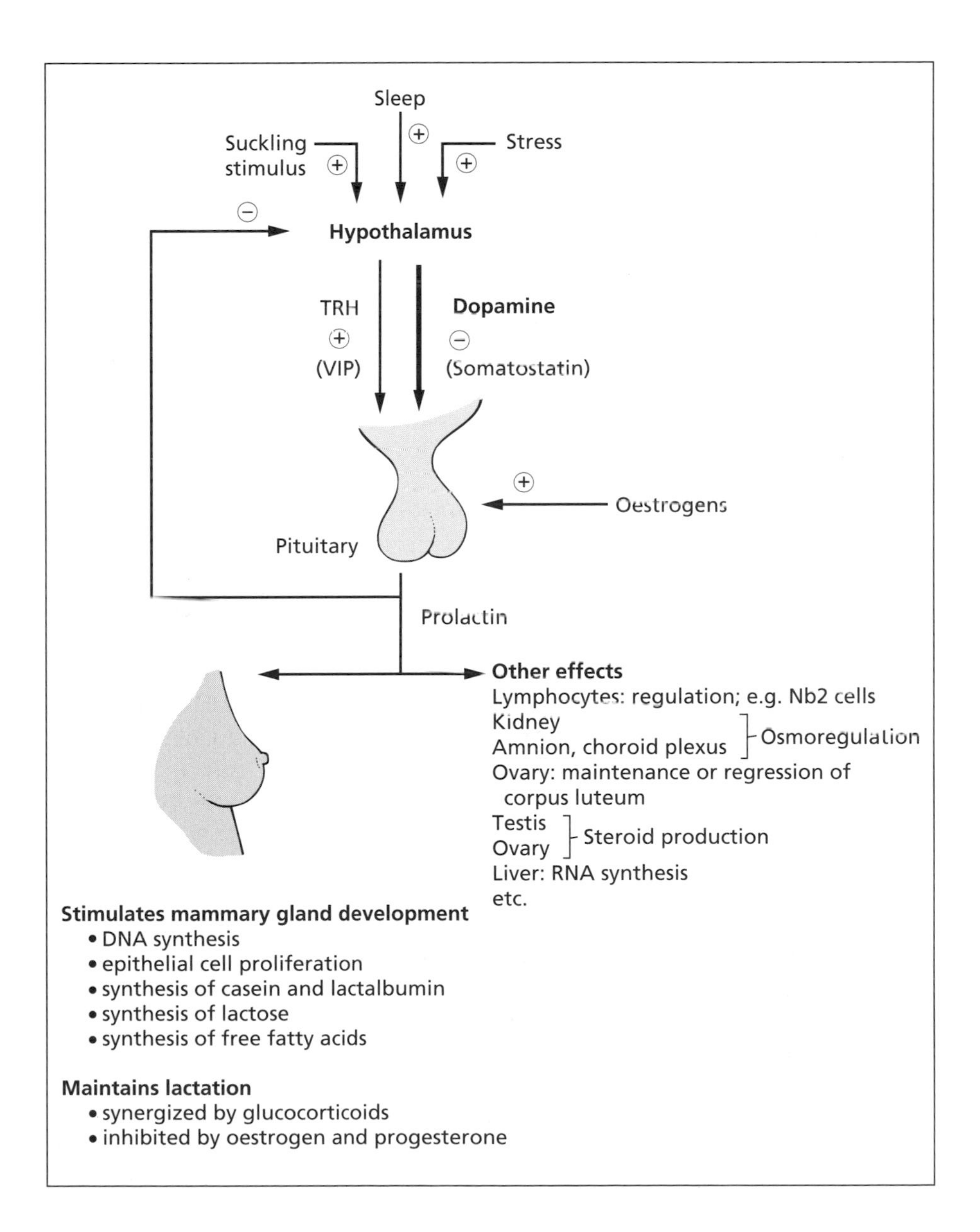

Figure 3.7 Summary of the regulation and effects of prolactin.

boys by testosterone. Some breast development happens in all pubertal boys, and gynaecomastia of puberty is not uncommon. It occasionally persists: if testosterone secretion is normal, mastectomy may be indicated. If it is not, a different series of diagnoses has to be considered.

Following childbirth, PRL and the adrenal steroids are essential for the initiation and maintenance of lactation. Hypophysectomy in experimental animals results in the immediate cessation of milk secretion, whereas adrenalectomy leads to a gradual reduction in milk secretion. The decrease in both oestrogen and progesterone after parturition is permissive for the initiation of lactation.

Many other actions have been attributed to PRL in both male and female mammals, but their physiological significance remains unclear (Fig. 3.7). Intriguingly, PRL-like molecules are not exclusive to mammals. In birds, the hormone stimulates crop-milk production (which forms the basis of an *in vivo* bioassay for PRL) and also nest-building activity. In reptiles, amphibians and teleosts, it acts as an osmoregulator. Over 100 actions have been associated with PRL when studied in different vertebrate groups.

Mechanism of action of PRL

The receptors for PRL are similar in structure to, and show regions of high homology with, the receptors for GH. They are single-chain glycoproteins with a molecular weight of ≈75 kDa that span the membrane once and are not linked to tyrosine protein kinase (see Fig. 2.7). As with GH, intracellular secondary signalling pathways are initiated by receptor dimerization (see Fig. 2.7) and the recruitment of tyrosine kinase (see Fig. 2.8).

Prolactin regulation

The major regulation systems are summarized in Fig. 3.7. PRL secretion is under the dominant negative control of dopamine. Thus, in the early pituitary transplant experiments (Table 3.2), PRL was unique in being the only hormone that increased in the circulation when transplanted to a site that was well vascularized but remote from the median eminence. PRL is released episodically, but the peaks are not as discrete as they are for GH. As with GH, the highest concentration is found at night and is dependent on sleep, but it is not associated with a specific sleep phase.

The most profound changes in the serum concentration occur during pregnancy and lactation. The concentration of PRL increases progressively, up to 10-fold, through pregnancy, remains elevated during lactation and is stimulated by suckling. The secretion rate declines during the later stages of lactation.

As with most of the other hormones of the anterior pituitary, stress (e.g. surgery, myocardial infarction and repeated venepuncture) stimulates PRL release. Pharmacological agents can also be used to stimulate release; for example, administration of L-α-methyldopa (which inhibits dopamine synthesis, and is used in the treatment of hypertension) results in increased circulating concentrations of PRL, and can induce loss of libido and lactation. Dopamine agonists, such as the precursor of dopamine, L-dopa (used in the treatment of Parkinson disease), inhibit PRL release. The ergot derivative, bromocriptine, is so powerful that it is used to treat the commonest secreting tumours of the pituitary, called prolactinomas. Many drugs used in the treatment of psychological disorders and many antiemetics stimulate the secretion of PRL because of their dopamine antagonist properties, and so induce lactation: thus, galactorrhoea can be an important side-effect of such treatment.

Assay

PRL is measured for routine clinical purposes by immunoassay. The commonest *in vivo* bioassay exploits the stimulation of cell proliferation in the crop sac of the pigeon. Cells in the walls of the crop sac, which are rich in protein and fat, are sloughed off the crop wall and regurgitated as a milk-like fluid. The bioassay measures crop-sac weight after injection of PRL. A highly sensitive *in vitro* bioassay relies on PRL stimulation of cultured cells of a rat lymphoma cell line, the Nb2 cells; both metabolism and proliferation are stimulated, as revealed by microculture tetrazolium assays (see Appendix 1, Table A1.2).

Adrenocorticotrophin (adrenocorticotrophic hormone, corticotrophin) and related peptides

Structure

ACTH is a peptide with 39 amino acid residues arranged in a single chain, with a molecular weight of 4500. The amino acid residues 1–24 are common to all species, but species-specific variations occur in the remaining residues. ACTH is one of a family of related peptide hormones derived from a larger precursor glycoprotein of molecular weight 31 000, known as pro-opiomelanocortin (POMC) (Fig. 3.8). Other products are α-, β-, and γ-MSH, lipotrophin molecules and β-endorphin. Lipotrophin was originally given its name because it was thought, mistakenly, to have fat-mobilizing activity. β-Endorphin is derived from β-lipotrophin; the name endorphin is derived from the endogenous morphine-like activities of this group of peptides. They have been found in many tissues, and may have a role in inhibiting signals to the brain arising from extreme stress or pain.

Effects of ACTH

The actions of ACTH are largely confined to the adrenal

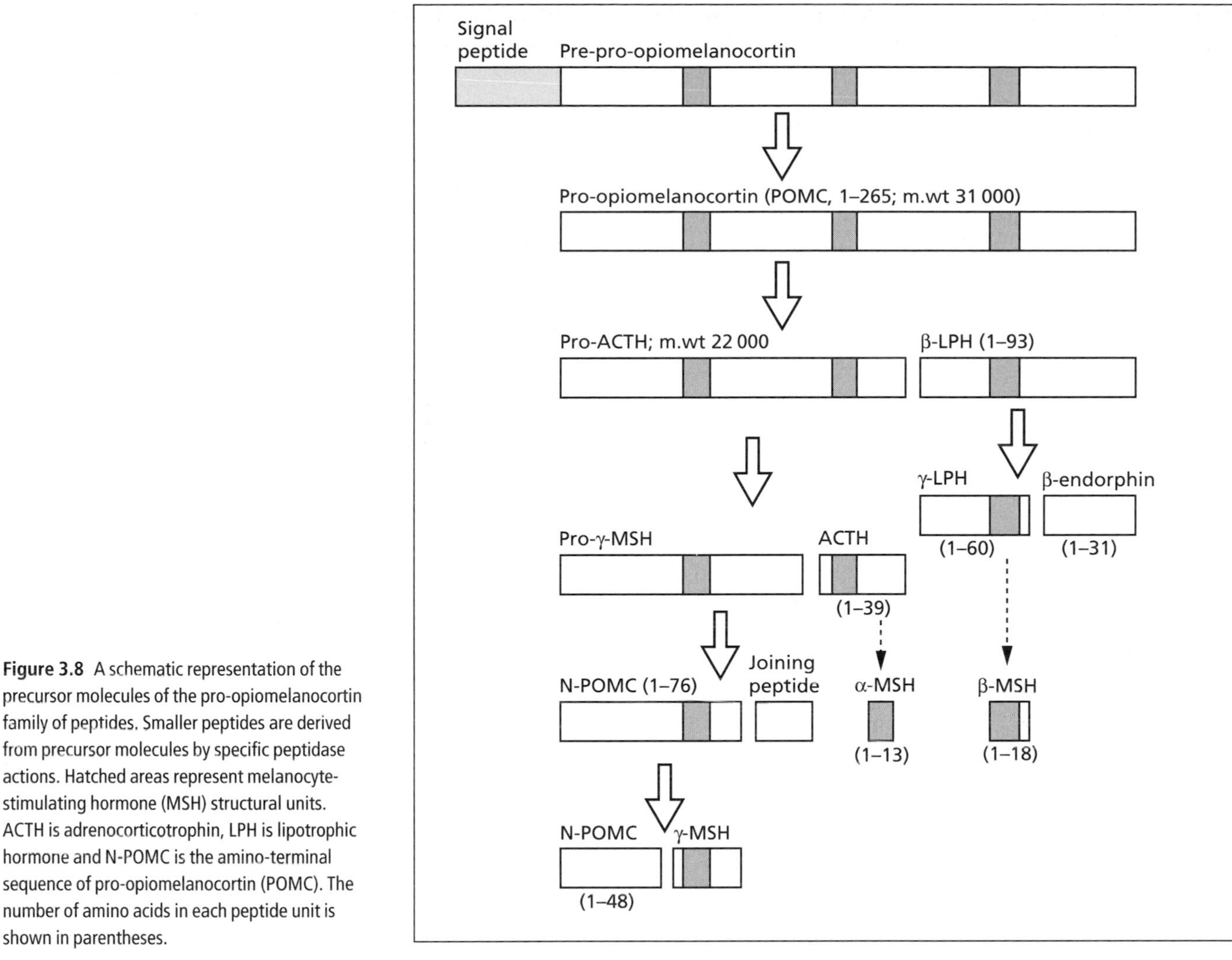

Figure 3.8 A schematic representation of the precursor molecules of the pro-opiomelanocortin family of peptides. Smaller peptides are derived from precursor molecules by specific peptidase actions. Hatched areas represent melanocyte-stimulating hormone (MSH) structural units. ACTH is adrenocorticotrophin, LPH is lipotrophic hormone and N-POMC is the amino-terminal sequence of pro-opiomelanocortin (POMC). The number of amino acids in each peptide unit is shown in parentheses.

cortex (see Chapter 4); it stimulates the conversion of cholesterol to pregnenolone in the zona fasciculata and zona reticularis. Administration of ACTH results in an increase in adrenal blood flow and cortical-cell protein synthesis. If the administration is prolonged, adrenal hypertrophy results. Because MSH is secreted with ACTH, darkening of the skin is a consequence of excessive ACTH secretion.

Mechanism of action of ACTH

ACTH stimulation of adrenal steroidogenesis is initiated with the binding of ACTH to receptors in the adrenocortical membrane and subsequent activation of adenylate cyclase (see Fig. 2.1). Ionic calcium enhances coupling of the stimulatory G-protein (G_s) subunit to adenylate cyclase. Enhanced mobilization of cholesterol and increased conversion of cholesterol to pregnenolone follows, as discussed in Chapter 4 and Appendix 3.

Control of secretion

Control of ACTH secretion is under the influence of hypothalamic CRH (Table 3.1), the secretion of which is in turn determined by blood cortisol acting by negative feedback at the hypothalamic level and by neural inputs from other brain centres (Fig. 3.9). CRH may be only a part of a releasing-factor system, and its action can be strikingly potentiated by other peptides, such as vasopressin. In addition, cortisol acts directly on the pituitary corticotrophs, and administration of glucocorticoids inhibits ACTH release in response to exogenously administered CRH. The most characteristic feature of ACTH secretion is its circadian rhythm, which is related to the light/dark cycle: the concentration of ACTH is lowest around midnight, increases until a morning peak, and thereafter slowly declines. Its rhythm is thus the reverse of that of GH. ACTH release is stimulated by stress, such as pain, fear, fever, or hypoglycaemia; the latter is a useful clinical test of ACTH reserve.

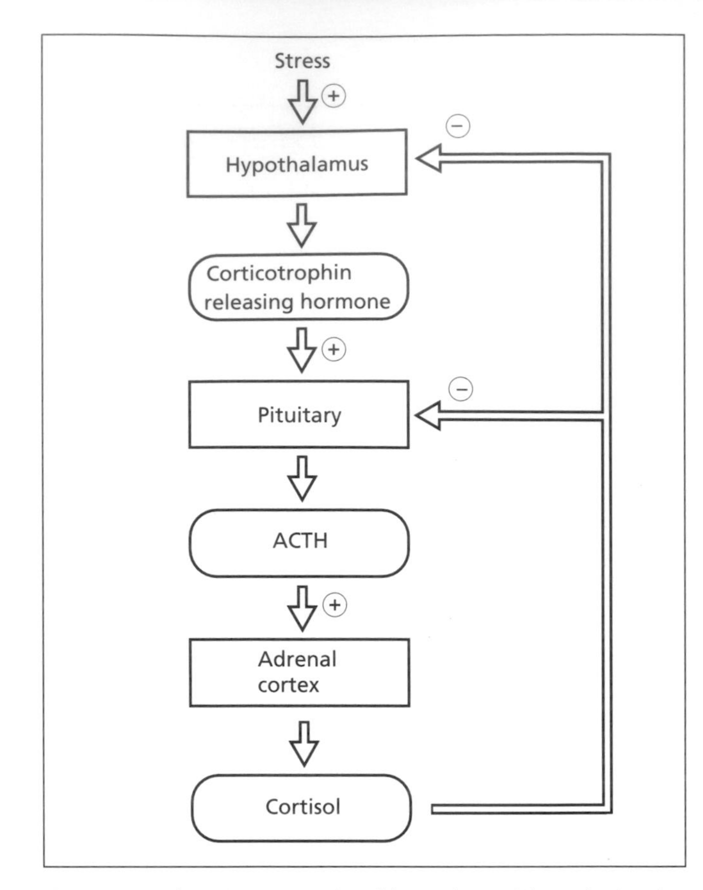

Figure 3.9 A schematic representation of the regulation of the production of cortisol from the adrenal cortex and of feedback regulation to the hypothalamus and pituitary.

Assay

Bioassays have played an important part in studies of the secretion of ACTH, since the actions of the hormone on the adrenal gland can be relatively easily measured. Hypophysectomized animals are usually used for this purpose, since the basal secretion from their adrenal glands is low. The output of steroids can be measured directly, but an indirect method has also been employed in which the depletion of the ascorbic acid content of the adrenal cortex, which accompanies steroidogenesis, is measured. Dispersed adrenal cells, immortalized ACTH-responsive Y1 cells, or slices of the adrenal gland in tissue culture, have been used for *in vitro* bioassays.

Immunoassays have been developed, some of which are directed against the amino (N)-terminal region (which is the part of ACTH that is important for biological activity) and some of which are specific for the carboxy (C)-terminal region of the molecule (which contains the species-specific but biologically inactive portion of the molecule). Highly sensitive two-site immunoradiometric assays (IRMAs) are also available that will measure only intact ACTH. Technical difficulties with the handling of samples for ACTH immunoassays have made it more usual to rely on cortisol measurements as an indirect indicator of ACTH levels.

Glycoprotein hormones secreted by the anterior pituitary: thyrotrophin (thyroid-stimulating hormone)

Structure

TSH-secreting cells (thyrotrophs) constitute about 10% of all cells in the anterior pituitary. TSH is composed of two subunits (α and β), both of which contain carbohydrate moieties. The molecular weight is about 30 kDa, and it varies slightly in different species. It should be noted that the structure of the α-subunit is similar for TSH, LH and FSH, but the β-subunits are different, and it is therefore this chain that confers hormonal specificity. It is possible to produce α- and β-subunit hybrids with, for example, the α-subunit derived from TSH and the β-subunit from LH. The resulting molecule will exhibit the biological activities of LH. Microheterogeneity of TSH is largely due to variation in the carbohydrate composition of the molecule.

Actions

TSH is the major physiological regulator of the thyroid gland (Fig. 3.3). It stimulates a wide range of metabolic parameters of the thyroid follicular cell, which are summarized in Table 3.5 and discussed in greater detail in Chapter 5. In normal circumstances, it is the major factor controlling the formation of thyroid hormones.

TSH stimulation of the thyroid follicular cell is initiated by the binding of the hormone to receptors on the basal surface of the cell and primarily by subsequent activation of adenylate cyclase (see Fig. 2.12). Cyclic AMP acts as the dominant second messenger.

Control of secretion

Negative-feedback control involving the hypothalamo-pituitary–thyroid axis was the first of these endocrine control systems to be established (Fig. 3.3). TRH stimulates the synthesis and release of TSH by the pituitary thyrotrophs. In turn, TSH stimulates hormonogenesis in the thyroid gland and release of the thyroid hormones, thyroxine (T_4) and triiodothyronine (T_3), which exert negative feedback on the pituitary and hypothalamus. The basal secretion of TSH is dependent on the tonic release of TRH by the hypothalamus. Focal hypothalamic lesions or transection of the pituitary stalk result in deficiency of TSH and subsequent hypothyroidism. Acute exposure to cold results in a temporary rise in TSH secretion.

The set point for regulation of the secretion of TSH appears to be determined by the level of TRH secreted by the hypothalamus, but it is likely that the primary site for negative-feedback control by thyroid hormones is at the level of the pituitary, where increased concentrations of thyroid hormone decrease the effectiveness of TRH action on the pituitary and hence inhibit TSH secretion. While TRH acts rapidly via cAMP to increase secretions of TSH, there is a long period before the inhibitory effects of thyroid hormones are observed. This is consistent with the view that the thyroid hormones act primarily by reducing the number of TRH receptors on the thyrotrophs. However, additional modulation of negative feedback in the thyrotroph may be provided by specific deiodinases (see Chapter 5).

Somatostatin also inhibits TSH secretion from the anterior pituitary and, in some species, e.g. the rat, oestrogens can reverse the inhibitory effect of thyroid hormones on the TSH response to TRH.

Assay

TSH is measured for routine clinical purposes by immunoassay. Several *in vivo* bioassay techniques have been developed for TSH that depend on stimulation of iodide uptake by the thyroid gland or release of T_3/T_4. *In vitro* bioassays have been devised that use various preparations of thyroid tissue, such as plasma membrane preparations, slices, or dispersed cells. More commonly, cultures of immortalized thyroid cell lines, such as the FRTL-5 cells derived from the rat thyroid or mammalian cells that have been transfected with the human TSH receptor, are now used. The responses measured include rises in intracellular cAMP, increased iodide uptake and incorporation of ^{3}H-thymidine, and also the bioreduction of tetrazolium salts. (For additional discussion, see Appendix 1.)

Glycoprotein hormones secreted by the anterior pituitary: gonadotrophins—luteinizing hormone and follicle-stimulating hormone

Structure

LH and FSH are secreted from the gonadotrophs, which make up 10–15% of the cells in the anterior pituitary. It is uncertain whether the two hormones are secreted by different cell types. As described for TSH, the glycoproteins LH and FSH are composed of two subunits (α and β), and have molecular weights of about 30 kDa (Table 3.3). Substantial microheterogeneity occurs, and it is largely due to variations in the carbohydrate components (see Chapter 1).

Table 3.5 Major stimulatory effects of thyrotrophin (thyroid-stimulating hormone, TSH) on thyroid follicular cells.

Early	Late
Adenylate cyclase	Iodide uptake
Endocytosis of colloid	Protein synthesis
Mitochondrial respiration and cell metabolism	DNA replication and mitotic activity

DNA, deoxyribonucleic acid.

Actions

LH acts in females to initiate steroidogenesis in the ovarian follicle, to induce ovulation and to maintain the secretory functions of the corpus luteum. In males, LH stimulates the Leydig cells of the testes to produce testosterone. FSH acts in females to stimulate the development of ovarian follicles and their secretion of oestradiol, while in males it stimulates spermatogenesis and the production of sex hormone–binding globulin. In both sexes, FSH also causes the secretion of a glycoprotein called inhibin, which exerts negative feedback on FSH secretion by the pituitary (see Chapter 6).

Control of secretion

GnRH (Table 3.1) is a positive regulator of both LH and FSH secretion. Their secretion is inhibited by high concentrations of gonadal steroids (i.e. testosterone or oestradiol), and FSH can also be inhibited by inhibin production (Fig. 3.10). Castration causes a marked rise in both the synthesis and the secretion of LH and FSH. Administration of androgens or oestrogens results in lower concentrations of gonadotrophins in plasma. Paradoxically, however, there is also a positive-feedback effect by sustained high concentrations of oestrogen, which leads to the sudden rise in LH release seen just before ovulation. LH secretion is pulsatile, with pulses occurring about every 90 min in response to pulses of GnRH. This pulsatile pattern is important for the action of this hormone, and significant changes may occur in some pathological conditions that are not detected by measurement of random basal levels of LH.

Assay

Both LH and FSH are measured by immunoassay for routine clinical use. *In vivo* bioassays for LH rely on the increase in prostate weight that is produced by testosterone, or on the depletion of the ovarian content of ascorbic acid or cholesterol, using hypophysectomized rats. FSH can be measured *in vivo* by its effects on rat or mice ovarian weight 4 days after administration of the hormone to hypophysectomized animals. An *in vitro* bioassay for FSH

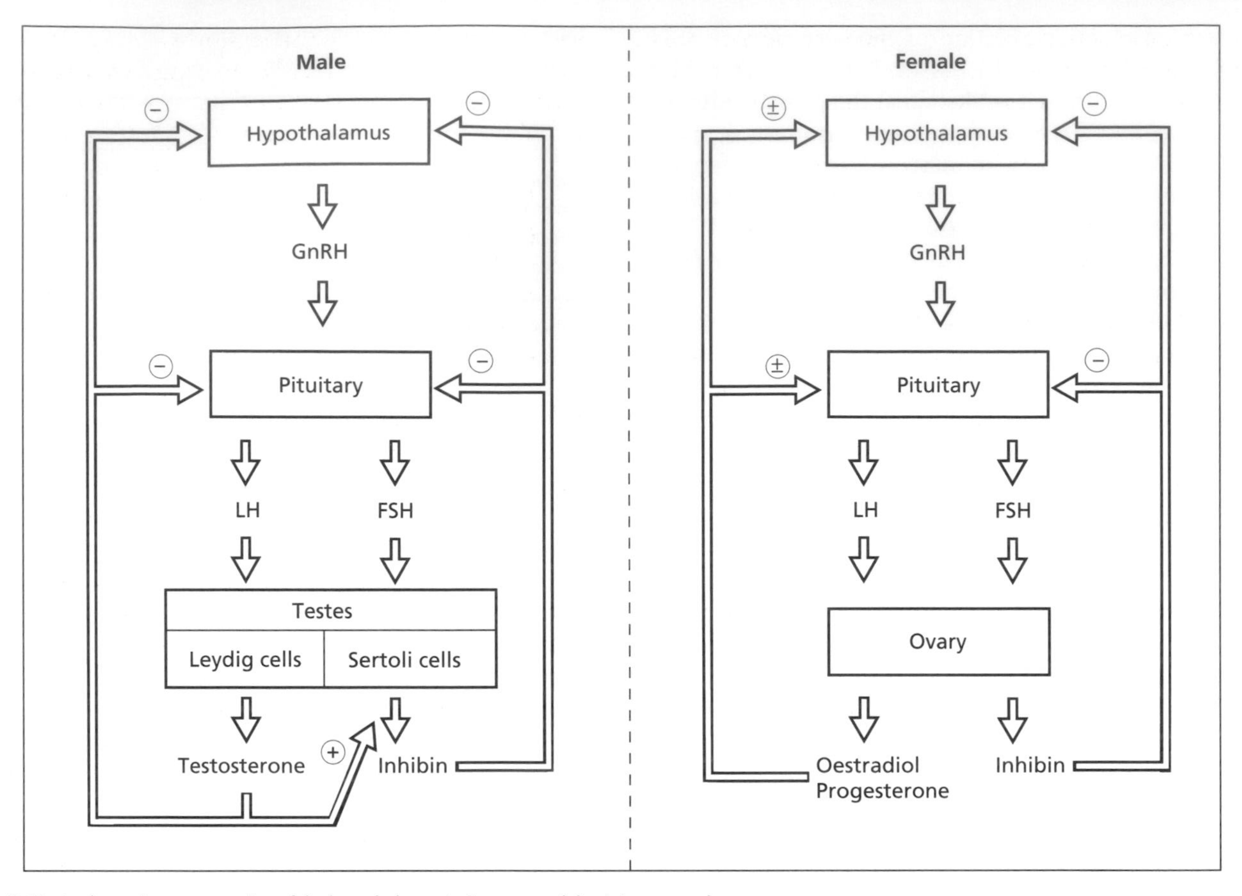

Figure 3.10 A schematic representation of the hypothalamopituitary–gonadal axis in men and women.

uses the increase in ^{3}H-thymidine incorporation into ovarian tissue maintained *in vitro*, and that for LH typically measures testosterone production from isolated Leydig cells. In addition, the responses, such as increased intracellular cAMP, can be used for an LH-responsive cell line, MA10. (For additional discussion, see Appendix 1.)

INAPPROPRIATE PRODUCTION OF ANTERIOR PITUITARY HORMONES

Disorders of oversecretion

Oversecretion is usually due to a benign tumour known as an adenoma. This may arise *de novo* in the pituitary gland, or result from a lack of suppression of the hypothalamic trophic hormone at the usual level. In Cushing disease, for example, there is a feedback abnormality, so that CRH and ACTH secretion are only suppressed at inappropriately high circulating levels of plasma cortisol. Continuous stimulation of the ACTH-producing cells of the pituitary gland by CRH results in a tumour: in days gone by, Cushing disease was treated by removal of the adrenal glands, and the basophil adenoma in the pituitary gland then grew without restraint, resulting in a condition of ACTH oversecretion called Nelson syndrome. It is now treated by trans-sphenoidal removal of the pituitary tumour.

The presence of a pituitary tumour may have local effects because of the position of the pituitary gland at the base of the skull and in close proximity to the optic nerves (Fig. 3.1). Pressure on the optic nerves may lead to loss of visual field, and restricted drainage of the cerebrospinal fluid (CSF) may lead to raised intracranial pressure, headaches and vomiting. If the tumour spreads laterally, it may invade the cavernous sinus and damage the oculomotor nerves, or it may extend into the sphenoid sinus, leading to a loss of CSF through the nose—a condition called CSF rhinorrhoea.

Advances in imaging techniques make the visualization of pituitary tumours very much easier, and magnetic resonance imaging of this area is particularly effective (Fig. 3.1). Treatment is always surgical in the first instance, and it is now common to operate through the nose and to perform an exploratory operation for the cure of the overproduction syndromes, even if imaging of the adenoma has not been entirely successful.

Tumours secreting excessive amounts of PRL, GH, or ACTH are commonest, but TSH and gonadotrophins are rarely produced in excess. Some pituitary tumours appear to be functionless, although they still contain numerous secretory granules and may be secreting pituitary hormones at a low level.

Effects of prolactin-secreting tumours

The commonest result of hyperprolactinaemia is a loss of reproductive function (see Chapter 6). The gonadal dysfunction is due to interference with the hypothalamopituitary–gonadal axis by the hyperprolactinaemia, through some mechanism not yet identified. Thus, in women, for example, the raised PRL inhibits both the normal pulsatile secretion of LH and FSH and the midcycle LH surge, resulting in anovulation.

The circulation of raised PRL itself may cause inappropriate secretion of milk, called galactorrhoea. This is classic in patients with primary hypothyroidism, because a lack of T_4 feedback leads to increased TRH secretion and to the generation of TSH, but TRH also stimulates PRL and FSH. Thus, in men, testicular volume increases in primary hypothyroidism and the breast may secrete milk; but this is more striking in women, because the FSH secretion that accompanies hypoprolactinaemia also results in breast stimulation by oestradiol from the ovaries.

The treatment of prolactinomas with bromocriptine, a dopamine agonist, is highly effective and surgery and/or radiotherapy are rarely required to control the tumours. Because of its inhibitory control, interruption of the hypothalamopituitary circulation by a tumour or by transection of the pituitary stalk secondary to trauma may lead to mild elevation of PRL concentrations. These are useful in diagnosis, but do not have clinical effects.

Effects of ACTH-secreting tumours: Cushing disease

Cushing syndrome is the name given to the symptom complex that results from excessive secretion of adrenocortical hormones (see Chapter 4). When excessive secretion of adrenocortical hormones is the result of the feedback abnormality of CRH–ACTH secretion mentioned above, this has been called Cushing disease. This is always due to the presence of an ACTH-secreting basophil tumour, even though it may be difficult to visualize on magnetic resonance imaging. In adult patients, it may be useful to catheterize the venous drainage of the pituitary gland and to administer CRH in order to determine the side on which the adenoma lies: in children, because of the mixing of pituitary venous blood, this is not a useful procedure, and it is arguable that localization of the pituitary adenoma by direct inspection by an experienced neurosurgeon is the logical way to proceed, once the diagnosis has been made. Making this diagnosis and separating Cushing disease from the other causes of Cushing syndrome is relatively straightforward in about 85% of cases, but it is sometimes extremely difficult to identify the cause, since none of the tests available give unequivocal answers (see Chapter 4).

Because ACTH is initially part of a much larger molecule (POMC) (Fig. 3.8), α-MSH is also cosecreted with ACTH in the situation of Cushing disease, and this results in hyperpigmentation of the skin.

Effects of GH-secreting tumours: gigantism and acromegaly

Growth in the fetal period and the first 8–10 months of life is largely controlled by nutritional intake; GH then becomes the predominant influence on the rate at which children grow. A person destined to become tall secretes GH continuously at rather higher circulating concentrations than his or her smaller peers. The consequence is that he or she grows rather faster than average and, year by year, gains height. When a GH-secreting tumour is present, this excessive growth rate continues throughout childhood and the years of puberty, and can lead to extremely tall stature—210 cm (7 ft) or more. If GH is secreted excessively after the growing ends of the bones have fused, a condition known as acromegaly will develop. The hands, feet and jaw become enlarged by thickening of the bones, and this is exaggerated by thickening of the soft tissues (Fig. 3.11). Excessive sweating is a common clinical feature; headaches and visual-field loss are not uncommon because of the pressure on the optic nerves.

Since GH causes an increase in glucose concentration, insulin production rises. Since insulin receptors are downregulated by hyperinsulinaemia (see Chapter 8), a condition of insulin resistance develops, and the patient may present with symptoms of diabetes mellitus. Removal of the pituitary tumour cures the diabetes.

Acromegaly is a dangerous condition because of these effects, but also because of hypertrophy of the heart and hypertension, which follows water retention.

GH is secreted in a pulsatile fashion (Fig. 3.5) and the hallmark of acromegaly or gigantism is the secretion of GH without the usual pulsatile pattern. It is relatively easy therefore to diagnose acromegaly, because there is never a time when GH is not present in the circulation. Also, IGFs are elevated secondarily to the unrestrained production of GH. GH secretion is usually suppressed by rising glucose levels (Fig. 3.6), such as after a meal; a classic test for the diagnosis of uncontrolled GH secretion is to administer glucose and to show that the GH levels do not fall.

In acromegalic subjects, for reasons that are not at all clear, the dopamine agonist bromocriptine is sometimes

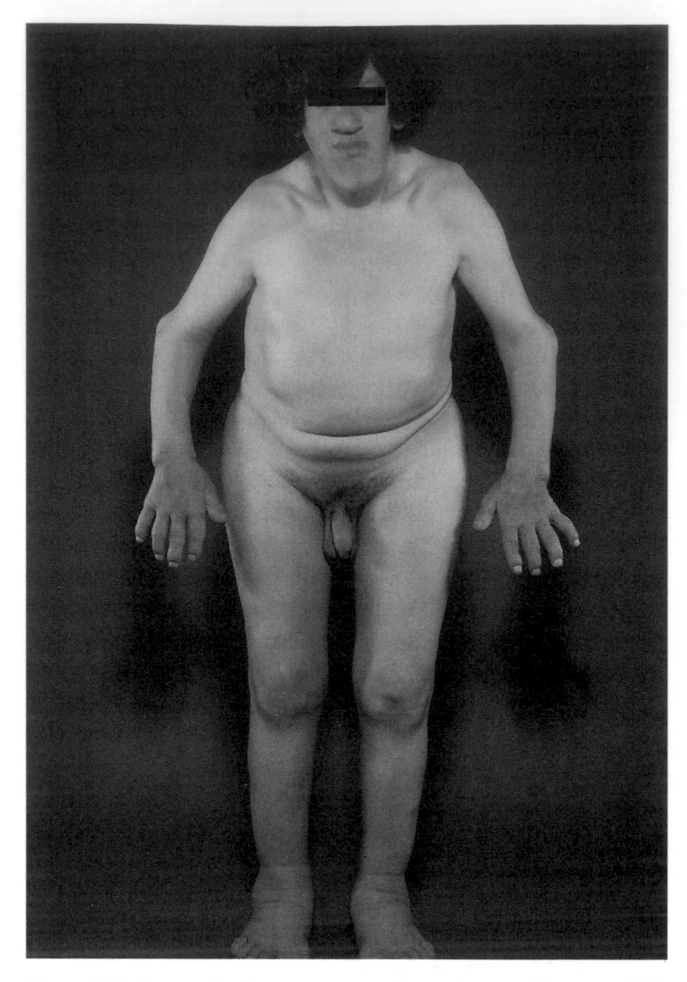

Figure 3.11 Acromegaly: the consequences of excessive growth hormone (GH) secretion in adult life. Note enlargement of the hands, feet and jaw. There is thickening of the soft tissues and fluid retention, which is manifested here by ankle oedema.

effective in reducing GH secretion. It is also possible to use long-acting somatostatin analogues to control unrestrained GH secretion, but the best treatment is undoubtedly the surgical removal of the GH-secreting adenoma.

Undersecretion of pituitary hormones

Reduced pituitary function, hypopituitarism, can result from many causes (Table 3.6). The hypothalamopituitary axis is particularly vulnerable to irradiation, and progressive loss of pituitary hormones is almost inevitable after cranial radiotherapy, even if a brain tumour is not close to the hypothalamopituitary axis. Gonadotrophin secretion is particularly vulnerable to trauma (which includes surgery), while GH secretion is especially susceptible to irradiation.

Table 3.6 Causes of hypopituitarism.

Causes
Impaired secretion of hypothalamic hormones
Disconnection of the hypothalamopituitary axis
Tumours
Trauma
Infections
Pituitary aplasia or hypoplasia
Pituitary destruction
Tumour
Surgery
Infarction
Irradiation

Effects of loss of GH secretion

In the adult subject, loss of GH secretion is a physiological part of the ageing process, and accelerated loss of GH secretion does not usually produce obvious clinical symptoms. In younger adults, but more particularly in children, loss of GH secretion leads to an obvious loss of growth rate and, less obviously, also to a loss of the metabolic functions of GH, leading to an increase in body fat and decreased muscle strength.

When GH secretion is diminished, the patients have a very characteristic physical appearance (Fig. 3.12). The child is short and fat, and the face is characteristic. This condition is eminently treatable using exogenous biosynthetic GH administered by daily subcutaneous injection—and the result in clinical terms is spectacular, with a small child growing slowly into a normal adult.

GH has to be given by injection, because the molecule would be degraded in the gastrointestinal tract. Because supplies of biosynthetic GH are unlimited (except by cost), GH has also been used in pharmacological amounts for the treatment of many other causes of short stature. The effects of this treatment on final heights have yet to be reported, but it is clear that the administration of GH in adequate dose will make any child grow more quickly in the short term.

Effects of loss of ACTH

The symptoms of loss of adrenocortical hormone secretion will be covered in Chapter 4. ACTH controls the secretion of both cortisol and adrenal androgens. For this reason, patients with Cushing disease have not only the effects of hypercortisolaemia, but also those of hyperandrogenaemia; conversely, patients with ACTH insufficiency suffer from the effects of cortisol deprivation (hypoglycaemia and weakness) and also those due to the loss of adrenal androgen secretion. In males, this is largely

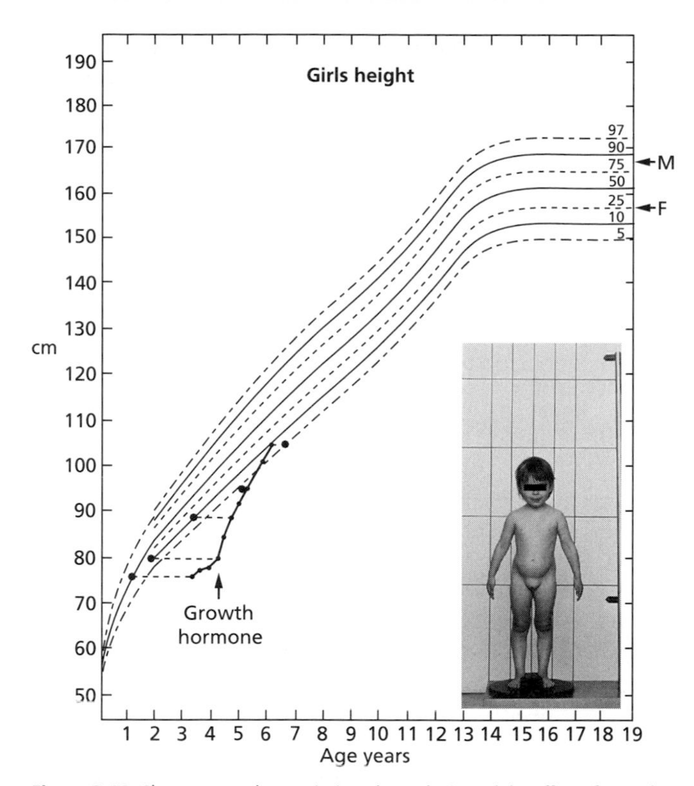

Figure 3.12 Short stature due to pituitary hypoplasia and the effect of growth hormone (GH) replacement. The height of this girl, who is suffering from GH deficiency, is shown compared to the population reference standards. With these, 50% of girls' heights lie below the 50th centile line and 5% below the 5th, etc. Her height for her chronological age (•) is greatly reduced, but her skeletal maturity (or bone age) is also delayed. As a consequence, her height plotted for her bone age (●) falls within the centiles of normality. (Bone age is determined by radiological examination of the epiphyses of the long bones in the hand: comparison is made with standard radiographs to assess skeletal maturity.) The finding that this girl's bone age is delayed means that she has the potential to attain an adult height appropriate for her family. This is because she could grow for longer than most children, owing to the delay in skeletal maturation and the fusion of her epiphyses. M represents the mother's height centile and F the father's. The appearance of this child is, in several respects, similar to that of the boy with Laron syndrome, who is suffering from GH resistance rather than deficiency (see Fig. 2.9). However, unlike the latter, her GH concentration was undetectable in a basal sample, and no secretion could be elicited by insulin-induced hypoglycaemia. Secretion of her other anterior pituitary hormones was normal. After GH replacement treatment was initiated, there was rapid catch-up, both of her height and skeletal maturity.

obscured by the testicular secretion of testosterone, but females with ACTH deficiency lack pubic and axillary hair and also sexual libido.

Effects of loss of gonadotrophin secretion

The secretion of GnRH is extremely vulnerable to calorie restriction. Thus, in patients with anorexia nervosa or in those who exercise excessively, GnRH secretion falls and this is the commonest reason for a loss of reproductive function. As mentioned previously, PRL-secreting tumours interfere with the hypothalamopituitary–gonadal axis, and the resulting gonadotrophin deficiency leads to secondary amenorrhoea in women and impotence and infertility in men; loss of gonadotrophin function in children leads to a failure to advance in puberty (see Chapter 6).

Many treatments are available for the management of abnormalities of reproductive function. For example, it is possible to use GnRH administered by subcutaneous pulsatile infusion, gonadotrophins or sex hormones (testosterone or oestradiol) to restore fertility.

Effects of loss of TSH

Congenital TSH deficiency is a rare problem, but any or all of the pituitary hormones may be lost in congenital pituitary hypoplasia or aplasia, which is particularly associated with loss of midline structures, including the optic nerves, leading to the combination of blindness and congenital hypopituitarism (septo-optic dysplasia). TSH deficiency causes the clinical signs of hypothyroidism (Chapter 5), although they are usually less marked than in primary thyroid disorders. Most newborn babies are screened for thyroid dysfunction, but because most of the screens employ the fact that a loss of T_4 leads to elevation of the TSH concentration, congenital hypothyroidism secondary to TSH deficiency is often missed, as the TSH concentrations are low.

Effects of loss of prolactin

There are no clinical symptoms associated with PRL deficiency, but this condition is extremely rare, because—as has already been indicated—PRL is the only pituitary hormone that is under inhibitory rather than stimulatory control. The condition therefore only occurs after pituitary destruction.

FUNCTIONS OF THE POSTERIOR PITUITARY GLAND (NEUROHYPOPHYSIS)

Oxytocin and vasopressin

The two hormones released from the posterior pituitary are oxytocin and vasopressin. Although they are both nonapeptides, with very similar structures (see Fig. 1.4), they have quite different physiological roles. Oxytocin, which literally means 'quick birth', is important for contraction of smooth muscles, such as those in the uterus during labour, and the myoepithelial cells that line the duct of the mammary gland (see Chapter 6). Vasopressin regulates water excretion and is a potent vasoconstrictor.

It is also referred to as antidiuretic hormone (ADH) or, in humans, arginine vasopressin (AVP); the latter terminology distinguishes the form found in humans (AVP) from that produced by pigs, lysine vasopressin, which is less potent in humans but has been used therapeutically.

As discussed earlier in this chapter, both oxytocin and vasopressin are packaged in granules as larger precursor molecules. This synthesis occurs in nerve cells of the supraoptic and paraventricular nuclei. The granules move down the axons, through the stalk, to the posterior pituitary. Each hormone, together with its associated neurophysin, is liberated by proteolysis from the larger precursor molecule.

The released hormones circulate in blood largely in an unbound form, and so are removed rapidly from the circulation, with a half-life of about 5 min. The kidney acts as the main site of clearance of the hormones.

Both oxytocin and vasopressin act on their target cells via G-protein-linked cell-surface receptors (see Fig. 2.1). Oxytocin and the V_1 class of receptors for vasopressin, which mediate its stimulation of vascular smooth muscle contraction, increase phosphatidylinositol (PI) turnover and thereby mobilize intracellular calcium (see Fig. 2.18). In contrast, the renal action of vasopressin, which is produced via the V_2 class of receptors, uses cAMP as the dominant intracellular messenger (see Figs 2.1 and 2.12).

Control of vasopressin secretion

The main physiological stimulus for the release of vasopressin is an increase in osmotic pressure in the circulating blood. Vasopressin causes retention of water by the kidney, which reduces plasma osmolality. This in turn acts as a negative-feedback signal on the hypothalamic osmoreceptors, which suppress vasopressin secretion.

In addition, there are a number of nonosmotic factors that can stimulate vasopressin release. For example, a fall in blood volume of 8% or more stimulates vasopressin release. In addition, alterations in blood volume also change the relationship between osmolality and the release of vasopressin. The fact that haemorrhage is a potent stimulus for the release of vasopressin could be important since at high concentrations the hormone has a vasoconstrictor effect. The response depends on baroreceptors located in the carotid sinus and the aortic area, and on plasma volume receptors present in the left atrium. In addition, a reduction in the arterial partial pressure of oxygen (Pa,O_2) and an increase in the arterial partial pressure of carbon dioxide (Pa,CO_2) stimulate the release of vasopressin. A number of hormones, including angiotensin II, epinephrine, cortisol, and sex steroids (oestrogen and progesterone), may also regulate the release of vasopressin. The effects of sex steroids may explain the fluid retention that can occur in the latter part of the menstrual cycle.

As with other hypothalamic hormones, the central nervous system plays an important part in the regulation of the release of neurohypophyseal hormones. The pain and trauma associated with surgery cause a marked increase in the circulating concentration of vasopressin, as do nausea and vomiting. Psychogenic stimuli may also be effective in releasing these neurohypophyseal hormones. The activity of the neurohypophyseal system is also influenced by environmental temperature; a rise in temperature stimulates vasopressin release before there is any change in plasma osmolality.

Actions of vasopressin

Vasopressin, in the concentrations that normally circulate, has its chief action in the kidney, where it reduces the flow of urine and leads the latter to become more concentrated. It acts on the final section of the distal convoluted tubule and on the collecting ducts to increase their permeability to water and hence its reabsorption, since the renal interstitium has a high osmolality. Vasopressin binds to the V_2 receptors on the peritubular surface of the collecting ducts, but produces its effect on the luminal membranes. Water leaves the cells partly via the lateral membranes, and enters the lateral intracellular spaces. The intracellular messenger for vasopressin action on the kidney is cAMP; vasopressin-sensitive adenylate cyclase has been demonstrated in the collecting duct and part of the distal convoluted tubule.

The effect of this hormone on water balance, through its action in the collecting duct, is truly remarkable. For example, a child weighing 30 kg needs to excrete a solute load of about 800 mosm/24 h: at the extreme of urinary dilution (50 mosm/kg), this load could be excreted in 16 L of urine, and at the extreme of concentration (1100 mosm/kg) in 727 mL.

Vasopressin action on blood vessels has been known for some time to be of pharmacological importance, and vasopressin or its analogues have been used to obtain haemostasis, for example, when there is severe bleeding from the gastrointestinal tract or postpartum haemorrhage. Measurements of cardiac output and total peripheral resistance in the conscious state show that physiological concentrations of vasopressin can exert potent vasoconstrictor actions.

Control of oxytocin secretion

Oxytocin circulates in very low concentrations and is normally undetectable in the blood, but it is elevated during parturition, during lactation and also during mating. During parturition, the concentration of oxytocin rises to peak values at the time of delivery of the fetus and expulsion of the placenta. Vaginal stimulation is an important factor controlling its release, though other factors, such as the fall in progesterone and the increase in oestrogen concentration, may play a part. If a balloon is inflated in the vagina, oxytocin is released; this response is known as the Fergusson reflex. A positive-feedback mechanism thus operates when a fetus moves down the birth canal. Under the influence of muscular contraction produced by oxytocin, there is vaginal distension, which stimulates still further secretion of oxytocin. Stimulation of the nipple also causes release of oxytocin during suckling and this leads to ejection of milk. Even the sight and sound of an infant can stimulate milk ejection, but stress inhibits the release of oxytocin and so reduces the flow of milk.

Actions of oxytocin

Oxytocin has two sites of action, namely the uterus and the mammary gland. By increasing the contraction of the uterus, it aids in the expulsion of the fetus and the placenta. In addition to a possible role in regulating the release of oxytocin, ovarian steroid hormones may influence its action by altering uterine sensitivity; progesterone appears to block and oestrogen appears to potentiate the response of the uterus to oxytocin. In the mammary gland, the myoepithelial cells surrounding the alveoli and ducts contract to expel milk from the alveoli and are sensitive to oxytocin. Oxytocin may also increase excretion of sodium; both oxytocin and vasopressin have been shown to act synergistically to promote sodium excretion.

Disordered secretion of the posterior pituitary

Syndromes of oxytocin excess and deficiency have not been described. Those arising from inappropriate secretion of vasopressin are discussed below.

Overproduction of vasopressin

Excess secretion of AVP may occur in any brain disorders such as trauma and infection, in patients with pneumonia and malignant disease, and in patients being treated with cytotoxic therapy and/or narcotics and analgesics. The result is retention of water, serum hypo-osmolality, hyponatraemia and inappropriately high urine osmolality. Symptoms are headache and apathy, progressing to nausea, vomiting, abnormal neurological signs and impaired consciousness. In very severe cases, there may be coma, convulsions and death, so this is not a situation to be taken lightly. Body oedema is not a feature of AVP excess, because free water is evenly distributed in all body fluid compartments. The only treatment is to restrict fluid intake and to replace sodium lost secondarily in the renal tubules. This is a difficult and dangerous situation.

Deficient secretion of vasopressin

Diabetes insipidus occurs when vasopressin secretion is reduced or absent. The term 'diabetes insipidus' stems from the days when physicians used to taste the urine and contrasted it with the condition of diabetes mellitus, in which the urine has a sweet taste. Patients with diabetes insipidus pass extremely large volumes of up to 20 L of urine in 24 h; this is of low specific gravity and low osmolality. This condition has to be distinguished from one caused by failure of the kidneys to respond to vasopressin, which is called nephrogenic diabetes insipidus. This rare condition is only inherited by males. This can be associated with a loss of the vasopressin (V_2) G-protein–coupled receptor. The germline mutation is on Xq2.8, and more than 100 mutations, all of which abolish a normal vasopressin response, have been found in different families. The obligate, heterozygote mother has random X inactivation, and exhibits varying degrees of polyuria and polydipsia. However, in an affected hemizygous male, plasma vasopressin, even when very high, is unable to increase urine concentration. Increased passage of dilute urine can also result from a psychological disturbance (psychogenic polydipsia), in which the patient drinks inappropriately large volumes of water.

Pituitary diabetes insipidus is most commonly produced by damage to the neurohypophyseal system. It can occur as a result of head injury or the growth of a tumour, and is sometimes called central diabetes insipidus, as opposed to nephrogenic diabetes insipidus discussed above. Isolated diabetes insipidus may also occur in the absence of any visible structural lesion, and in some of these cases it may be caused by an autoimmune process that destroys the vasopressin neurones.

A patient with diabetes insipidus is unable to reduce the flow of urine when deprived of water, and the plasma osmolality consequently rises. If a vasopressin radioimmunoassay is available, diagnosis is best confirmed by monitoring hormone concentrations after an infusion of hypertonic saline. Alternatively, a water-deprivation test may be used. Because of the inability to concentrate urine, the flow of dilute urine continues, and the patient loses weight. If body weight falls by 5% during the course of the deprivation test, the test must be terminated and the patient allowed to drink, to avoid dangerous dehydration. During a water-deprivation test, the osmolality of urine specimens of a patient with diabetes insipidus will not differ by more than 50 mosm/kg. In a normal subject the plasma osmolality ranges from 275 to 295 mosm/kg, while the range of urine osmolality is wide, from 40 to 1000 mosm/kg. After water deprivation, the urine osmolality will normally rise to exceed 800 mosm/kg, while the plasma osmolality remains below 295 mosm/kg. In contrast, the urine of patients with diabetes insipidus will be less concentrated than plasma, and the osmolality of plasma will rise above 300 mosm/kg. Patients with nephrogenic diabetes insipidus will not respond to vasopressin. Therefore they can be distinguished by administration of exogenous vasopressin or a synthetic analogue at the end of a water-deprivation test.

The management of diabetes insipidus due to AVP deficiency is relatively straightforward, involving administration of analogues of AVP, specifically desmopressin, which is highly effective. It is sometimes also used in normal children who suffer from nocturnal enuresis (bed-wetting), and it is something of a mystery how such patients avoid the syndrome of AVP excess outlined above.

OUTLINE OF BIOCHEMICAL TESTS OF ANTERIOR PITUITARY FUNCTION

The short-lived hypothalamic hormones, which are secreted into the portal vessels and regulate anterior pituitary function, are not routinely measured. Five of the six hormones secreted by the anterior pituitary are measured on a large scale by immunoassay of serum samples. Because of technical difficulties when handling specimens for the measurement of ACTH, there tends to be more restricted use of direct immunoassays of this hormone, greater reliance being placed on the immunoassay of cortisol to assess adrenal status.

The results from the immunoassays of the anterior pituitary hormones are interpreted in the knowledge of the feedback systems discussed previously. For example, in primary hypothyroidism, when circulating thyroid hormones are low due to defective thyroid function, the levels of TSH will be elevated due to lack of negative feedback and the response to exogenously administered TRH will be exaggerated. Alternatively, with secondary hypothyroidism (i.e. pituitary underactivity), both TSH and thyroid hormones are low, and there will be no response to exogenously administered TRH. Because of difficulties in interpreting the results of immunoassays of thyroid hormones, reliance is often placed on TSH immunoassays when assessing patient thyroid status (see Fig. 5.10).

An elevated level of LH in a man will reflect Leydig-cell hypofunction, and an elevated level of FSH reflects impaired spermatogenesis. In a woman, raised levels of LH and FSH indicate ovarian failure. Low levels of gonadotrophins are naturally encountered in both sexes, and thus hypogonadotrophin hypogonadism has to be diagnosed biochemically by the concomitant findings of a low sex-steroid hormone concentration and an inappropriately low concentration of LH and FSH.

Two of the three commonest functional tumours of the anterior pituitary—those secreting excessive amounts of PRL or GH in an autonomous manner—can be identified by the direct measurement of sustained levels of these hormones by immunoassay. Regression of the tumour in response to therapy can then be monitored by the decline in the levels of these hormones. The first biochemical indication of an ACTH-producing tumour could be persistently elevated serum cortisol levels, with an absence of diurnal fluctuation, and high levels of cortisol in the urine.

One of the difficulties in the interpretation of the direct measurement of anterior pituitary hormones, such as GH, is the pulsatile nature of their release into the circulation. This renders the interpretation of random samples impossible. To avoid this problem, dynamic tests of anterior pituitary secretion have been devised. Basically, there are two types: provocative tests, which are used to investigate suspected pituitary hypofunction, and suppression tests, which are used to monitor overactivity. Examples of provocative tests are shown in Table 3.7 and Fig. 3.6b, and an example of a suppression test is given in Fig. 3.6a, where the result of an oral glucose tolerance test is shown.

Table 3.7 Examples of provocative tests of the anterior pituitary.

Normal response	
TRH	↑ TSH and PRL at 30 min These decline at 60 min unless there is a hypothalamic lesion
GnRH	↑ LH and FSH at 30 min
Insulin	Induces hypoglycaemia ↑ GH at 30 min (see Fig. 3.6b). ↑ Cortisol (in response to ACTH).
Exercise	↑ GH after 10 min exercise

ACTH, adrenocorticotrophin hormone (adrenocorticotrophinc); FSH, follicle-stimulating hormone; GH, growth hormone; GnRH, gonadotrophin-releasing hormone; LH, luteinizing hormone; PRL, prolactin; TRH, thyroid-stimulating hormone-releasing hormone; TSH, thyroid-stimulating hormone (thyrotrophin).

CHAPTER 4

The Adrenal Gland

SUMMARY

The adrenal gland consists of an inner medulla and an outer cortex. The cortex has three clearly distinct cell types, each performing a different function. The outer layer of cells in the zona glomerulosa synthesizes aldosterone and releases this steroid hormone in response to stimulation by angiotensin II or to increases in potassium concentration. Aldosterone has potent mineralocorticoid activity and is involved—along with other hormonal and neural systems—in regulating sodium balance and blood pressure. The adrenal cortex also contains two other cell types in the zona fasciculata and zona reticularis, which respond to adrenocorticotrophin and yield cortisol and androgenic hormones, respectively.

In the medulla, the hormones epinephrine and norepinephrine are stored in granules. These require cholinergic, preganglionic sympathetic stimulation for release of their contents into the circulation. Epinephrine stimulates glycogenolysis and an increase in circulating free fatty acids, while norepinephrine is more potent in the latter action. Both hormones are vasoactive, although only norepinephrine increases mean blood pressure.

INTRODUCTION

The presence of the adrenal glands was noted in 1564 by Bartolommeo Eustachio. Little was known of the function of the adrenal gland until Thomas Addison described the effects of adrenal insufficiency in 1855, with the unusual association of increased pigmentation of the skin and progressive fatigue. In 1894, Oliver and Schaffer at University College, London, extracted a substance from the medulla that could raise systolic blood pressure. The pressor agent was epinephrine (adrenaline), which was isolated, chemically characterized and synthesized between 1900 and 1904. Demonstration of the properties of epinephrine made it seem that the medulla was more important than the cortex. However, it was eventually shown that the converse is true, and patients dying of Addison disease were successfully treated with extracts from the adrenal cortex.

MORPHOLOGY

Anatomy

The adrenal glands are small, triangular in shape and bilaterally positioned on the superior poles of the kidneys. Each gland is highly vascularized and weighs between 4 and 6 g in the normal adult, depending on age; the glands are usually heavier in females than in males. The outer cortex occupies 80–90% of the gland and is yellow, due to its high lipid content; the inner part, the medulla, is reddish brown.

Cytology of the cortex

There are three morphologically distinguishable concentric

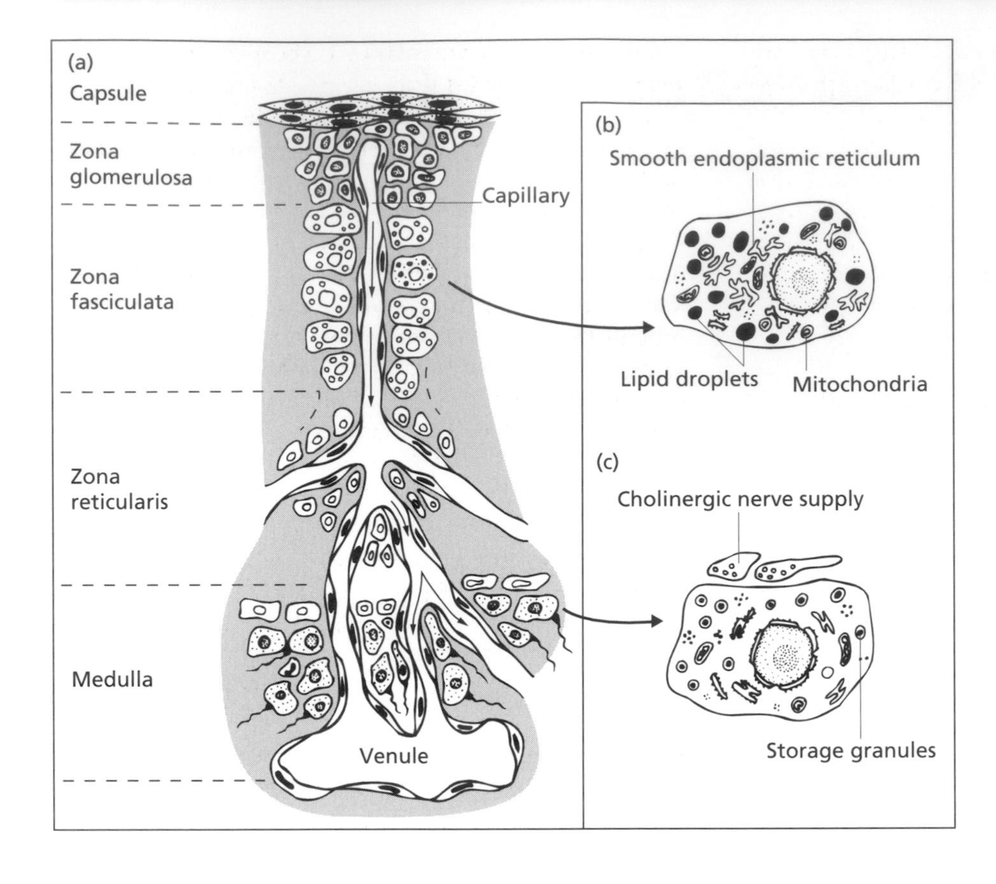

Figure 4.1 (a) A section through the cortex and medulla of the adrenal gland. The capsule surrounds the gland, and capillaries run through the cortex and empty into a medullary venule. The three zones of the cortex are shown: the thin outer zona glomerulosa; the thick central zona fasciculata; and the inner zona reticularis. The medulla consists of chromaffin cells and a cholinergic nerve supply. (b) The cytology of a zona fasciculata cell. Note the large number of lipid droplets and the extensive smooth endoplasmic reticulum associated with mitochondria. (c) The cytology of a medullary chromaffin cell. Note the numerous membrane-bound storage granules of catecholamines and the synaptic terminals of its cholinergic nerve supply (see also Fig. 4.13).

zones within the adrenal cortex: the glomerulosa, the fasciculata and the reticularis (Fig. 4.1). This zonation is functionally important, because aldosterone comes from the zona glomerulosa, while cortisol comes mainly from the zona fasciculata and sex steroids from the zona reticularis.

The outer zone, the zona glomerulosa, lies under a fibrous capsule and makes up 5–10% of the cortex. In humans, its cells are closely packed and form small, ill-defined clumps, but in other species the cells are arranged in a continuous layer. The glomerulosa cells possess the general characteristics of steroid-producing cells (see Fig. 1.6).

The middle cortical zone, the zona fasciculata, forms about 75% of the volume of the adrenal cortex. Its cells are larger than those in the zona glomerulosa and are arranged in long cords disposed radially with respect to the medulla; the cords are separated by the straight cortical capillaries. Fasciculata cells also exhibit the general characteristics of steroid-producing cells (see Fig. 1.6).

In the zona reticularis there is an anastomosing network of short cords of cells with interdigitating capillaries. The cells of the zona reticularis have characteristic features. Under the light microscope, their acidophilic properties reveal two kinds of cell, one a deeply staining, compact cell and the other a less intensely stained, clear cell; these tinctorial differences probably reflect differing physiological states. Ultrastructurally, there is a less extensive smooth endoplasmic reticulum and there are fewer lipid droplets than in the zona fasciculata, with more lysosomes and larger lipofuscin granules, which increase in number with age. The mitochondria tend to be more elongated and have both short and long tubular cristae. Cell contacts between cortical cells in all the zones involve desmosomes, but in the zona fasciculata and zona reticularis, large and numerous gap junctions are found, functionally coupling the cortical cells.

Cells of the zona glomerulosa migrate continuously centrally through the zona fasciculata to the zona reticularis, which differentiates in children aged 6–8 years. The purpose of this migration is not clear, but the secretory product of an individual cell certainly changes as it migrates.

Cytology of the medullary chromaffin tissue

Histologically, the medulla is composed of chromaffin cells. These are named from their capacity to show a brown coloration when exposed to an aqueous solution of potassium dichromate; this is thought to be due to the oxidation of catecholamines to a brown-pigmented polymer.

Chromaffin cells tend to be columnar in shape and are arranged in anastomosing epithelioid cords, separated by vascular spaces. The cells tend to be polarized, with their long axes at right angles to the adjacent fenestrated capillaries. Ultrastructurally, the most prominent feature of the cells is the abundance of membrane-bound, electron-dense granules, which are probably the store of the catecholamines, norepinephrine and epinephrine. Each chromaffin cell is innervated by a cholinergic, preganglionic sympathetic neurone.

The paraganglia. These are small groups of chromaffin cells that are histologically similar to those of the adrenal medulla and have the same embryological origin. Similar chromaffin granules are found in these cells, which contain norepinephrine. The paraganglia are widely scattered in the retropleural and retroperitoneal tissues, some being associated with sympathetic ganglia and others with parasympathetic nerves. Whether or not they release catecholamines into the circulation under normal circumstances is uncertain. They are, however, occasionally the site of growth of a tumour, a phaeochromocytoma, that can secrete catecholamines into the general circulation.

Blood and nerve supply

The blood supply of the adrenal gland (Fig. 4.2) is derived from a circle of different arteries arising from the superior, middle and inferior adrenal arteries. The small vessels from these trunks pierce the capsule and break up into a plexus. Three kinds of vessel arise from this: the capsular vessels, the cortical vessels and the medullary arterioles. The cortical vessels descend from the capsular plexus and form the capillary bed that supplies the cortical parenchyma. The straight capillaries between the fasciculata finally anastomose in the zona reticularis and then empty into the medullary vascular bed. The medullary arterioles penetrate the cortex and supply the medullary tissue directly. Thus, the medulla has a double blood supply—a systemic one via the long medullary arterioles and a secondary one derived from the cortical capillaries, which may be likened to a portal system.

Medullary venules collect the blood, which empties into the central vein. This originates in the tail of the gland and is surrounded by a cuff of cortical tissue, where it indents the medulla from below in the body of the gland. Longitudinal muscle columns of the central vein can obstruct the smaller veins entering it by shortening and swelling. Overflow of blood then occurs by an alternative route, the alar veins at the wings of the gland, which also drain the zona reticularis plexus. Emissary veins between the alar veins and others running along the surface of the gland serve as an additional regulator of blood flow.

The central vein of the right adrenal empties into the inferior vena cava, while on the left side it drains into the left renal vein. Thus, much of the blood the medulla receives is rich in the corticoid hormones that are necessary for the production of epinephrine. Further, the hormones of the adrenal can be stored in its vascular channels to be released in spurts as the muscle of the central vein contracts or relaxes. This complex circulation probably plays an important role in regulating steroid synthesis.

The innervation of the gland is derived from the splanchnic nerves, which arise from lateral-horn preganglionic sympathetic neurones at spinal cord levels T8–T11. Some of these preganglionic fibres synapse with postganglionic sympathetic neurones in the coeliac ganglion, the fibres of which innervate the blood vessels in the adrenal. Other preganglionic splanchnic fibres enter the medulla, ramify in the tissue and end in cholinergic synapses on the chromaffin cells, which are the equivalent

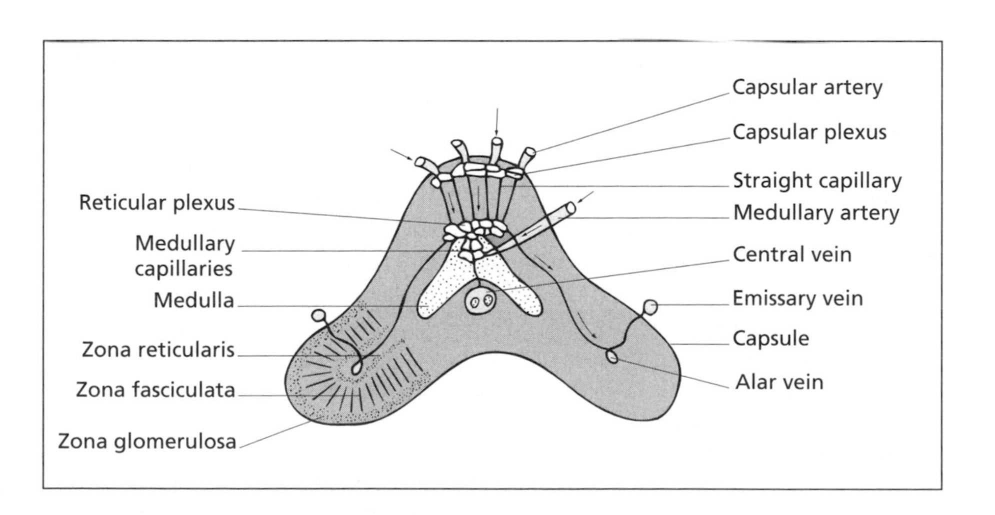

Figure 4.2 A section through the centre of the human adrenal gland, showing the capsule, the cortex and its three zones (zona glomerulosa, zona fasciculata and zona reticularis), as well as the central medulla. Also shown is the gland's blood supply. Arteries pierce the capsule and form a capsular plexus. From this arise the straight capillaries, which run between the columns of zona fasciculata cells and eventually anastomose to form the reticular plexus of capillaries in the zona reticularis. These in turn empty into the medullary capillaries, which eventually fuse to form venules that run into the large central vein. Note that some cortical blood can escape via the alar veins into the emissary vein. The medulla also has a direct arterial supply, which runs from the capsular arteries directly to the medullary capillaries.

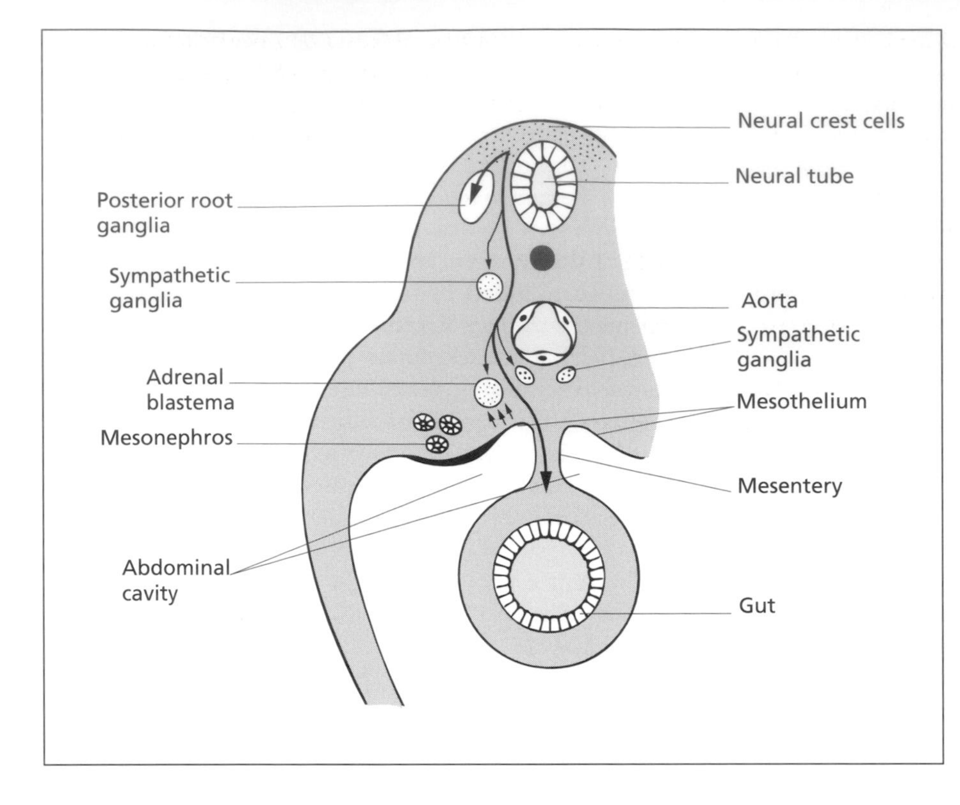

Figure 4.3 The development of the adrenal gland. The cortex is derived from the mesothelium lining cavity. The cells invade (↖) the underlying stroma and form a compact mass, the adrenal blastema. Neural-crest cells migrate ventrally; some give rise to posterior-root ganglia and sympathetic ganglia, while others invade the adrenal blastema and form the medulla of the gland. Note also the neural tube, aorta, mesonephros, mesentery and gut.

of postganglionic neurones. The cells of the adrenal cortex, however, do not have a secretomotor innervation.

Embryological development

The adrenal gland is derived from ectodermal neural-crest cells, which form the medulla, and from mesodermal cells, which give rise to the cortex (Fig. 4.3).

Medulla

In the human, cells originating from the neural crest migrate from each side of the neural tube towards the dorsal aorta, where they position themselves laterally and just posterior to it during the fifth week of development. Most of the cells form a bilateral chain of segmentally arranged sympathetic ganglia, but some of the neural-crest cells, called phaeochromaffinoblasts, invade the medial aspect of the developing adrenal cortex, position themselves in its centre and eventually become the adrenal medulla. These cells do not form nerve processes, although they are the equivalent of postganglionic neurones. They differentiate into two kinds of chromaffin cells, which synthesize and secrete norepinephrine and epinephrine, respectively. During fetal life, the chromaffin cells secrete only norepinephrine, but just before birth some cells begin to synthesize epinephrine.

Cortex

The adrenal cortex originates from mesothelial cells located at the cranial ends of the mesonephros; these lie between the root of the mesentery and the developing urogenital ridge. During the fifth week of development, these cells proliferate and invade the underlying retroperitoneal mesenchyme. They form an acidophilic mass of cells, which are penetrated on their medial aspect by the phaeochromaffinoblasts at about the seventh week of development. The mesothelial-derived cells form the primitive fetal cortex. In the human, a second wave of mesothelial-derived cells proliferate, surround the fetal cortex and eventually form the cortex of the adult gland. As is explained later, the function of the fetal and adult or 'definitive' cortex is very different. Mesenchymal cells that surround the fetal cortex differentiate into fibroblasts and lay down the collagenous capsule. The blood and nerve supplies of the gland also develop during this period. At the end of fetal life, the adrenal gland is about 20 times larger relative to other organs than it is in the adult, and it is large even compared with the kidney.

Postnatally, the fetal cortex regresses and has usually disappeared by the end of the first year of life, being replaced by the adult cortex. The glands decrease in size by about a third during the first months after birth and do not regain their size at birth until adult life. Complete absence of both glands is rare, as is the existence of true accessory glands, consisting of both cortex and medulla. However, ectopic adrenal cortical tissue alone occurs frequently, as do patches of medullary tissue. These isolated groups of cells may be found in the adult spleen or retroperitoneally, for example, below the kidneys, along the aorta, in the pelvis or associated with gonadal structures. Functionally, ectopic adrenal tissue, whether of cortical or medullary origin, is of no significance unless it becomes hyperplastic or malignant; then its location may become very important.

Zonation of the cortex begins during late fetal life. The zona glomerulosa and zona fasciculata are present at birth, but the zona reticularis is not obvious until the end of the sixth year. Differentiation of the cells in the cortex and the development of function in the fetus appear to be under the control of adrenocorticotrophin (ACTH) secreted by the fetal pituitary gland. In the adult, following hypophysectomy or suppressive doses of cortisone, the cells of the zona fasciculata and zona reticularis, which are ACTH-dependent, regress, but those of the zona glomerulosa do not.

Role of the fetal cortex

In vitro studies of primate adrenals and estimation of steroids in umbilical venous blood show that the fetal adrenal is capable of steroid production at an early stage of gestation, but the function of the gland is not known. Since it does not contain 3β-hydroxysteroid dehydrogenase activity (Fig. 4.4), it produces mainly dehydroepiandrosterone sulphate (DHEAS), which provides the substrate for oestrogen synthesis by the placenta (see Fig. 6.12).

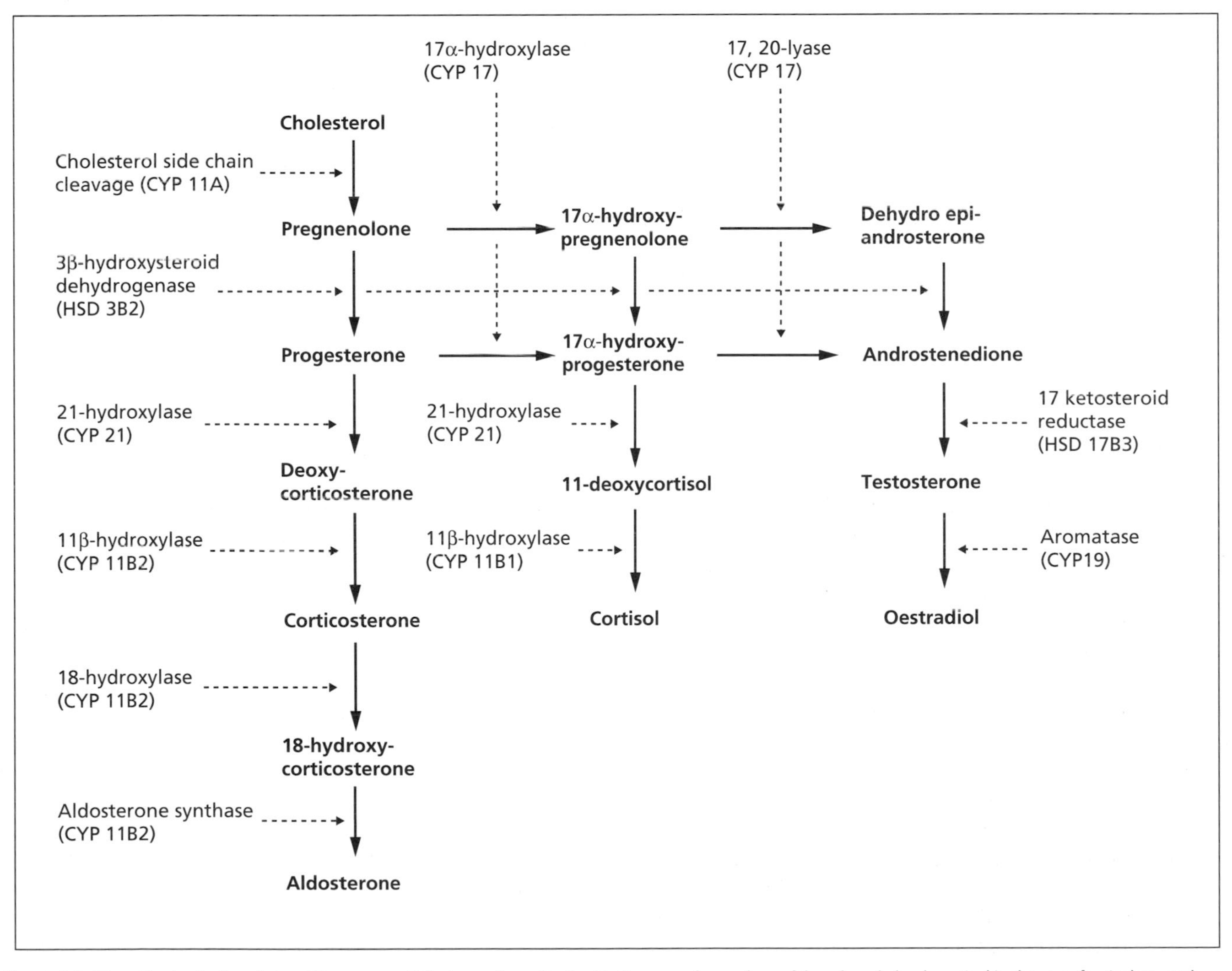

Figure 4.4 Biosynthesis of adrenal steroid hormones. Aldosterone is synthesized in the zona glomerulosa of the adrenal gland, cortisol in the zona fasciculata, and dehydroepiandrosterone and androstenedione in the zona reticularis. Testosterone is synthesized in the testes and ovary; it is converted to oestradiol in the ovary. For further details, see Appendix 3.

It cannot synthesize progesterone, glucocorticoids, or androstenedione. Glucocorticoids—presumably obtained from the mother or synthesized from placental progesterone by the fetus—are, however, involved in a number of important processes in fetal tissues, which may be due to their interactions with other growth factors. Examples of these development-promoting effects are:

1 Production of surfactant from type II cells of the alveoli of the lung, a lack of which leads to the respiratory distress syndrome in newborn infants.

2 Development of hypothalamic function and of the hypothalamopituitary axis.

3 The sequential changes of placental structure and the ionic composition of amniotic and allantoic fluids during development.

4 The initiation of the endocrine changes in the fetus and mother that are responsible for parturition.

5 The development of hepatic enzymes, including those involved in gluconeogenesis.

6 Induction of thymic involution.

FUNCTION OF THE ADRENAL CORTEX

The division of the cortex into separate layers is very important, since the zones produce different steroids; aldosterone, for example, is produced only in the zona glomerulosa. Figure 4.4 summarizes the pathways of steroid biosynthesis in the adrenal cortex.

Cholesterol—the starting-point for all steroid hormone biosynthesis (see Appendix 3)—is obtained mostly from circulating low-density lipoprotein, and only very little is synthesized locally from acetate. As Fig. 4.4 shows, cholesterol is modified by a series of hydroxylation reactions. Five of the enzymes (CYP11A, CYP17, CYP21, CYP11B1 and CYP11B2) are members of the cytochrome P450 superfamily of haemoproteins; they are called P450 because they show a characteristic shift in light absorbance from 420 to 450 nm upon reduction with carbon monoxide. The enzymes of the CYP11 family are located in the mitochondria, and the remainder are located in the endoplasmic reticulum, so the substrates have to move around the cell for the process of steroidogenesis to be complete.

The nomenclature of the enzymes and the genes encoding them have been revised, so that the same code shown in Fig. 4.4 applies to the gene when italicized capitals are used (e.g. *CYP*11A) and to the enzyme when ordinary capitals are used (e.g. CYP11A).

In Appendix 3, there is an amplified discussion of these biosynthetic pathways that emphasizes the structural changes taking place to the steroid molecule at each of the steps shown in Fig. 4.4.

Function of the zona fasciculata

This area of the adrenal cortex is the main source of cortisol, which is the most important glucocorticoid hormone in humans. There is relatively little cortisol storage, and active synthesis is required when the need for hormone increases. Most cortisol is converted in the liver to inactive cortisone; in plasma, the ratio of cortisol to cortisone in the adult is about 1 : 2. Cortisol is bound to a binding globulin, and in case of need, cortisone can be converted to cortisol and bound cortisol can be freed.

Effects of cortisol

Changes in carbohydrate, fat and protein metabolism. The metabolic effects of cortisol generally oppose those of insulin and vary with the target tissue: in muscle, adipose and lymphoid tissue it is catabolic, but in liver it stimulates the synthesis and storage of glycogen. Cortisol increases the concentration of glucose in blood by stimulating gluconeogenesis in the liver and to a lesser extent decreasing the utilization of glucose in other tissues. The increased blood glucose is available for the production of glycogen and is important in maintaining liver glycogen during prolonged fasting. The increase in liver glycogen after administration of corticosteroids provides the basis of a bioassay of glucocorticoid activity.

These effects on metabolism are produced by cortisol binding to intracellular receptors (see Figs 2.1, 2.20–2.23) and increasing transcription of specific genes, which leads to the increased synthesis of the appropriate enzymes. For example, key enzymes involved in hepatic gluconeogenesis are stimulated, and there is an increased availability of amino acids, which are derived from protein catabolism in several tissues (Fig. 4.5). In the liver, protein anabolism occurs. However, the net effect is one of negative nitrogen balance. The energy required for gluconeogenesis is obtained by breakdown of fats and the release of fatty acids.

Cortisol also stimulates the appetite, so that when there is excess cortisol, as in Cushing syndrome, there is central obesity with an increase in body fat. The reason for the redistribution of adipose tissue is not understood.

Anti-inflammatory effects. In addition to its effects on metabolism, cortisol also acts on body defence mechanisms to suppress tissue response to injury. It thus has an anti-inflammatory action, which has been extensively used therapeutically. The first example of this was the discovery, in the late 1940s, that cortisone could be used to treat rheumatoid arthritis. When treating inflammatory conditions, steroids such as prednisolone are particularly useful, because they have good anti-inflammatory/immunosuppressive actions but relatively low potencies

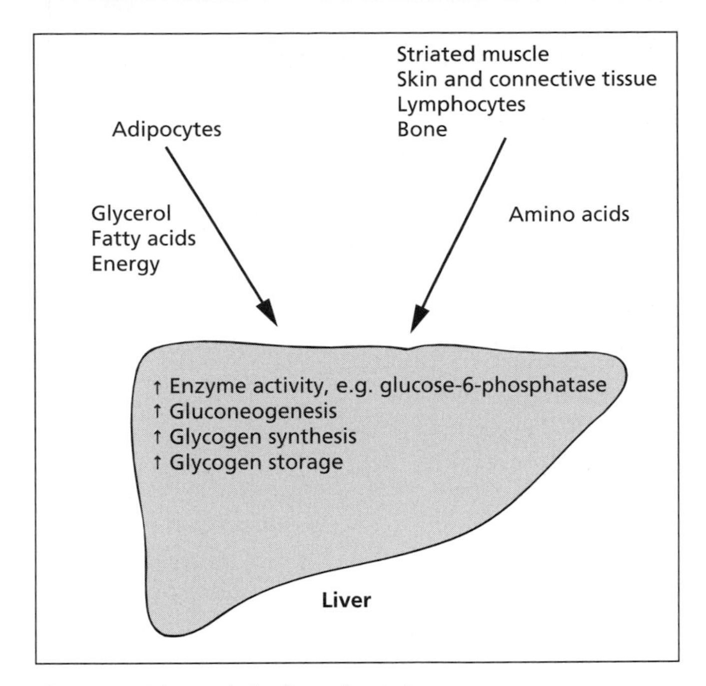

Figure 4.5 Major metabolic effects of cortisol.

as mineralocorticoids. Cortisol in moderately high concentrations leads to a reduction in the size of lymph nodes and to involution of the thymus. The tissue shrinkage is rapid and dramatic. This situation is an unusual example of a hormone acting as a cytosolic agent, with the cortisol activating a programme for apoptosis. It reduces the number of lymphocytes in blood and so decreases antibody production. It thus impairs both cellular and humoral immunity and thereby renders patients susceptible to infection.

Other effects. Although cortisol is predominantly a glucocorticoid, it does have mineralocorticoid effects when present in large amounts; it can help to maintain extracellular fluid volume and prevent the shift of water into cells, and it also supports tissue perfusion, which may be important during stress. Cortisol has a number of other effects that become apparent only if it is present in excess. It sensitizes arterioles to the action of norepinephrine (resulting in hypertension) and has permissive effects on the action of norepinephrine on carbohydrate metabolism (resulting in hyperglycaemia and glucose intolerance). In addition, it can stimulate secretion of acid by the stomach and increase activity in the central nervous system to produce euphoria or even mania.

Secretion of cortisol

Regulation. The anterior pituitary, through secretion of ACTH, controls the activity of the zona fasciculata and zona reticularis (see Chapter 3). ACTH interacts with G-protein–linked cell-surface receptors (see Fig. 2.1), and via adenylate cyclase (see Fig. 2.12) it stimulates the production of cortisol by increasing cholesterol side-chain cleavage to form pregnenolone. This is the rate-limiting step in cortisol synthesis (Fig. 4.4). A small pulse of ACTH increases glucocorticoid production within 5 min, and it then wanes over the next 10 min. However, if the stimulation is continued over a longer period of time, cytoplasmic lipid droplets and ascorbic acid in the fasciculata cells decrease, and eventually the zona fasciculata and zona reticularis will increase in thickness.

In hypophysectomized animals, lack of ACTH leads to shrinkage of the zona fasciculata and zona reticularis to less than half of their original thickness, and it also leads to almost complete abolition of cortisol and adrenal androgen synthesis. The cells lose lipid droplets, the smooth endoplasmic reticulum dwindles, and the concentration of ascorbic acid in the cells falls, for reasons that are not clear. These changes in the cortical region of the adrenal clearly illustrate the 'trophic' nature of the actions of ACTH on the structure and function of the zona fasciculata and zona reticularis.

Negative feedback of cortisol on secretion of adrenocorticotrophin. The end-product of the action of ACTH, namely cortisol, has a direct inhibitory action on the pituitary (see Fig. 3.9). It also exerts a negative-feedback action on the hypothalamus, to inhibit the release of corticotrophin-releasing hormone (CRH). The secretion of CRH can be stimulated by emotion, stress and trauma.

There is a circadian rhythm of hypothalamopituitary activity operating during the sleep/wake cycle. As a result, the concentration of cortisol in plasma in humans is minimal around midnight and rises to a maximum between 6 and 8 a.m., thereafter falling slowly during the day. Superimposed on these trends is an episodic pattern of release, with fluctuations lasting for periods of several minutes. Since the adrenal–pituitary feedback system is not very well 'damped', large swings in the concentrations of ACTH and cortisol in the circulation can readily occur. However, if the system is suppressed for a long time, for example by the administration of exogenous steroid, it can take months for the synthesis and release of ACTH, and hence of cortisol, to be restored.

Measurement of secretion rate. It will be appreciated that the importance of a hormone in controlling a given process will depend not only on the biological potency, i.e. the biological effect as a function of the molecular concentration of that hormone, but also on its secretion rate, i.e. the amount of hormone secreted over a given time period (Fig. 4.6). *In vitro*, this can be measured when isolated adrenal glands are incubated. In experimental animals,

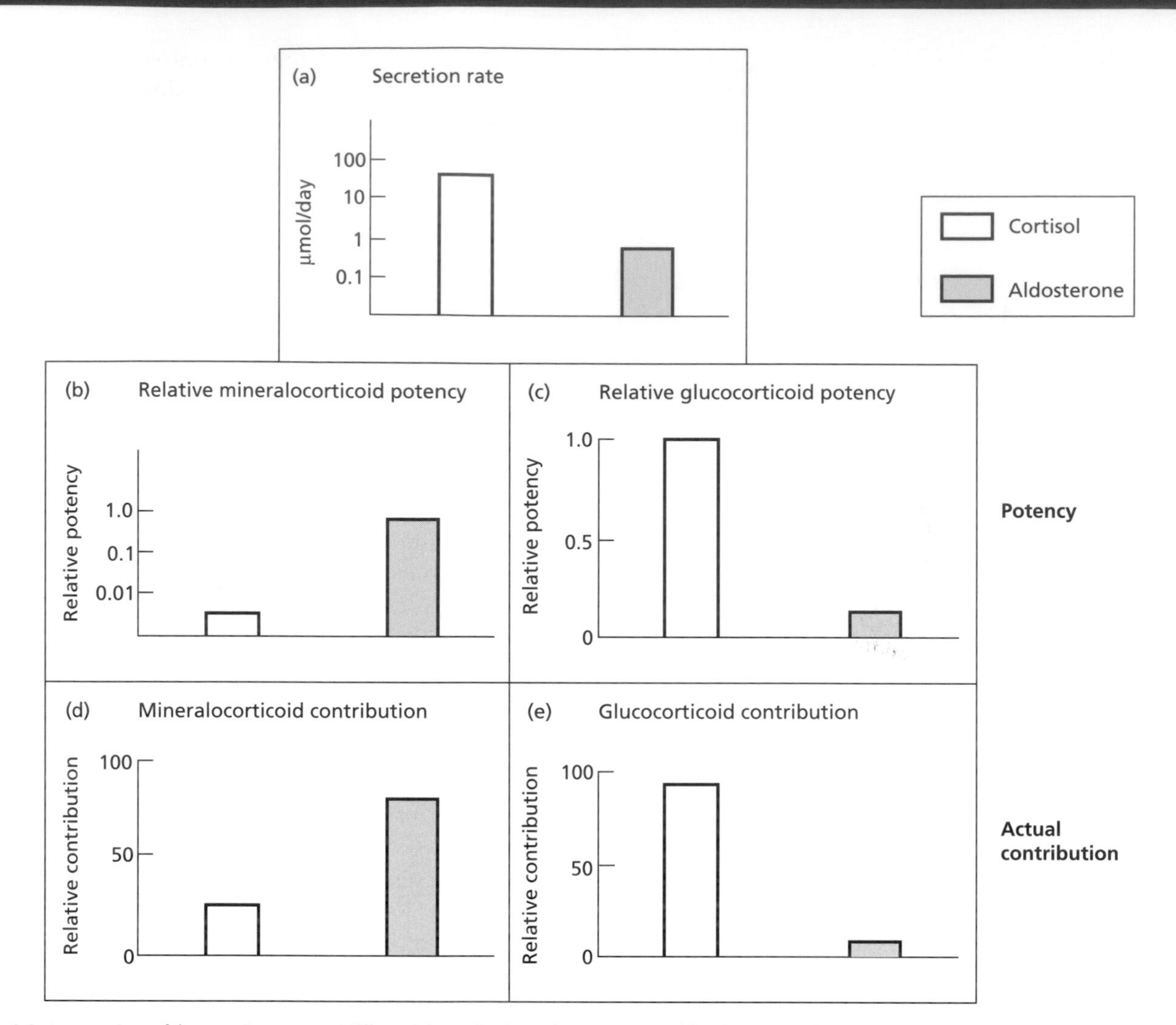

Figure 4.6 A comparison of the secretion rates and differential contributions of cortisol and aldosterone on glucocorticoid and mineralocorticoid activities. Cortisol is secreted at a much higher rate than aldosterone (a). As a consequence, although its relative potency as a mineralocorticoid is relatively low (b), it can still make a significant contribution to overall mineralocorticoid activity (d). Glucocorticoid activity (c and e) was measured as the ability to increase glycogen in liver, whereas mineralocorticoid effects (b and d) were measured in terms of the ability to reduce the ratio of the excretion of sodium to the excretion of potassium in urine. Clearly, aldosterone is much more potent in this respect.

the secretion rate can be established *in vivo* by collecting the venous effluent from the adrenal gland over a period of time and measuring the amount of hormone in that blood. In humans, it is possible to estimate the secretion rate by measuring the excreted metabolites in urine.

Transport of circulating cortisol

In plasma, there is a specific corticosteroid-binding globulin (transcortin), which is a glycoprotein with a molecular weight of 52 000, synthesized in liver. About 80% of the circulating cortisol is bound to this protein, and serum albumin can bind an additional 15%. If the concentration of cortisol is increased so that the specific binding sites are saturated, then much of the surplus is carried by albumin. Transcortin-bound cortisol is protected from metabolism and inactivation in liver. The affinity of transcortin for progesterone is also high, but it is much lower for aldosterone, and as a consequence this steroid has a relatively short half-life in the circulation. It does not bind the synthetic steroid dexamethasone. If the concentration of the binding proteins is elevated, then the total concentration of the hormone in plasma will be increased. This happens in pregnancy and following oestrogen treatment (e.g. contraception or treatment for cancer of the prostate). Thus, it is necessary to take account of the concentration of binding globulins when considering the physiological significance of a total steroid concentration determined in plasma.

Function of the zona glomerulosa

Aldosterone is produced exclusively in the zona glomerulosa (see Appendix 3). This is the most potent mineralocorticoid produced by the adrenal.

Cellular actions of aldosterone

Aldosterone binds to specific intracellular mineralocorticoid receptor proteins (see Figs 2.20–2.23) within its target cells. These then function as hormone-activated transcription factors, which enhance the expression of the appropriate genes by interaction with their hormone-response elements. As discussed in Chapter 2, the mineralocorticoid receptor is unusual in that it binds both cortisol and aldosterone with equal affinities. Despite the higher concentration of cortisol, aldosterone is the dominant mineralocorticoid, because aldosterone-responsive cells are protected by the effect of the enzyme 11β-hydroxysteroid dehydrogenase (11β-HSD), which converts the cortisol to cortisone, which is not active on the mineralocorticoid receptor (see Fig. 2.25). Congenital deficiency of 11β-HSD results in the syndrome of 'apparent mineralocorticoid excess' (AME), which is a cause of mineralocorticoid hypertension. Curiously, the consumption of large quantities of liquorice can lead to an acquired deficiency of 11β-HSD, due to the inhibitory effects of glycyrrhetinic acid, which is present in liquorice, on 11β-HSD. The condition is manifested as a mineralocorticoid excess state, with hypertension and hypokalaemia.

Effects of aldosterone

The main sites of action of aldosterone are in the distal tubule and the collecting ducts of the kidney, where it increases sodium reabsorption (so promoting retention of sodium) and increases the excretion of potassium and hydrogen ions. Sodium reabsorption is linked to the secretion of potassium and hydrogen ions by a cation-exchange mechanism. Aldosterone raises blood pressure, partly by increasing plasma volume and partly by increasing the sensitivity of the arteriolar muscle to vasoconstrictor agents. The response of an individual to administered aldosterone is observed only after a lag period of about 1 h, during which there is synthesis of a specific aldosterone-induced protein that promotes sodium transport. If administration of aldosterone is continued, the ability to excrete excess sodium is regained after 1–3 weeks, depending on sodium intake; this 'escape phenomenon' is almost certainly the result of readaptation of the feedback control system that is responsible for the regulation of the rate of reabsorption of filtered sodium in the proximal tubule.

Secretion of aldosterone

Despite the rate of aldosterone secretion being about 100 times lower than that of cortisol, it is responsible for about 80% of the mineralocorticoid activity of the adrenal glandular secretion (Fig. 4.6). Aldosterone is cleared more rapidly from the circulation than cortisol, having a half-life of 20–30 min, as opposed to 100 min for cortisol. This rapid clearance is in part explained by the fact that it is bound only to a limited extent by carrier proteins in the circulation. The circulating concentration of aldosterone is normally about 300 pmol/L, which is about a thousand times lower than that of cortisol.

In animals maintained on a low-sodium diet, the secretion of aldosterone increases. The zona glomerulosa can double in thickness in 3 weeks. Initially, lipid is lost from the glomerulosa cells, but this is gradually restored as the cells hypertrophy, with an increase in the amount of smooth endoplasmic reticulum, the Golgi complex and the number of mitochondria. Conversely, in animals maintained on a high-sodium diet, the secretion rate falls, and there is a decrease in the thickness of the glomerulosa by about 50%; cytoplasmic lipid content is reduced, while lysosomal bodies (autophagic vacuoles) are usually increased.

The renin–angiotensin system. This is the most important regulator of the secretion of aldosterone. It had been shown in the late 1890s that extracts of renal tissue could produce hypertension in experimental animals, and in 1936 Goldblatt demonstrated that constriction of one renal artery (producing renal ischaemia) caused a slow rise in arterial pressure. This effect is due to the action of a substance called renin (Fig. 4.7), which is secreted by special cells in the juxtaglomerular region of the nephrons in the kidney (Fig. 4.8). These juxtaglomerular cells are found surrounding the afferent arteriole just before it enters the Malpighian corpuscle and breaks up into the glomerular capillaries. They are epithelioid in nature and replace the smooth-muscle cells of the afferent arteriole at this point. They synthesize the proteolytic enzyme, renin, which is stored intracellularly in granules. Adjacent to the juxtaglomerular cells are those of the macula densa, which is a specialized part of the distal tubule. The juxtaglomerular cells and the macula densa form the juxtaglomerular apparatus. Release of renin is activated by a fall in plasma fluid volume; it is discharged from the cells by exocytosis and then diffuses into the lumen of the arterioles and thus into the circulation, where it has a half-life of about 20 min.

Renin is a proteolytic enzyme that splits a leucine–valine bond (Fig. 4.7); its usual substrate is a circulating

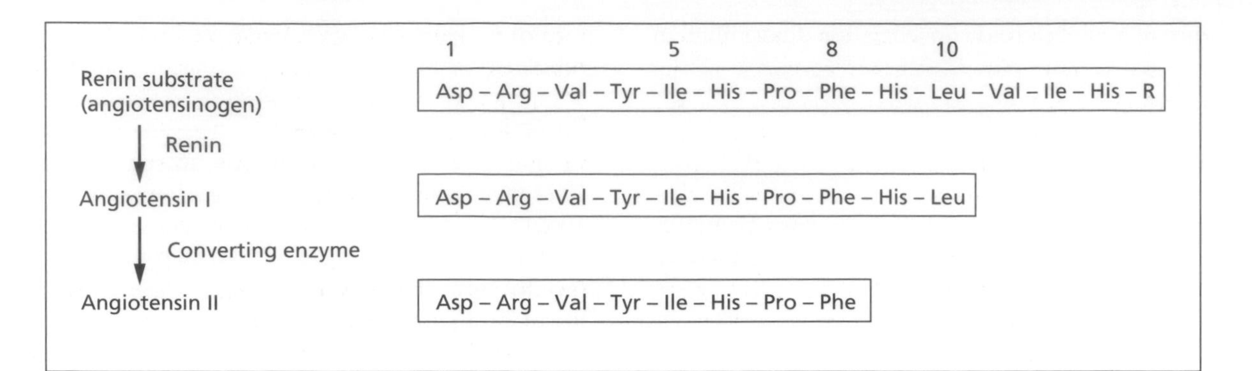

Figure 4.7 The human renin–angiotensin system. Note that R in the substrate represents the rest of the α_2-globulin.

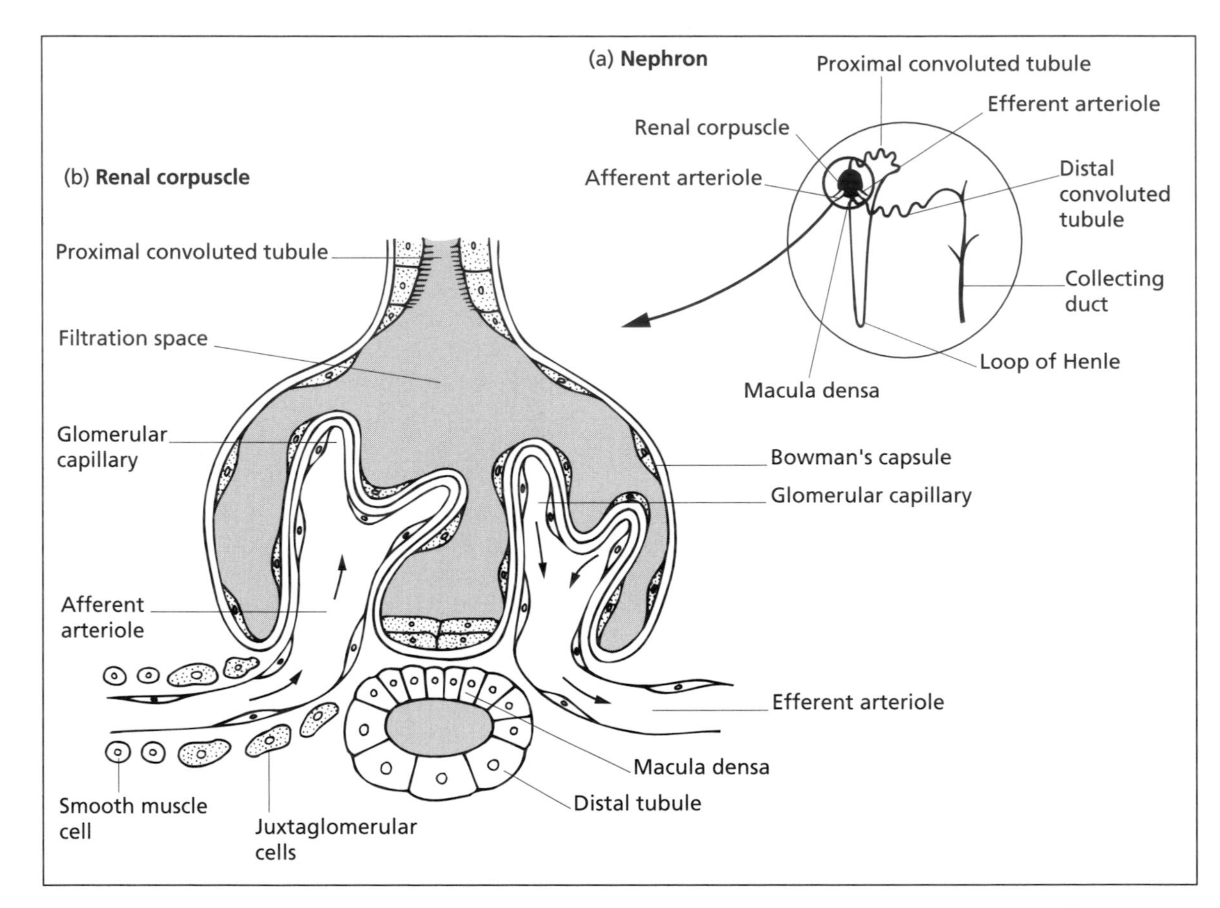

Figure 4.8 (a) The structure of a nephron. Note the renal corpuscle and its blood supply with an afferent and efferent arteriole. From the renal corpuscle arises the proximal convoluted tubule, which straightens out to form the descending limb of the loop of Henle. The ascending limb forms the distal convoluted tubule before emptying into a collecting duct. Where the distal tubule lies between the afferent and efferent arterioles, it forms the macula densa. (b) The detailed structure of a renal corpuscle, its blood supply and the juxtaglomerular apparatus. Note the afferent and efferent arterioles. Between them lie the glomerular capillaries, which are surrounded by Bowman's capsule. The filtration space empties into the beginning of the proximal tubule. The juxtaglomerular apparatus consists firstly of the juxtaglomerular cells, containing renin granules; these cells replace the smooth-muscle cells of the afferent arteriole. In addition, the closely packed cells of the distal tubule form the second component of the juxtaglomerular apparatus, the macula densa.

α_2-globulin (angiotensinogen or renin substrate), which is made in the liver. Renin cleaves a decapeptide from angiotensinogen. The decapeptide is angiotensin I, which is largely biologically inactive, but is converted in several tissues to angiotensin II, an octapeptide and the most potent pressor substance known; it raises both systolic and diastolic blood pressures, and so pulse pressure does not alter. The lung is the primary site of conversion of angiotensin I to angiotensin II, where its endothelial cells contain the appropriate endopeptidase, known as angiotensin-converting enzyme (ACE).

Normally, in humans, angiotensinogen is present in adequate concentrations, and the supply of renin is rate-limiting for angiotensin II production. For this reason, plasma renin is usually used to reflect changes in plasma angiotensin II concentration, since the latter is more difficult to measure, and its half-life in the circulation is only about 1 min.

Angiotensin II acts directly on the zona glomerulosa cells to stimulate aldosterone secretion. Since it also acts on peripheral arterioles, it helps maintain blood pressure both directly and indirectly. During sodium depletion, angiotensin II has a particularly potent effect on the renal circulation, as it reduces the rate of glomerular filtration and in consequence reduces renal excretion of sodium. When injected in minute quantities directly into the hypothalamus of animals, it increases thirst, causing polydipsia. Since angiotensin II does not cross the blood–brain barrier, this effect may not be physiologically significant; however, renin has been found in brain tissue, and so there may be local production of angiotensin II. Renin, or at least a closely related substance, is also present in the uterus and in salivary glands, but renin disappears from the circulation almost completely after nephrectomy, so that the kidney must be the main source of circulating renin.

Regulation of the production of renin. Three factors control the secretion of renin by the kidney (Fig. 4.9). One of these is neural; the juxtaglomerular apparatus of the kidney is richly supplied by sympathetic neurones, and destruction of this nerve supply leads to a blunting of the renin response to sodium depletion. The second important factor is the flux of sodium across the macula densa of the distal tubule. When the flux is high (as, for example, when sodium is plentiful), the secretion of renin is suppressed, and it is clear that normally the renin–angiotensin system is not important in maintaining blood pressure in the sodium-replete state. However, when the animal is sodium-depleted, renin secretion increases, and the effects of sodium on aldosterone production from the adrenal are largely mediated via the renin–angiotensin system. This is essential for maintenance of blood pressure during sodium depletion. The third factor regulating renin production is the mean transmural pressure (as opposed to the pulse pressure); when the transmural pressure is high, renin secretion is suppressed, and when it is low, the secretion of renin is stimulated. Another regulatory factor

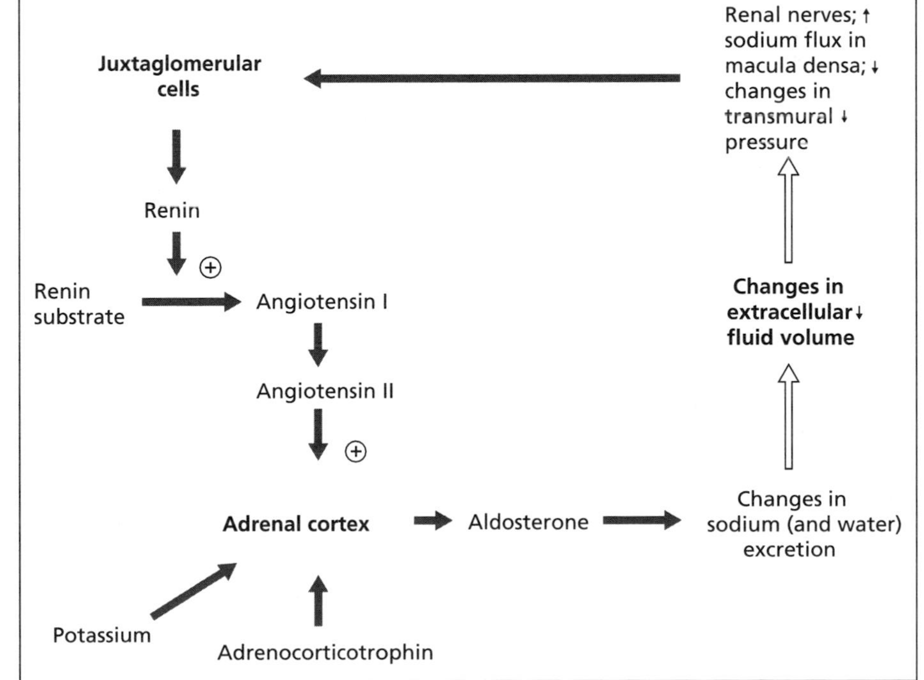

Figure 4.9 The factors that interact to control the secretion of aldosterone and renin and regulate extracellular fluid volume and total body sodium and water. For example, a fall in extracellular fluid volume produces increased activity in renal nerves, reduced sodium flux in the macula densa and a fall in transmural pressure (as shown by the thin arrows (↑ ↓)). These activate the juxtaglomerular apparatus, which, through increased renin production, leads to more angiotensin and so stimulation of aldosterone secretion, which helps restore extracellular fluid volume.

is the concentration of angiotensin II itself; it has been shown that infusion of angiotensin II into the renal circulation will sharply reduce the secretion of renin, due to a short-loop feedback system.

Plasma potassium has only a weak effect on the production of renin, and what effect it does have is actually antagonistic to the direct effect that changes in potassium have on the secretion of aldosterone by the glomerulosa cells. For example, a low concentration of potassium in the plasma sharply reduces aldosterone secretion, but at the same time it has a small but definite stimulatory effect on renin production. Because potassium can have a direct action on the adrenal as well as an effect on production of renin, there can be a dissociation between the production of aldosterone and the amount of renin present in some situations.

Interplay of factors regulating the secretion of aldosterone. Angiotensin II, potassium and ACTH can directly stimulate the rate of secretion of aldosterone (Fig. 4.9), as can melanocyte-stimulating hormone (MSH), while somatostatin and atrial natriuretic peptide (see below) can inhibit aldosterone secretion. The effects of potassium can be seen when plasma volume is constant: then, small changes of potassium within the physiological range affect aldosterone secretion. The dependence of the aldosterone secretion rate on plasma volume is mediated by the renin–angiotensin system, which can override any opposing changes in the plasma concentration of potassium and ACTH. For example, the secretion of aldosterone rises during the morning (because of the fall in plasma volume on assuming an upright posture), even though the secretion of ACTH falls during the day. Injection of ACTH can stimulate aldosterone production, but this effect lasts only 24–48 h even if ACTH is administered repeatedly. This is because the aldosterone-producing cells no longer respond to ACTH. This is not due to salt retention affecting the glomerulosa cells, since it can occur on a low-sodium diet. Lack of ACTH as a result of hypophysectomy or disease does not significantly reduce the zona glomerulosa, in contrast to the zona fasciculata or reticularis; aldosterone production is maintained. Overproduction of aldosterone is not a consequence of prolonged excessive secretion of ACTH.

Atrial natriuretic peptide. A number of physiological experiments have indicated the existence of natriuretic substances (i.e. substances that increase the excretion of sodium). In 1981, de Bold and his colleagues showed that extracts of the atrium of the heart could increase the excretion of sodium and of water. The atrial muscle cells (cardiocytes) synthesize a peptide that is stored in secretory granules. This peptide has been isolated from both the left and the right atria. The secretory granules contain a prohormone with 126 amino acids, while the secreted form of the hormone has only 28 amino acids, with an intrachain disulphide bond. The gene encoding the peptide has been cloned and expressed in eukaryotic systems, and a synthetic peptide has been made. After secretion by the heart into the bloodstream, the peptide is rapidly removed from the circulation. Specific membrane receptors for the peptide, which are coupled to guanylate cyclase, have been found in the glomeruli and in the medullary collecting ducts of the kidney, in the zona glomerulosa of the adrenal cortex and in peripheral arterioles. The cells of the zona glomerulosa express an isoform of phosphodiesterase that is activated by cGMP. This leads to a reduction in intracellular cAMP and aldosterone secretion. For reasons that are not clear, atrial natriuretic peptide also accumulates in the paraventricular nuclei of the hypothalamus.

A graded release of atrial natriuretic peptide occurs in response to increased stretching of the isolated rat heart. In intact animals, a graded increase in blood volume also stimulates a progressive release of the hormone. Increase of sodium intake and of water can both stimulate the discharge of the secretory granules containing the peptide from heart muscle. The response to atrial natriuretic peptide is best studied in conscious animals, since anaesthesia itself affects renal handing of salt and water. Atrial natriuretic peptide causes a fall in plasma renin and in the concentration of circulating aldosterone, and it increases renal blood flow. It promotes the excretion of water, possibly by inhibiting the action of antidiuretic hormone. The increase in sodium excretion is due largely to a rise in the rate of glomerular filtration and also to inhibition of sodium reabsorption in the medullary collecting duct. Atrial natriuretic peptide relaxes vascular smooth muscle and inhibits vasoconstriction produced by angiotensin II. Although it is clear that atrial natriuretic peptide in animals is a potent hormone, its precise role in humans still remains to be established. It may act as an acute response system for improving cardiac haemodynamics. At present, little is known about its role in pathophysiology.

Production of sex steroids in the adrenal cortex

The production of sex steroids (androgens in the male and oestrogens and progestogens in the female) is mainly from the gonads, and it is therefore considered in Chapter 6. However, the adrenal cortex—in particular, the zona reticularis—contributes by production of DHEAS and androstenedione (Fig. 4.4). These are referred to as pre-androgens, and they can be converted to testosterone in peripheral adipose tissue. The role of sex steroids produced as a result of adrenocortical activity is not entirely clear; their synthesis is important to growth of body hair in females and may become more important in disease. Before the onset of puberty in a normal child, the secretion of DHEAS rises sharply. This coincides with the maturation of the zona reticularis and is called adrenarche. It is responsible for promoting a growth spurt in middle childhood. Sometimes pubic and axillary hair and apocrine sweat develop at this time of life, but usually not until signs of true puberty appear, with breast development and testicular enlargement.

DIAGNOSIS AND MANAGEMENT OF CLINICAL DISORDERS

There are three adrenocortical groups of steroids to be considered: mineralocorticoids, principally aldosterone; glucocorticoids, principally cortisol (used in treatment as hydrocortisone); and the sex steroids, principally DHEAS. Mineralocorticoid secretion is under the control of the renin–angiotensin system, and glucocorticoid and sex steroid secretion is under the control of ACTH, or possibly in respect of the latter, of an ACTH-related peptide also under the control of CRH.

Overproduction of adrenocortical steroids

Cortisol

Cortisol may be produced in excess as the result of CRH drive of ACTH secretion (a CRH-producing tumour); ACTH drive of cortisol production (an ACTH-producing tumour, most frequently found in the lung); a feedback problem, such that CRH–ACTH drive is reduced only by inappropriately high levels of cortisol; and adrenal tumours, which produce cortisol. The commonest cause of the symptom complex called Cushing syndrome is the administration of steroid medications, i.e. an iatrogenic cause. The effects of excess cortisol are summarized in Table 4.1.

The appearance of a patient with Cushing syndrome is shown in Fig. 4.10. The central obesity, thinning of the skin and bruising, through capillary fragility, are all direct results of cortisol overproduction. There is glucose intolerance in such patients, who are often hypertensive and whose bones and muscles become wasted through protein catabolism promoted by overproduction of cortisol. If adrenal androgens are also secreted in excess, as they are in a patient suffering ACTH-driven cortisol overproduction, the patient may also show signs of androgen excess, such as frontal baldness, acne and hirsutism. Males may experience a reduction in testicular volume, since the adrenal androgens reduce pituitary gonadotrophin secretion, and females may have enlargement of the clitoris, called clitoromegaly.

Cushing syndrome can make patients extremely ill, and the diagnosis of its cause can be very difficult. If ACTH levels are undetectable, it is probable that the hypercortisolaemia has its origin in the adrenal glands, or that the cause is iatrogenic (medication). If ACTH levels are high, the probability is that there is an ACTH-secreting tumour. It is the moderate elevation of ACTH seen in Cushing disease—which is by definition due to ACTH from the pituitary—which is most difficult to be certain about. The differentiation is critical, because ACTH from a tumour requires computed tomography (CT) scanning of the chest and abdomen to seek the source of the tumour—whereas, in Cushing disease, a basophil adenoma of the pituitary gland requires magnetic resonance imaging (MRI) and pituitary adenomectomy by the transnasal route. Where the cause is of adrenal origin, adrenal remedies are required, by either pharmacological or surgical means. Metyrapone, which inhibits 11-β hydroxylase, can be used to block cortisol overproduction. It will also reduce aldosterone synthesis (Fig. 4.4). There is then the danger of Nelson syndrome, due to a subsequent rise in

Table 4.1 Changes due to increased glucocorticoid activity.

Basic action	Effects in excess (Cushing syndrome)
Increased glucogenesis, hepatic	Diabetes mellitus
glycogenesis and protein catabolism	Muscle wasting; easily bruised, thin skin; thin (osteoporotic) bones that easily fracture
Increase and redistribution of body fat	Central obesity, moon facies, buffalo hump, relatively thin limbs
Involution of lymphatic and thymic tissue and reduced inflammatory response	Susceptibility to infection
Increased secretion of acid by the stomach	Predisposition to gastric ulcer
Suppression of release of adrenocorticotrophin	Persistently suppressed adrenocorticotrophic hormone
Na^+ retention; redistribution of body fluids	Hypertension

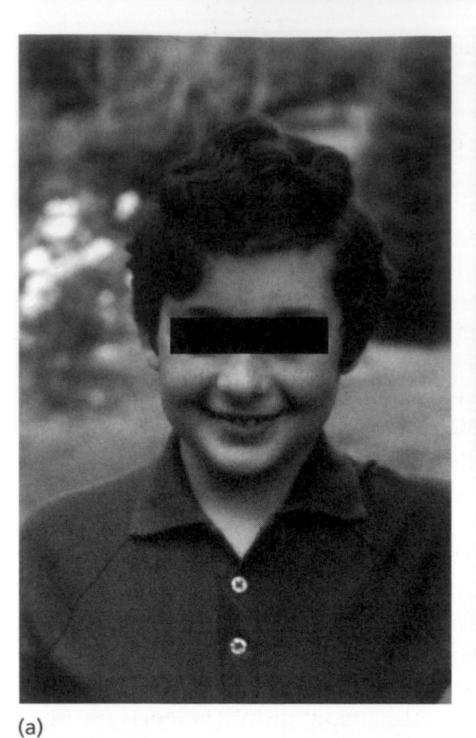
(a)

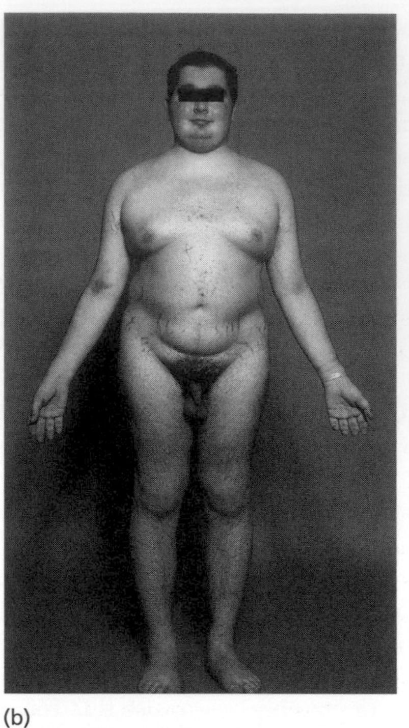
(b)

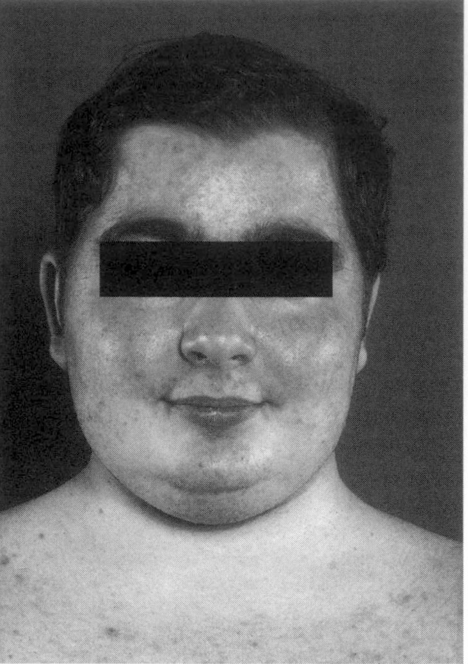
(c)

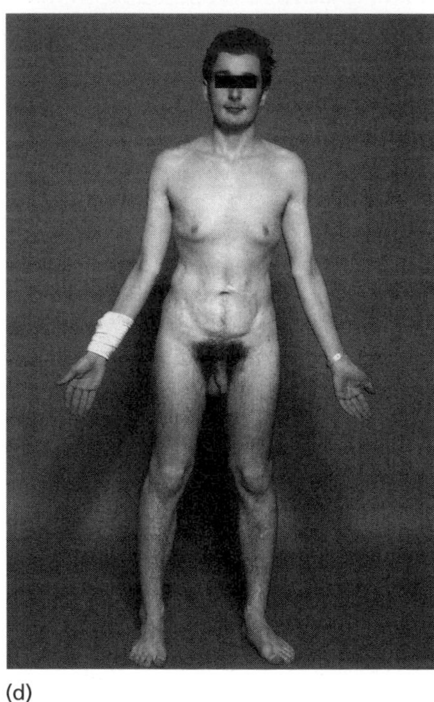
(d)

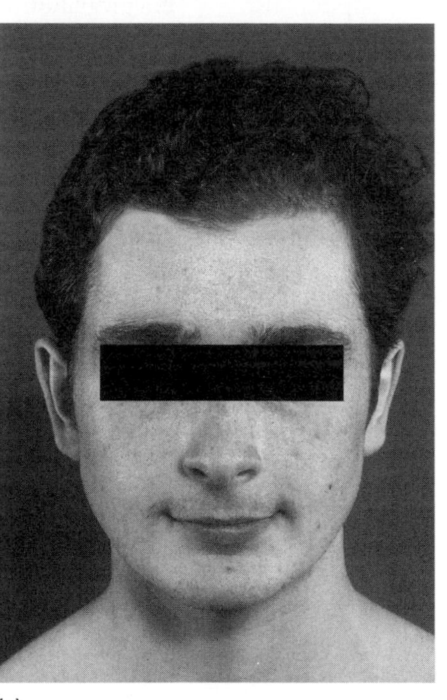
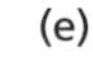
(e)

Figure 4.10 The effects of excess cortisol secretion secondary to a pituitary adenoma in a patient. His appearance at 6 years was normal (a), but it changed progressively during childhood. By age 15 (b and c), he had florid signs of cortisol excess, with a round face, greasy skin, severe acne, truncal obesity with stretch marks (striae) and bruising from a venepuncture site on the right arm. One year after transphenoidal adenomectomy (d and e), now aged 16, he had lost his obesity, and he is shown after an operation to remove excess abdominal skin. He has regained his normal facial appearance, without either acne or an excessively greasy skin.

ACTH and MSH production from the pituitary. This leads to pigmentation of the skin and increases the risk of a pituitary tumour.

Androgen excess

The symptoms of hyperandrogenaemia outlined above can be extremely distressing, and the cause is usually the ACTH drive of conversion of cholesterol to DHEAS in the zona reticularis. A more sinister cause is an adrenal adenoma or carcinoma, and the distinction between benign and malignant tumours in the adrenal gland is extremely difficult. Therapy for adrenal carcinoma is difficult, dangerous and often ineffective, so the distinction from a pituitary cause of adrenal androgen excess is important.

Mineralocorticoid excess

Retention of sodium leads to hypertension, and when mineralocorticoid steroids are produced in excess, the signs and symptoms of raised blood pressure (headaches, blurring of vision and cerebral vascular accidents) are clear. Cortisol has a weak mineralocorticoid action, but if it is present in very large amounts, that action can be important. Excess ACTH can probably also cause hypersecretion of mineralocorticoids, by enhancing the incorporation of cholesterol into the adrenal cortex.

More common causes of mineralocorticoid excess are a tumour producing aldosterone (or other mineralocorticoid hormones), or excessive renin secretion. One important cause of this is an apparent reduction of renal pulse pressure by narrowing of the renal artery (renal-artery stenosis) or of the aorta (coarctation), leading to hyperreninaemia and excessive mineralocorticoid secretion. Since hypertension is very common, and as a mineralocorticoid cause of it is rather rare, physicians need to be on their guard, because the treatment is quite different.

Aldosterone excess can be treated with the aldosterone antagonist, spironolactone.

Undersecretion of adrenal hormones

If the adrenal glands are removed or destroyed by an autoimmune process, inflammatory disease (classically tuberculosis), or haemorrhage, patients become extremely ill. The loss of sodium reabsorption in the distal tubule leads to low concentrations of sodium in the blood, accompanied by high concentrations of potassium. Hypotension leads ultimately to severe collapse—but this may take some time to develop, because hypocortisolaemia leads to an inability to excrete a water load, so that the patients retain water through this mechanism while losing it through the other.

Such patients complain of a multiplicity of symptoms, but especially of tiredness and weakness. They become anorexic and may vomit as a result of glucocorticoid deficiency. Because anorexia and vomiting are common presentations of anorexia nervosa, with or without bulimia (and this occurs in up to 10% of females at one or other time of life), the confusion with the diagnosis of Addison disease (adrenal failure) can be marked.

The majority of cases of Addison disease are of autoimmune aetiology. In autoimmune adrenalitis, varying degrees of lymphocytic infiltration can be observed, together with disruption of the cortical histology and/or cortical atrophy. There is a strong human leucocyte antigen DR3 (HLA–DR3) association, but the nature of the autoantigen or autoantigens involved remains unknown.

In classic Addison disease, ACTH is secreted in large amounts and cosecreted with α-MSH, so that patients become hyperpigmented, especially in skin creases, on scars and inside the mouth. The combination of hyperpigmentation and hypotension in a patient complaining of nonspecific symptoms should alert the physician to the possibility of Addison disease.

When ACTH secretion fails for any reason, patients have glucocorticoid and androgen deficiencies. Such patients will not, of course, become pigmented, but they do report a striking loss of body hair, especially females. Girls with ACTH deficiency may go normally through the gonadotrophic events of puberty, but develop no pubic hair because they have no adrenal androgens. Boys have sufficient testicular testosterone to make up for the loss of adrenal androgen secretion.

Treatment

Since aldosterone has a short plasma half-life, it is itself unsuitable for mineralocorticoid replacement therapy. 9α-Fluorocortisol (fludrocortisone acetate, trade name Florinef) is therefore used. Hydrocortisone is prescribed to replace cortisol. Doses have to be tailored to the patient's size, but the administration of treatment is much less difficult than making the diagnosis—although this is not difficult if the possibility crosses the physician's mind. Replacement of adrenal androgens in women is also possible, although rather rarely performed except in endocrine centres.

Congenital adrenal hyperplasia (CAH)

A particularly fascinating bridge between physiology and clinical medicine is offered by the group of conditions that go under the name of congenital adrenal hyperplasia. The feature in common is that there is a block in the biosynthesis of cortisol anywhere from cholesterol through the various enzymatic steps shown in Fig. 4.4 and Fig. A3.2 to cortisol. The response of the body to such a block is to increase endogenous CRH–ACTH drive of cholesterol incorporation into the adrenal gland (causing the hyperplasia of the name). What follows clinically is entirely predictable from the level of the block, particularly since the same enzymatic systems are involved in the testes and ovary for the elaboration of sex steroids as they are in the adrenal gland (Table 4.2).

Thus, for example, in the case of a baby with an abnormality of cholesterol transport due to a defective steroid acute regulatory (StAR) protein (see Appendix 3), there is no delivery of cholesterol to the side-chain cleavage enzyme, and as a consequence no steroids can be produced. Such a baby will not have been able to differentiate as a male, even if there are testes present, but such testes will produce anti-Müllerian hormone (see Chapter 6); the baby will be born with a short vagina and absent uterus

Defect	Ambiguous genitalia in genotypic Males	Females	Salt loss	Hypertension	Puberty
StAR protein	+	–	+	–	Absent
3β-hydroxysteroid dehydrogenase	+	+	+	–	Absent
17α-hydroxylase	+	–	–	+	Absent
21-hydroxylase	–	+	+	–	Precocious
11β-hydroxylase	–	+	–	+	Precocious

StAR, steroid acute regulatory (protein).

Congenital adrenal hyperplasia (CAH) may present with: ambiguity of the genitalia; a salt-losing crisis in the newborn period; hypertension; precocious puberty in males; signs of androgen excess in females; bilateral cryptorchidism and breast development in puberty, i.e. females raised inappropriately as males. These are all indications to think of in the diagnosis, which may be confirmed by demonstrating: (1) a low or normal cortisol concentration in the presence of elevated adrenocorticotrophic hormone (ACTH) concentrations; (2) the presence of precursor steroids in blood in abnormal concentrations (e.g. 17α-hydroxyprogesterone); (3) the identification of urinary steroid metabolites in abnormally high or low quantities, which will enable the enzymatic block to be defined.

Table 4.2 Varieties of congenital adrenal hyperplasia (CAH) and their effects.

and Fallopian tubes, since in a female these develop from the Müllerian duct. At birth, he will be apparently female, but will rapidly lapse into a salt-losing crisis, become profoundly ill and die unless steroids are administered. This condition is known as congenital lipoid adrenohyperplasia, since it is characterized by an accumulation of lipid droplets in the cells of the adrenal cortex. This is the most serious form of CAH, and it can be modelled with mice that are StAR protein knockouts. There are no known pathologies associated with defective side-chain cleavage enzyme.

Contrast this with the effects of 11β-hydroxylase (CYP11B1) deficiency. Such a patient will be unable to make cortisol, but CRH–ACTH drive will force the overproduction of deoxycorticosterone, a mineralocorticoid that can lead to malignant hypertension. There will also be excessive production of sex steroids, leading to masculinization of a female fetus *in utero* (Fig. 4.11), or to precocious puberty in a boy exposed to excessive androgen stimulation. This is another example of a cause of hypertension that needs to be excluded, especially in a young patient and especially if there are other signs of androgen activity.

All varieties of enzymatic block have been recognized, and Table 4.2 shows the clinical effects of the loss of the various enzyme systems. The most common is due to a deficiency of 21-hydroxylase, accounting for some 90% of the cases. Identification of the enzyme deficiency depends on measuring circulating steroids and identifying those that are deficient and those that are produced in excess. For example, there is an accumulation of progesterone and 17α-hydroxyprogesterone if there is a deficiency of the 21-hydroxylase.

For all of these conditions, treatment is available with either mineralocorticoid or glucocorticoid replacement, or

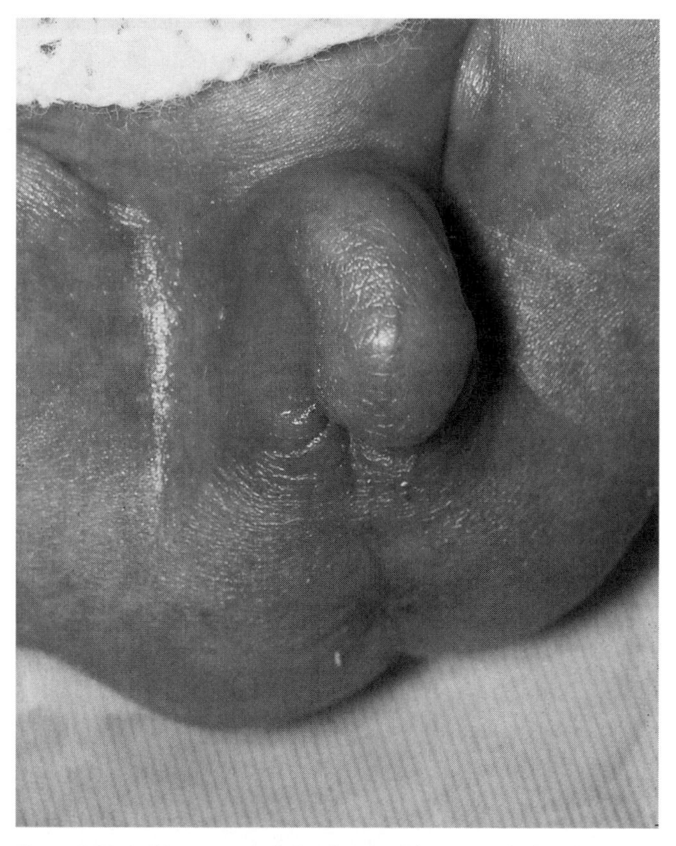

Figure 4.11 Ambiguous genitalia in a female with congenital adrenal hyperplasia. This girl was masculinized *in utero* and presented at birth with clitoral hypertrophy, fusion of the labia and a urogenital opening at the base of the phallus. At the age of one week, she developed hyperkalaemia (serum K^+ 5.2 mmol/L) and would have had a salt-losing crisis if mineralocorticoid replacement and salt had not been given. She subsequently underwent clitoral reduction and plastic surgery to the vagina (vaginoplasty), but will need further examination under anaesthesia, as well as genital reconstruction, before puberty.

both, and some of them will, of course, require sex-steroid treatment at puberty. The consequences of making the wrong diagnosis are very considerable for the individual patient.

OUTLINE OF BIOCHEMICAL TESTS OF THE HYPOTHALAMIC–PITUITARY–ADRENAL AXIS

Because of technical difficulties with the measurement of ACTH by immunoassay, the first-line test is usually the immunoassay of cortisol. Cortisol exhibits a diurnal variation (Fig. 4.12), and thus blood sampling is always performed at an identified time of day, e.g. 8 a.m.

Tests for adrenal hypofunction (Addison disease)

The diagnosis of primary adrenal failure is based on a depressed or absent cortisol response to an injection of a synthetic form of ACTH, Synacthen (tetracosactrin). First, a short form of the test is carried out. At 8 a.m., a baseline sample is taken, together with samples 30 and 60 min after Synacthen administration (250 μg i.m.). A normal result would show a baseline cortisol > 190 nmol/L, with an increment of ≈300 nmol/L. Should an impaired response be obtained, a longer form of the test can be carried out, to distinguish primary from secondary adrenal failure. Synacthen (1 mg depot, i.m.) is given for 3 days, and serum cortisol is determined at 8 a.m. each day and also on day 4. For primary adrenal insufficiency, the serum cortisol will remain low, e.g. < 100 nmol/L. With secondary adrenal insufficiency (hypothalamic or hypopituitarism), which may have caused partial adrenal atrophy, the longer-term, higher doses of Synacthen would restore adrenal function, so that the serum cortisol can reach at least 200 nmol/L above baseline.

Pituitary failure can also be identified by ACTH determination, if available, or by the impaired cortisol response to hypoglycaemia induced by insulin.

Tests for adrenal hyperfunction

Cushing syndrome/disease

In Cushing disease, the raised cortisol is secondary to excessive pituitary ACTH production. Raised ectopic ACTH, or a primary adrenal defect with overproduction of glucocorticoids and possibly mineralocorticoids, together with adrenal androgens, is referred to as Cushing syndrome.

Biochemical investigation requires: (i) the demonstration of elevated baseline serum cortisol and loss of diurnal variation; and (ii) identification of the cause. The first two tests will be measurement of cortisol in a 24-h urinary collection and a dexamethasone suppression test. Dexamethasone is a synthetic glucocorticoid that binds to

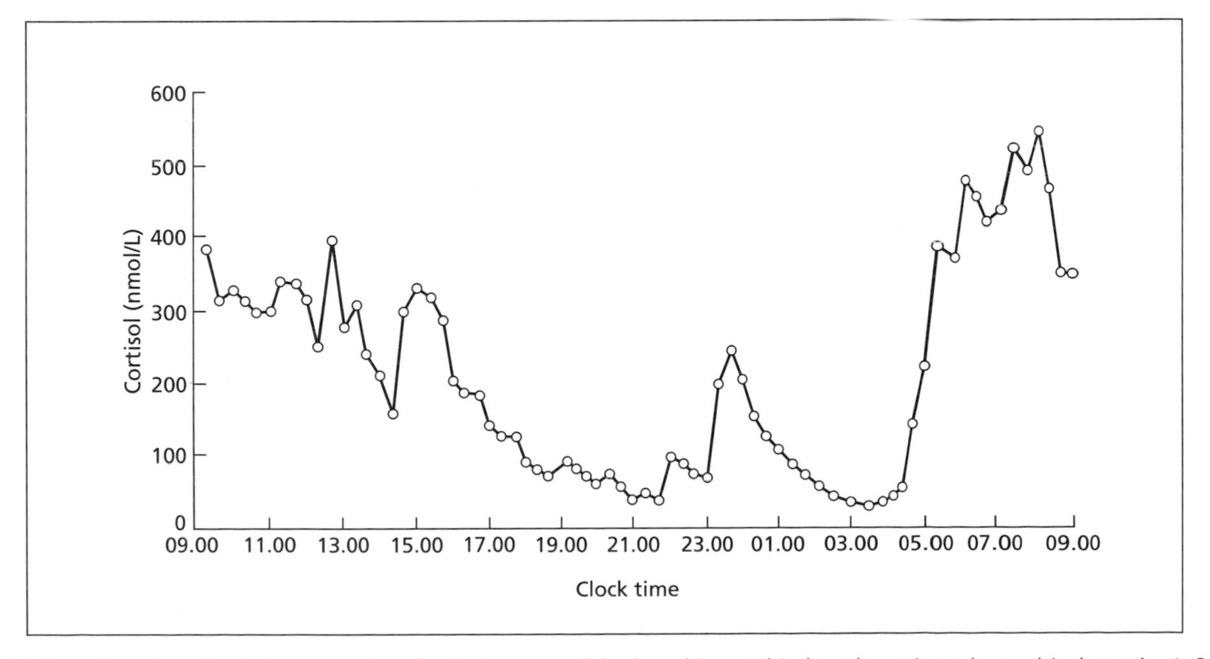

Figure 4.12 Typical diurnal variation in the concentration of cortisol in serum with levels reaching a peak in the early morning and a trough in the evening. In Cushing syndrome, the concentrations may not necessarily be greatly elevated, but the diurnal variation seen here is lost.

Table 4.3 Additional factors that can increase serum cortisol and complicate the differential diagnosis of Cushing syndrome.

- Stress
- Obesity—a diurnal variation is usually retained
- Alcoholism—the cortisol falls on removal of alcohol abuse
- Depression—a response to insulin-induced hypoglycaemia, i.e. a rise in plasma cortisol is retained, whereas in Cushing syndrome this *increase* in cortisol is suppressed

cortisol receptors in the pituitary and thus would normally suppress ACTH release. It does not cross-react in the cortisol immunoassay. An excretion of excessive cortisol (e.g. > 300 nmol/24 h) would be consistent with enhanced serum cortisol. Dexamethasone (1 mg orally at bedtime) would be expected to reduce 8 a.m. serum cortisol the following day to < 50 nmol/L in a normal subject. In Cushing disease, the pituitary is still susceptible to negative feedback by glucocorticoids, but is less sensitive than normal. Thus, if the initial dexamethasone-suppression test failed to reduce the serum cortisol, an increased dose (e.g. 2 mg four times daily for 2 days) should be tested. A large reduction in serum cortisol, e.g. 50%, will result if the adrenal hyperfunction is secondary to overproduction of ACTH by the pituitary (Cushing disease). In Cushing syndrome caused by adrenal tumours or ectopic ACTH, no response to dexamethasone would be expected. The ectopic production of ACTH is demonstrated by immunoassay of ACTH. Several situations can complicate the investigation of Cushing syndrome (Table 4.3).

Excess aldosterone

Primary hyperaldosteronism (Conn syndrome) is rare and is due to hyperactivity of the cells of the zona glomerulosa. A more common cause of hyperaldosteronism is excessive renin secretion. A differential diagnosis can be made with the measurement of these two analytes. In primary hyperaldosteronism, the concentration of renin will be low, while in secondary hyperaldosteronism, the concentration of renin (and therefore angiotensin II) is high.

FUNCTION OF THE ADRENAL MEDULLA

The principal hormones of the adrenal medulla are catecholamines, and in the adult 80% of the catecholamine content consists of epinephrine (see Fig. 1.3); the remaining 20% is norepinephrine. The adrenal medulla thus differs from the sympathetic nervous system, which only releases norepinephrine. While the adrenal medulla is not vital for survival, it does contribute to the response to stress.

Much of the volume of the cytoplasm of the cells in the medulla is occupied by granules, which are the storage sites of the catecholamines (Fig. 4.13). They also contain proteins, some of which are soluble; at least 12 such soluble proteins have been identified, including dopamine β-hydroxylase, which can be either soluble or bound to the granule membrane. The remainder of the soluble proteins are called chromogranins, and they are found within the matrix of the granule. The storage granules also contain phenylethanolamine *N*-methyl transferase, which is important in the methylation of norepinephrine, i.e. its conversion to epinephrine. In the granules, adenosine 5′-triphosphate (ATP) forms a loose, high-molecular-weight complex with the catecholamines. The membranes of the chromaffin granules are characterized by their high levels of lysolecithin.

Each chromaffin cell is innervated by a cholinergic, preganglionic sympathetic neurone, which releases acetylcholine. These synapses are the terminations of fibres carried in the splanchnic nerves, whose cell bodies lie mainly between T3 and L3. Acetylcholine stimulates the release of catecholamines from the chromaffin cells by depolarizing them; an accompanying influx of calcium ions (Ca^{2+}) occurs, which leads to the membrane of the granules fusing with the plasma membrane. Exocytosis of the granule contents then occurs. The contents are released into the extracellular space, where they diffuse into the local blood supply. This process is known as 'stimulus–secretion coupling'. The granule membrane then seals off, detaches itself from the cell membrane and is ready for recycling again. It is also possible that catecholamines may leak out of the granules and leave the cell by diffusion through the plasma membrane.

The chromaffin cells of the adrenal medulla also synthesize and store a number of opioid peptides, particularly met-enkephalin and leu-enkephalin. The sequences of these two opioid peptides are tyr–gly–gly–phe–met and tyr–gly–gly–phe–leu, respectively; thus they differ only in the carboxy-terminal residues, and it is from these that they derive their names. They are formed by proteolytic cleavage of proenkephalin A, which consists of 267 amino acids; within that sequence are six copies of met-enkephalin and one of leu-enkephalin. The structure of enkephalin A was deduced from analysis of the sequences of bases in a complementary deoxyribonucleic acid (cDNA) prepared from the adrenal medulla. An additional sequence of a signal peptide with 24 amino acids was also identified in the DNA, thus giving the structure of preproenkephalin A.

There are two important groups of large opioid peptides—those that begin with a met-enkephalin sequence, followed by additional amino acid residues on the carboxy-terminal side; and those that begin with the

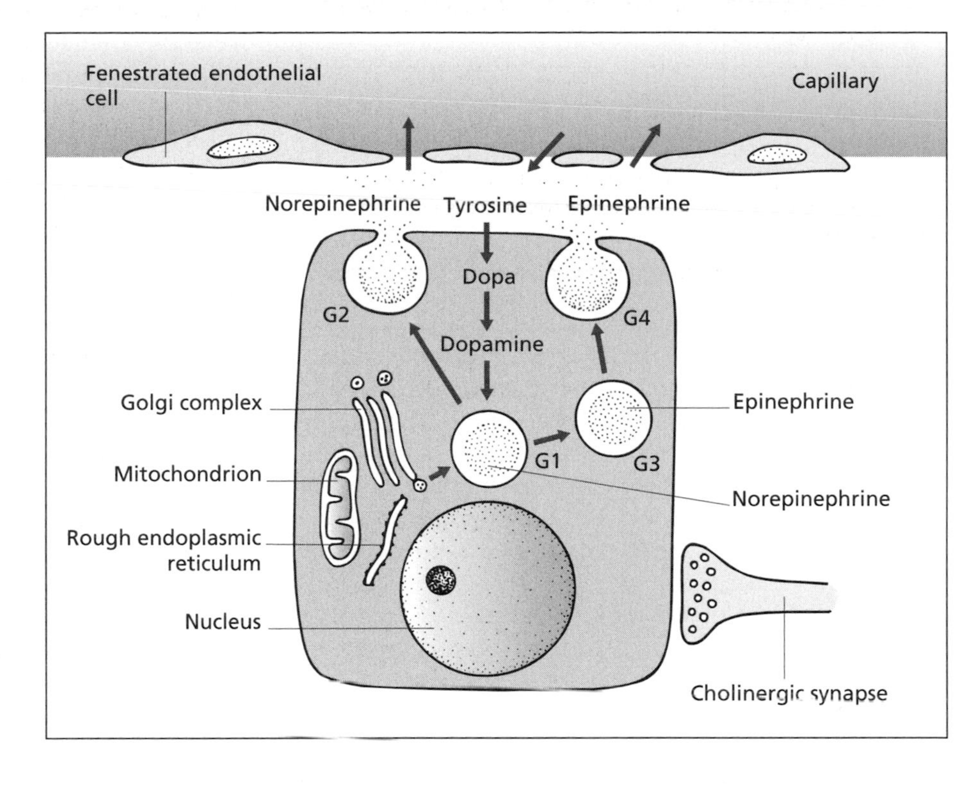

Figure 4.13 The synthesis, storage and release of catecholamines in the adrenal medullary chromaffin cell. The protein components of the storage granules (G), including the chromogranins, are synthesized on the rough endoplasmic reticulum and packaged in the Golgi complex to form the granule. Tyrosine enters the cell and is enzymatically converted to 3,4-dihydroxyphenylalanine (dopa) and then 3,4-dihydroxyphenylethylamine (dopamine) in the cytoplasm (Fig. 1.3). Dopamine enters a granule (G1) and is converted by the enzyme dopamine β-hydroxylase to norepinephrine. The norepinephrine can then be released exocytotically (G2), and it then diffuses into the local fenestrated capillary. Alternatively, norepinephrine can be further converted by phenylethanolamine *N*-methyl transferase to epinephrine in a different storage granule (G3), where it can also be released exocytotically (G4). Each cell has a cholinergic synapse where acetylcholine is released, which initiates the train of events leading to exocytosis. The nucleus and a mitochondrion are also shown. Although the cell in this diagram is shown secreting both of the catecholamines, chromaffin cells usually only secrete either norepinephrine or epinephrine.

sequence of leu-enkephalin. The former group (those containing the met-enkephalin pentapeptide) includes α-, γ- and β-endorphins, with 16, 17 and 31 amino acids, respectively. They are found in β-lipotrophin, which is formed from pro-opiomelanocortin along with ACTH in the pituitary (see Fig. 3.8). These met-enkephalins are derived from residues 61–76, 61–77 and 61–91 of β-lipotrophin, respectively.

Prepro-opiomelanocortin has 284 amino acids, including the 20 residues in its signal peptide. The opioid peptides containing leu-enkephalin include the dynorphins, with 8, 17 or 29 amino acid residues; α-neo-endorphin, with 9 amino acid residues; and β-neo-endorphin, with 10 amino acid residues. These are present in nerve fibres and may also be found in the adrenal medulla; they are neurotransmitters that can bind to opioid receptors without removal of the carboxy-terminal extension. They are all contained within and derived from a single precursor protein, called prodynorphin (or proenkephalin B). Thus, there are three distinct parent proteins, namely enkephalin A, opiomelanocortin and dynorphin, each with a distinct family of peptides that can be formed from them.

In the adrenal medulla, met-enkephalin and leu-enkephalin are packaged with chromogranin A and epinephrine, norepinephrine and other peptides, with which they are cosecreted. The roles of the adrenal enkephalins remain to be established. Leu-enkephalin reacts particularly with δ-opioid receptors (associated with inhibition of activation of adenylate cyclase), while met-enkephalin binds preferentially to the receptors that are associated with the classic effects of morphine, such as analgesia. The secretion of enkephalins from the adrenal medulla may account for the ability of runners to overcome pain and the production of a euphoric state over long distances, through the action of endogenous analgesics.

Secretion of catecholamines

The synthesis of norepinephrine and then of epinephrine from tyrosine occurs in four steps (Fig. 4.14). The first step, the conversion of tyrosine to 3,4-dihydroxyphenylalanine (DOPA) by tyrosine hydroxylase, is the rate-limiting one. Regulation of this enzyme is controlled by negative feedback in the adrenal. Norepinephrine and dopamine reduce the activity of tyrosine hydroxylase by combining with its cofactor, tetrahydropteridine. The conversion of norepinephrine to epinephrine by phenylethanolamine *N*-methyl transferase requires the presence of a high concentration of glucocorticoids, which is provided by the

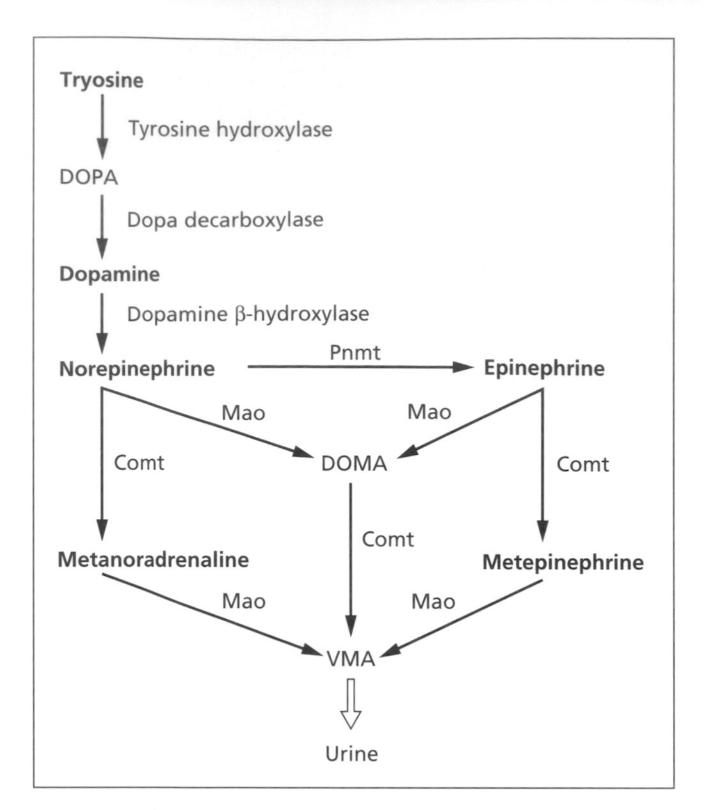

Figure 4.14 The synthesis and degradation of the catecholamines, norepinephrine and epinephrine. Dopa, 3,4-dihydroxyphenylalanine; dopamine, 3,4-dihydroxyphenylethylamine; Pnmt, phenylethanolamine *N*-methyl transferase; Mao, monoamine oxidase; Comt, catechol-*O*-methyl-transferase; DOMA, 3,4-dihydroxymandelic acid; VMA, vanillylmandelic acid (3-methoxy-4-hydroxymandelic acid).

portal vein system already described, within the adrenal gland.

In addition to the action of acetylcholine on chromaffin cells, histamine, 5-hydroxytryptamine and acetylcholine-like substances (such as nicotine and carbachol) can also cause release of these hormones. Any substance that increases the activity of the vasomotor centre in the medulla oblongata in the brain stem will also indirectly provoke release of catecholamines. The output of these hormones can be changed in a number of different ways. Thus, α-methyltyrosine reduces hormone synthesis by inhibiting the rate-limiting step dependent on tyrosine hydroxylase. In contrast, treatment with reserpine depletes the vesicles of their hormone content; administration of ganglion-blocking drugs, such as hexamethonium, will impede access of acetylcholine to the nicotinic receptors on the adrenal medullary cells and so decrease catecholamine secretions.

There is some evidence to suggest that the proportions of epinephrine and norepinephrine released will differ according to the emotional circumstances; fear may provoke a preferential increase in plasma epinephrine concentration, while anger favours an increase in norepinephrine concentration. However, the relative contributions of the sympathetic nervous system and the adrenal medulla to the rise of norepinephrine are difficult to separate.

The fate of epinephrine and norepinephrine

Uptake in cells is also important in terminating the actions of the two hormones. Norepinephrine, in particular, can be taken up into postganglionic sympathetic nerve terminals (uptake 1), where it can then be metabolized by monoamine oxidase. Most of the norepinephrine taken up in this way from the circulation will enter the storage vesicles, where it becomes available for reuse as a neurotransmitter. Epinephrine, and to a lesser extent norepinephrine, can also be removed by nonneuronal uptake (uptake 2); and since no storage occurs in such tissues—for example, in platelets—the hormones will be almost wholly metabolized if taken up in this way.

Metabolism plays a minor role in terminating the action of circulating epinephrine and norepinephrine. The enzymes involved in this are catechol-*O*-methyl transferase and monoamine oxidase, and among the many end-products, the main one is vanillylmandelic acid (VMA). These two enzymes are distributed widely throughout the body, particularly in the liver. Catechol-*O*-methyl transferase is found in nonneuronal tissue in association with its cofactor, *S*-adenosyl methionine, whereas monoamine oxidase occurs in mitochondria in both neuronal and nonneuronal tissues. The two hormones are found in urine; 5% is unchanged, but 95% represents metabolites of epinephrine and norepinephrine. Removal of the adrenal medulla leads to loss of all urinary epinephrine.

Effects and mode of action of catecholamines

Epinephrine increases systolic blood pressure but reduces diastolic blood pressure, so that there is little change in mean pressure. Tachycardia occurs and gut motility is reduced, with secondary closure of the sphincters. Epinephrine is a bronchodilator and can also cause piloerection. Topical application of high concentrations of epinephrine onto the conjunctivae causes dilatation of the pupil (mydriasis). The systemic effects of norepinephrine are rather different; it raises both systolic and diastolic pressure and so increases the mean blood pressure; it causes bradycardia, which is reflex and can be blocked by prior administration of atropine; it has much less effect in reducing gut motility than epinephrine, and it does not produce bronchodilatation. However, like epinephrine, norepinephrine causes piloerection and dilatation of the pupils.

The metabolic effects of epinephrine are also important. It promotes hepatic glycogenolysis, which leads to the production of glucose-6-phosphate. This in turn leads to hyperglycaemia and lactic acidaemia, due to further metabolism in the liver and muscle, respectively (see Chapter 8). Epinephrine also increases the plasma concentration of free fatty acids. Norepinephrine is much less potent than epinephrine in producing hepatic glycogenolysis, but is more potent in causing mobilization of free fatty acids.

The difference between the effects of epinephrine and norepinephrine are partially explained by the existence of two populations of receptors on the surface of effector cells, referred to as α- and β-adrenoreceptors. The receptors have been defined on the basis of their blockade by certain other synthetic pharmacological agents. This blockade (antagonism) therefore provides a convenient method of classifying these receptors, although the physiological significance of α- and β-type activities has not yet been resolved. Interaction with α-adrenoreceptors produces effects that are predominantly excitatory, while with β-adrenoreceptors the effects are predominantly inhibitory. Both the α- and the β-adrenoreceptors can be further subdivided into α_1-, α_2-, β_1- and β_2-receptors, on the basis of the relative potencies of a series of adrenergic agonists. Norepinephrine interacts only with α- and β_1-receptors, cannot cause bronchodilatation and is less potent on the gut. In blood vessels, only norepinephrine has vasoconstrictor actions, but in those blood vessels that have α- and β_2-receptors, epinephrine can cause dilatation in low concentrations. In studying the effects of injected norepinephrine, consideration of the reflex changes is important, since norepinephrine reflexly reduces sympathetic activity, while also increasing vagal activity.

Metabolically, as opposed to neurologically, the β-adrenoreceptor is closely associated with the adenylate cyclase system. In both cardiac and bronchial muscle, containing β_1- and β_2-adrenoreceptors, respectively, administration of epinephrine increases the production of cyclic adenosine 5′-monophosphate (cAMP). Both α- and β-adrenoreceptors are classic G-protein–linked receptors (see Figs 2.12 and 2.13). Both the β_1- and β_2-adrenoreceptors activate the adenylate cyclase catalytic subunit (see Fig. 2.13). However, agonists binding to the α_2-adrenoreceptors interact with an inhibitory α-subunit of the G-protein, which results in inhibition of adenylate cyclase activity, whereas those binding to the α_1-receptor activate phospholipase C (see Figs 2.12 and 2.18).

ADRENOMEDULLARY DYSFUNCTION

Adrenomedullary deficiency

Failure of the adrenal medulla is very uncommon. It causes hypotension and, more importantly, hypoglycaemia, but the hormones of the adrenal cortex are more important in this respect, and adrenomedullary replacement is not required after adrenalectomy or adrenal destruction by haemorrhage.

Adrenomedullary hyperfunction

Tumours secreting catecholamines cause hypertension, which may be episodic or sustained. It is usually due to a tumour of neural-crest origin, such as a phaeochromocytoma or neuroblastoma. There may be an association with other endocrine neoplasia (multiple endocrine neoplasia syndrome type 2). Diagnosis requires the measurement of blood catecholamines and/or their urinary metabolites and localization of their origin. Treatment requires surgical removal of the tumour, with the assistance of an especially experienced anaesthetist, and the patient must be carefully prepared to block against the effects of catecholamines. It will be clear that the key to making such a diagnosis is to think of it during the differential diagnosis and not to dismiss hypertension simply as a phenomenon of ageing.

CHAPTER 5

The Thyroid

SUMMARY

Thyroid hormones have general, as opposed to tissue-specific, effects and are required for the maintenance of co-ordinated growth and development in the young and for basal metabolism. They bind to specific receptors in the cell nucleus, and induce transcription of the genes responsive to thyroid hormones.

Thyroid hormone production is regulated by the hypothalamopituitary–thyroid axis. Both thyroid hormones—thyroxine and triiodothyronine—are synthesized by the thyroid gland, and the gland is unique in that there is a large store of the hormone in an extracellular depot contained within the follicles of the gland. Dietary iodide is required for the synthesis of thyroid hormones, and the thyroid is the only tissue that can both concentrate and organify ingested iodide. Thyroid hormones are bound to proteins in blood, with only a small fraction circulating as free hormone. The majority of thyroxine is converted peripherally, by the target cells, to the biologically more potent thyroid hormone triiodothyronine—80% of triiodothyronine being obtained by this route, as opposed to direct production by the thyroid gland. This peripheral conversion is due to two contrasting 5′-monodeiodinases, which probably provide an additional system for the regulation of triiodothyronine levels.

Unlike other hormones, thyroid hormone levels are kept remarkably constant, and thyroid physiology is organized at many different levels to achieve this stability. Thus, apart from the hypothalamopituitary–thyroid axis, there are 'stores' of hormones in the thyroid follicles and bound to circulating binding proteins. In addition, thyroxine acts primarily as a prohormone for triiodothyronine. In circumstances liable to reduce available triiodothyronine, such as when an individual enters an iodine-deficient region of the world, these systems act as a buffer to maintain the individual euthyroid over a long period.

INTRODUCTION

The thyroid gland is a discrete organ situated just caudal to the larynx and adherent to the front of the trachea. It is named after the shield commonly used in ancient Greece, since this approximately describes its gross morphology, which consists of two flat, oval-shaped lobes joined by an isthmus. The characteristic feature of the gland is its ability to concentrate iodide from the bloodstream and synthesize thyroxine (T_4) and triiodothyronine (T_3). The gland is dependent on a constant supply of dietary iodide, and when the element is scarce the thyroid enlarges to form a goitre. In geographical areas of severe iodide limitation, which are estimated to affect at least 800 million people world-wide, both endemic goitres and mental retardation due to cretinism are encountered, and iodide supplementation programmes have therefore been set up to try to alleviate this situation.

In the late nineteenth century, associations were made between a number of clinical symptoms and thyroid malfunction. Thyroid atrophy was linked to sporadic cretinism in infants, and to the classical features of myxoedema in adults. In 1891 in Newcastle, the successful treatment of a myxoedematous patient with an extract of sheep thyroid was reported; this was the first example of hormone replacement therapy.

The importance of dietary iodide in relieving endemic goitre was progressively understood in the last century, and led to the idea that the thyroid produced an iodine-containing compound. Kendall isolated an iodine-containing substance from thyroid tissue in the USA in 1914, but it was almost 20 years later that Pitt-Rivers and Harrington in London determined the structure of the first thyroid hormone to be so recognized. This was T_4, which contains four iodine atoms per molecule. In 1952, Gross and Pitt-Rivers identified a second thyroid hormone, T_3, in human serum. The dominant significance of T_3 in thyroid physiology has been recognized only comparatively recently.

In 1956, Doniach, Roitt and Campbell in London associated antithyroid autoantibodies with certain forms of hypothyroidism; this was the first description of an autoimmune phenomenon in humans. Coincidentally, Adams and Purves in Dunedin associated an unusual thyroid stimulator with the hyperthyroidism of Graves disease—later found to be another autoantibody, now known as a thyroid-stimulating antibody (TSAb).

MORPHOLOGY

Development

In the human embryo, the early stages of development of the thyroid gland and parathyroid glands are closely associated. Thyroid development commences at day 24 as a midline thickening and then as an outpouching of the endodermal floor of the pharyngeal cavity. This primordium of the thyroid eventually forms a sac-like diverticulum between the first and second pharyngeal pouches (Fig. 5.1a). At about 1 month of development, when the fetus is nearly 4 mm in length, the diverticulum comprises a solid mass of cells, and weighs about 1–2 mg. By the sixth to seventh week, it is clearly bilobed, and as the embryo elongates and the tongue grows forward, the thyroid descends the neck but remains attached to its point of origin by a narrow canal, the thyroglossal duct. During the fifth and sixth weeks of development, the distal ends of the third and fourth paired pharyngeal pouches differentiate into the primordia of the four parathyroid glands (Fig. 5.1a). Caudal movement of the developing thyroid brings it down to the level of parathyroid glands IV, which do not appreciably alter their position relative to the thyroid. However, parathyroid glands III bud off from the pharyngeal body during this time, pass the parathyroids IV in their caudal descent, and come to rest on the posterior surface of the thyroid gland. Parathyroids IV thus become the superior, and parathyroids III become the inferior, parathyroid glands in humans, lying on the posterior surface of the thyroid gland.

The lower (ventral) portion of the fourth pharyngeal pouches, the ultimobranchial bodies, come into contact with the thyroid anlagen, and eventually a fusion of the two organs occurs, with a mixing of the two cell types. These latter cells become the C-cells of the thyroid gland, making up about 10% of the adult cell mass of the gland, and they secrete the hormone calcitonin (see Chapter 7). The thymus is derived from cells that arise from the ventral portion of the third pharyngeal pouch and migrate caudally with the thyroid and parathyroids. If the parathyroids or ultimobranchial bodies do not become attached to or incorporated into the thyroid, they form ectopic glands.

Normally, the thyroglossal duct ruptures, and the cells atrophy or are resorbed by the second month, leaving only a small dimple (the foramen caecum) at the junction of the middle and posterior third of the tongue; persistent thyroglossal duct tissue may give rise to cysts (Fig. 5.1b). Cells in the lower portion of the duct differentiate into thyroid tissue, forming the pyramidal lobe of the gland as an upward, finger-like extension. The thyroid develops laterally into two distinct lobes connected by a narrow isthmus of thyroid tissue at the midline. The lobes come to rest on either side of, and slightly behind, the trachea, with the isthmus running across its front, just below the larynx in humans and most mammals; this therefore provides a convenient landmark for locating the thyroid gland.

By the seventh week of development, when connection of the human thyroid to the pharynx is lost, the cells of the thyroid are grouped into clusters. At about 11 weeks, a central lumen appears in each cluster, completely surrounded by a single layer of cells. Although the thyroid is functionally capable of trapping iodide and releasing hormone at this stage, it does not actually respond to pituitary secretion of thyrotrophin until this occurs at around week 22.

Abnormalities

Developmental abnormalities of the thyroid are common. The thyroglossal duct fails to atrophy or is only partially resorbed in approximately 15% of the population, and so may be present in the adult, yielding a midline pyramidal lobe of active thyroid tissue. In the same way,

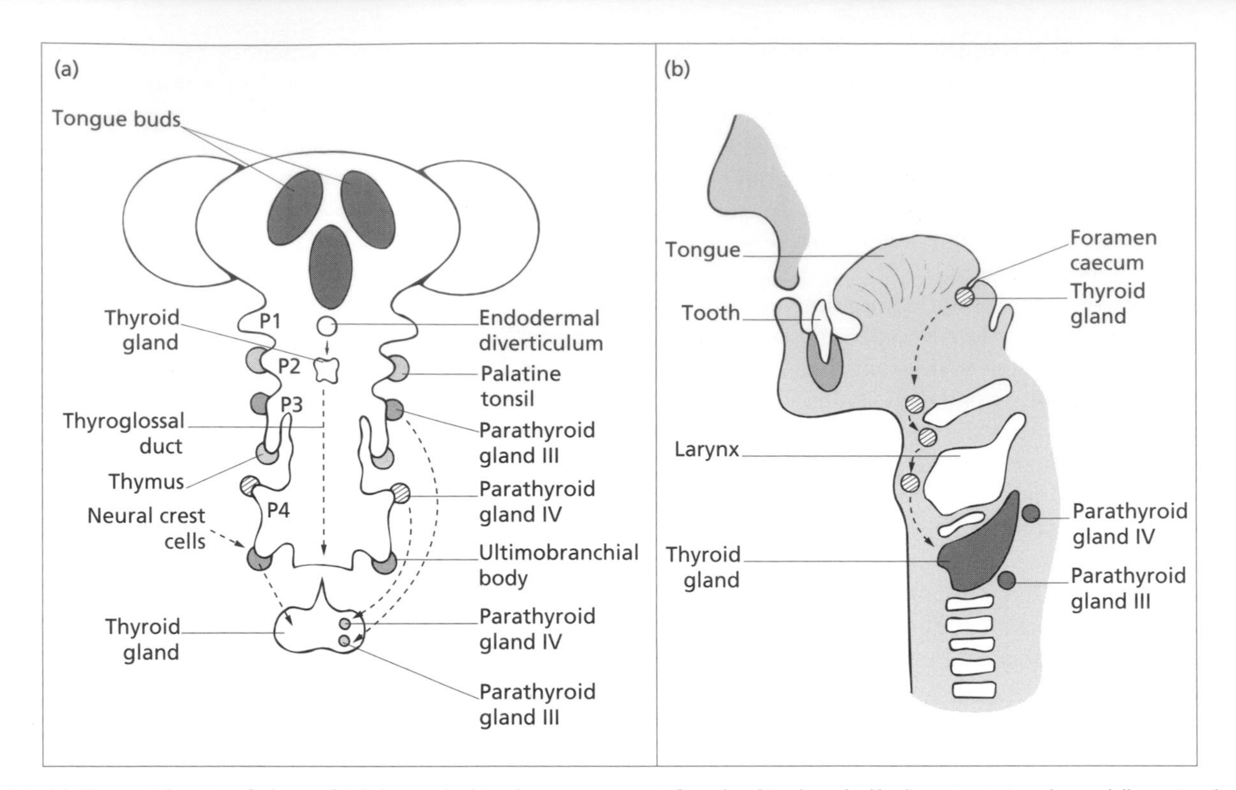

Figure 5.1 (a) A horizontal section of a human fetal pharynx, looking down on its floor, and showing the origin of the thyroid and parathyroid glands. The thyroid originates as an endodermal diverticulum in the floor of the pharynx at the level of the first pharyngeal pouch (P1). It moves caudally (- -►), becoming bilobed, but remaining for some time attached to its origin by the thyroglossal duct. As the thyroid moves caudally, paired cell masses detach themselves from the third (P3) and fourth (P4) pharyngeal pouches, respectively, become positioned on the thyroid's posterior surface, and form the parathyroid glands III and IV. Neural-crest cells, which have invaded the fourth pharyngeal pouch (P4) to form the ultimobranchial bodies, migrate into the caudally moving thyroid and form its C-cell component. The origins of the thymus, palatine tonsils and tongue buds are also shown. (b) The thyroid gland and its caudal migration (- -►) to just below the larynx. Its point of origin in the tongue persists as the foramen caecum. Common sites of thyroglossal cysts (⊘) are also shown, and the position of paired parathyroid glands III and IV are indicated (●). A developing tooth is also shown. (After K.L. Moore, *The Developing Human*, W.B. Saunders, Philadelphia)

developmental abnormalities of the isthmus may occur, which are not noted until the gland is investigated later in life. If the thyroid fails to descend to the correct level, or else descends too far, the thyroid gland may be found in sublingual or intrathoracic positions. Absence of the left lobe is also observed in some individuals, owing to development of only a single thyroid lobe. Usually, these developmental abnormalities do not affect thyroid function, and it is only during investigation of thyroid dysfunction that they may be found. Occasionally, congenital complete absence of the thyroid occurs; this requires immediate detection and treatment with thyroid hormone in order to minimize the severe and largely irreversible neurological damage that could occur to the infant.

The thyroid gland

The adult human gland weighs 10–20 g, and is usually smaller in regions of the world in which supplies of dietary iodine are abundant. It is nearly always asymmetrical, with the right lobe often twice the size of the left one. The thyroid is usually larger in women than men, and it enlarges during puberty, in pregnancy, during lactation and in the latter part of the menstrual cycle. Seasonal changes have also been reported between summer and winter; a decrease in thyroid mass frequently occurs in winter.

The gland is enclosed by two connective-tissue capsules. The outer is not well defined, and attaches the thyroid to the trachea. On the posterior surface of the thyroid, the two pairs of parathyroids are situated between the two capsules. From the inner capsule, trabeculae of collagen fibres pervade the gland and carry nerves and a rich vasculature to the cells (Fig. 5.2). In humans, the sympathetic and parasympathetic supply to the gland appears to regulate the rich vascular system. Secretomotor fibres to follicular cells have not been convincingly demonstrated. The arterial blood supply arises from the external carotids and subclavians, and enters the gland via the superior and

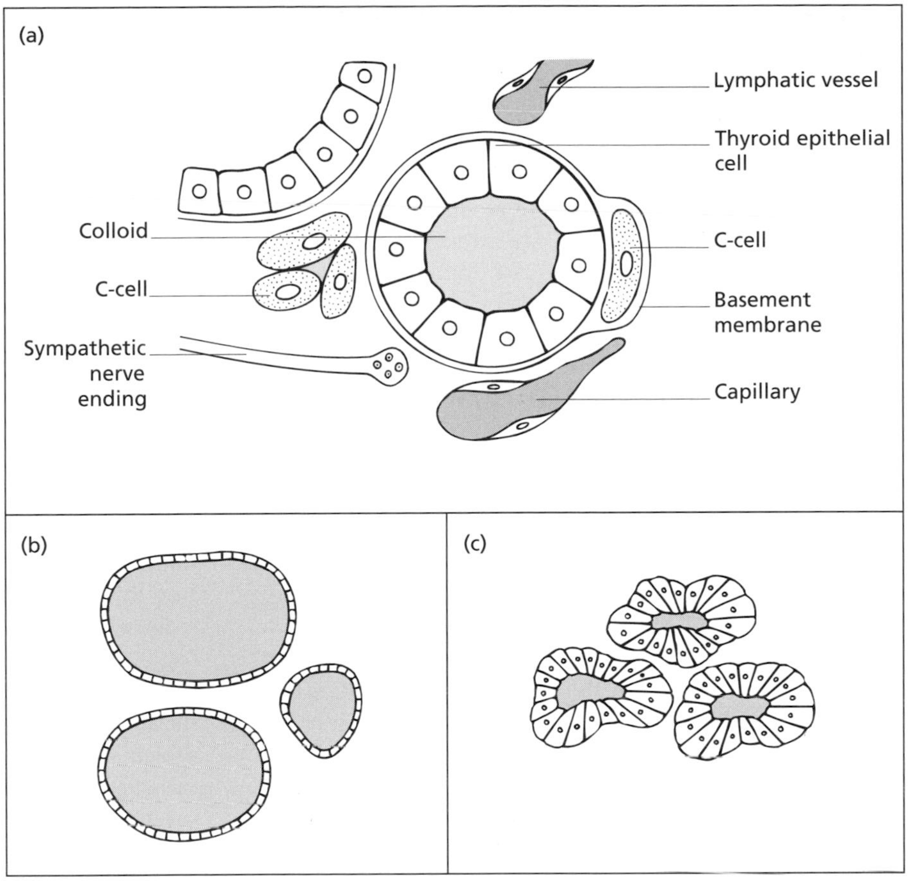

Figure 5.2 The histological components of the mammalian thyroid gland. (a) Euthyroid follicles are shown, consisting of hollow spheres of cuboidal, epithelial cells, the lumens of which are filled with gelatinous colloid in which are stored the thyroid hormones in the form of thyroglobulin. Surrounding each follicle is a basement membrane enclosing C-cells in a parafollicular position. In the interfollicular stroma are found fenestrated capillaries, lymphatic vessels and sympathetic nerve endings. (b) Underactive follicles are shown, with flattened thyroid epithelial cells and increased colloid. (c) Overactive follicles are shown, with tall, columnar epithelial cells and reduced colloid.

inferior thyroid arteries, respectively. The thyroid has a blood flow that has been estimated to range from 4 to 6 mL/min/g of tissue, which is nearly twice that of the kidney. In conditions of severe hyperplasia, greater flow rates may occur and may be evidenced by a trill or by an audible bruit when a stethoscope is placed on or near an overactive gland.

Histology

The functional unit of the gland is the thyroid follicle or acinus (Fig. 5.2). This consists of cuboidal epithelial (follicular) cells arranged as roughly spheroidal sacs, the lumen of which contains colloid. The latter is composed almost entirely of the iodinated glycoprotein called thyroglobulin, which yields an intensely pink positive result on periodic acid–Schiff (PAS) staining. The normal human follicle varies in diameter from 20 to 900 μm, and many thousands are present in the gland; several follicles are usually grouped together in arbitrary units, separated by blood vessels and connective tissue. As is typical of epithelial cells, they are enveloped by a basement membrane that surrounds each follicle. The basement membrane anchors the follicles to the connective tissue. The parafollicular calcitonin-secreting C-cells lie between this membrane and the follicular cells.

A loose framework of reticular fibres holds the follicles together, and an abundance of short, fenestrated capillaries surround them (Fig. 5.2). An extensive network of lymphatic vessels is also present, and small amounts of thyroglobulin are absorbed by this lymph system. Postganglionic sympathetic nerve fibres from the middle and superior cervical ganglia supply blood vessels and control the blood flow through the gland. By this means, they alter the delivery rate of thyrotrophin (thyroid-stimulating hormone, TSH), iodide and other metabolites—e.g. amino acids, etc.—to the gland cells. Preganglionic parasympathetic fibres from the vagus also enter the gland; adrenergic nerve terminals may be associated principally with mast cells in the thyroid, but it is impossible to rule out a direct, although probably minor, effect of the biogenic amines on thyroid follicular cells.

When the gland is normal but underactive, as occurs in an iodine-deficient hypothyroid state, the follicles are distended with colloid and the acinar cells are thin and flattened, with little cytoplasm visible under the light microscope. In an overactive gland, the acinar cells are tall and columnar, and colloid may be seen within some cells under the light microscope. Different follicles appear to be activated to different extents, as evidenced by differing densities of staining of the luminal colloid and colloid droplets in surrounding cells. Under the electron microscope, large pseudopodia and an extensive network of microvilli, which is characteristic of epithelial cells, may be observed at the apical or colloid end of the active cells.

CIRCULATING THYROID HORMONES

Chemical structure

The structures of the iodothyronine hormones produced by the thyroid, and some other important metabolites, are shown in Fig. 5.3. Thyroxine (or 3,3′,5,5′-tetraiodothyronine) is frequently abbreviated to T_4, and triiodothyronine is abbreviated to T_3, with the numbers representing the number of iodine atoms attached to each thyronine residue. A biologically inactive iodothyronine called 'reverse T_3'' (rT_3)—3,3′,5′-triiodothyronine—may be found in significant concentrations in human serum. For example, rT_3 rises in the serum of patients with the 'sick euthyroid' syndrome, when T_3 itself is low (see p. 95).

Once the serum iodothyronine concentrations have settled to constant values, which occurs about 3 days after birth, little change occurs in the normal individual throughout the remainder of life, except perhaps for a very slight decline in T_4 with age in some individuals.

Thyroid hormones in the circulation

T_4 and T_3 are strongly bound to serum proteins; about 0.015% of the total circulating T_4 and 0.33% of the total serum T_3 are present in the free form. T_3 is bound slightly less strongly to each of the three principal serum binding proteins than T_4, and the binding affinity of both iodothyronines decreases from thyroxine-binding globulin (TBG) to thyroxine-binding prealbumin (TBPA) to serum albumin, which is a relatively nonspecific binder of circulating thyroid hormone present in the circulation.

Drugs can also compete with iodothyronines for binding to the serum proteins, and may therefore elevate the free thyroid hormone concentrations and cause the control mechanisms to lower the total iodothyronine concentrations in serum. Typical of such drugs are the salicylates, the hydantoins used in the treatment of epilepsy, or anti-inflammatory drugs such as diclofenac, the structures of which resemble that of the iodothyronine molecule. In order to monitor thyroidal status by biochemical measurements of the circulating concentrations of iodothyronine hormones in the presence of altered serum binding protein concentrations, two courses of action are possible. Either a correction for the altered serum concentrations of thyroid hormone binding proteins is required, or direct

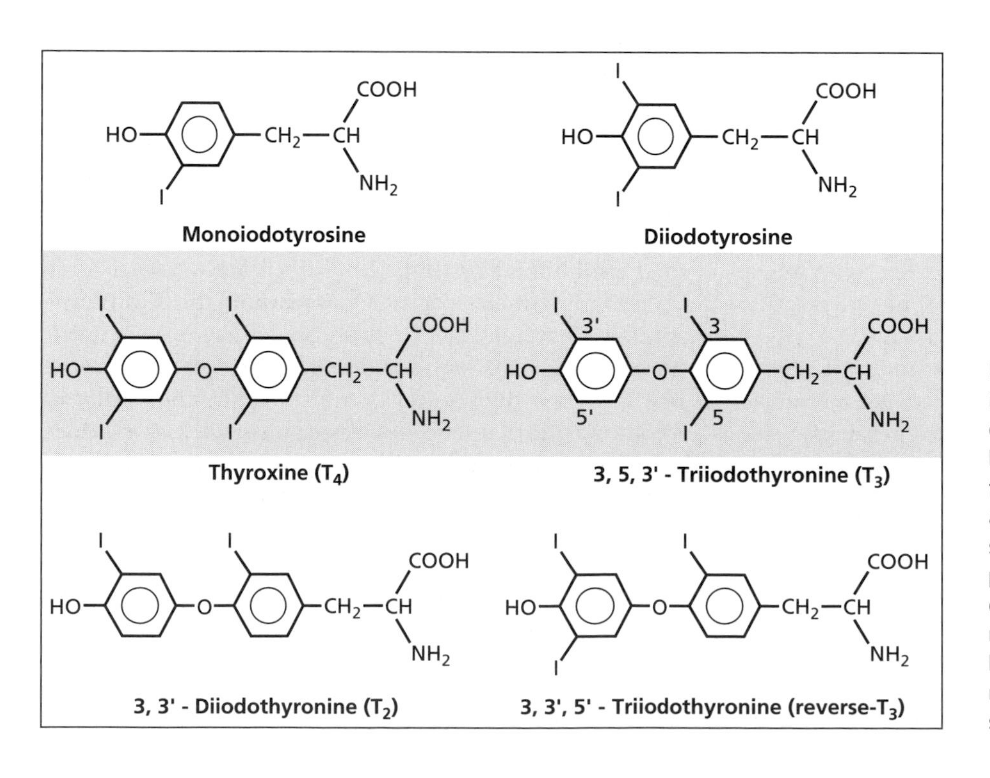

Figure 5.3 Structures of intrathyroidal iodoamino acids. Monoiodotyrosines and diiodotyrosines are precursors of the thyroid hormones (see text). Thyroxine (T_4) and triiodothyronine (T_3) are the two biologically active forms of the thyroid hormones. T_3 is secreted by the gland, but is mainly formed peripherally from T_4 by specific enzyme deiodination. 'Reverse T_3' and T_2 are inactive metabolites formed by deiodination of the thyroid hormones by peripheral tissues of the body. The numbering of critical positions is shown on the structure of T_3.

measurements of the free hormone concentrations must be performed. Nowadays, the latter is the usual strategy.

Kinetics

Studies on the kinetics of release and metabolism of iodothyronines show that T_3 has a shorter half-life (about 1–3 days) than T_4 (about 5–7 days), and rT_3 is cleared very rapidly, with a half-life of about 5 h. Depending on the biological response monitored, estimates of the relative potency of the two hormones show that T_3 is two to 10 times more active than T_4. However, the total serum concentration of T_3 is only about 2% of that of T_4—i.e. about 2 nmol/L for T_3 vs. approximately 100 nmol/L for T_4 (see Appendix 1).

Free thyroid hormones

The differential binding to serum proteins results in free T_3 concentrations being about 30% those of free T_4 (see Appendix 1). In spite of the higher concentrations of T_4 in serum, T_3 is turned over in the body at a faster rate.

The majority of cells appear not to take up the binding proteins from the serum, and so these cells can only respond to free thyroid hormones. Under most normal circumstances, the serum binding proteins remain at relatively constant concentrations, and measurements of the total thyroid hormone concentrations therefore mirror the levels of the free thyroid hormones present. However, in conditions in which serum binding protein concentrations are altered, the total thyroid hormone concentrations no longer reflect the free hormone concentrations in serum. This arises because altered binding protein concentrations in serum cause a change in the fraction of circulating free thyroid hormones, and the hypothalamopituitary–thyroid control mechanisms readjust to maintain the concentrations of iodothyronines that are free. Thus, when binding protein concentrations fall, as can occur in starvation or in some disease states (e.g. liver disease or renal failure), less total iodothyronine is required to maintain adequate free concentrations at the euthyroid level. Conversely, when liver synthesis of binding proteins is increased—for example, by steroid action on the liver during pregnancy, or when oral contraceptives are taken—then more total thyroid hormone is required to maintain the concentrations of free iodothyronines in the circulation.

EFFECTS AND MECHANISM OF ACTION OF THYROID HORMONES

General effects

The study of the mechanism of action of the thyroid hormones has been difficult. Constant exposure of cells of an adult animal to thyroid hormones implies that there is an essential requirement of iodothyronines for the maintenance of normal metabolic functions, but virtually the only definitive action of the thyroid hormones in intact animals is recognized to be an effect on increasing the basal metabolic rate (BMR). Although several short-term effects of the thyroid hormones have been observed at various subcellular sites, it is now recognized that the principal and probably primary site of action of the iodothyronine hormones is on the cell nucleus. Most of the actions of the thyroid hormones are mediated by T_3.

Cellular effects

Nuclear site of action

Thyroid-hormone receptors are nuclear acidic proteins associated with chromatin, which can bind to specific deoxyribonucleic acid (DNA) sequences when activated. As discussed previously (Chapter 2), they are a member of the superfamily of steroid–thyroid hormone receptors, which have been cloned and show homology with the *erb*-A oncogene (see Fig. 2.21). The binding affinities of T_3 and T_4 to this nuclear receptor in the liver reflect their differing potencies as metabolic stimulators, with T_4 having a much lower affinity than T_3. After hormone binding, the hormone–receptor complex induces transcription of the genes that are responsive to thyroid hormones. This is brought about by activation of a DNA domain known as the thyroid hormone response element (TRE), which is located close to the promoter region of the target gene (see Fig. 2.24). Note that, unlike many other members of this superfamily of receptors, thyroid-hormone receptors do not form stable complexes with heat-shock proteins in their inactive state (see Fig. 2.22). In addition, there is considerable evidence that association with the TRE can occur when the receptor is in its 'resting state', i.e. in the absence of thyroid hormones.

Thus the thyroid hormone receptors are hormone-responsive transcription factors, which contain both hormone-binding and DNA-binding regions. Following binding of the thyroid hormone, a physical change occurs to the receptor protein, which allows the DNA-binding region to activate the TRE of the target gene. This interaction with the hormone-response element can either enhance or inhibit the initiation of transcription by ribonucleic acid (RNA) polymerase. In this way, the thyroid hormones can activate genes, as with growth hormone (GH) production by the pituitary, or repress genes, as with negative feedback of TSH production by the thyrotrophs. The activated receptors are thought to interact with the TREs either as monomers, as homodimers, or as heterodimers formed with receptors for retinoic acid and other 'auxiliary' proteins. This requirement for co-operative action probably forms an important basis for tissue specificity of the responses, and receptors for retinoic acid may be important modulators of those for thyroid hormones.

Two cellular proto-oncogenes, c-*erb*-α and β, have been shown to code for two groups of thyroid-hormone receptors, designated α- and β-receptors, respectively. The β-gene can be transcribed from two promoters to yield β_1- and β_2-receptor isoforms. There is marked tissue-specific expression of these receptor isoforms, with the α_1 and β_1 forms being fairly widely distributed. However, the β_2-receptor is restricted to the anterior pituitary and specific regions of the brain. In addition, an alternative form of the α-receptor, the α_2-receptor, has been described. This may dominate in some tissues that are unresponsive to thyroid hormones, such as the adult rat brain. The α_2-receptor, which is produced by alternative splicing of c-*erb*-α, cannot bind thyroid hormones. However, it can bind to the TRE, albeit only weakly. Since this binding is not followed by target-gene activation, this isoform can, if present in a sufficiently high concentration, block gene induction by the α_1 thyroid-hormone complex. This can consequently act as a mechanism for repression of cell responsiveness to thyroid hormones. Such tissue-specific distribution of the thyroid-hormone receptor isoforms may well account for the differences in the responsiveness of tissues to thyroid hormones within a given species.

Because of the nuclear site of action, the effects of thyroid hormones are delayed in onset. It is usually several hours after an injection of T_3 or a day or two after T_4 before a biological expression of the response to hormone action is observed *in vivo* (Fig. 5.4). Subsequent to activation of the TRE, the earliest intracellular change to be detected is an increase in nuclear RNA, with later increases in ribosomal RNA, followed by increased protein synthesis. This leads to rises in specific enzymes, shown as increased amino acid incorporation/mg ribosomal RNA in Fig. 5.4, and ultimately a rise in liver weight.

Mitochondrial actions. Thyroid hormones are not now thought to uncouple oxidative phosphorylation, as was once postulated. The general metabolic increases that give rise to an enhanced BMR are most likely to be due to an increase in the intracellular concentrations of enzymes involved in catabolic processes within the body; this is suggested because no convincing evidence has yet been presented for allosteric or conformational effects of the thyroid hormones at physiological concentrations on the affinity constant (K_M) or the reaction rate (v_{max}) of the many enzymes so far examined.

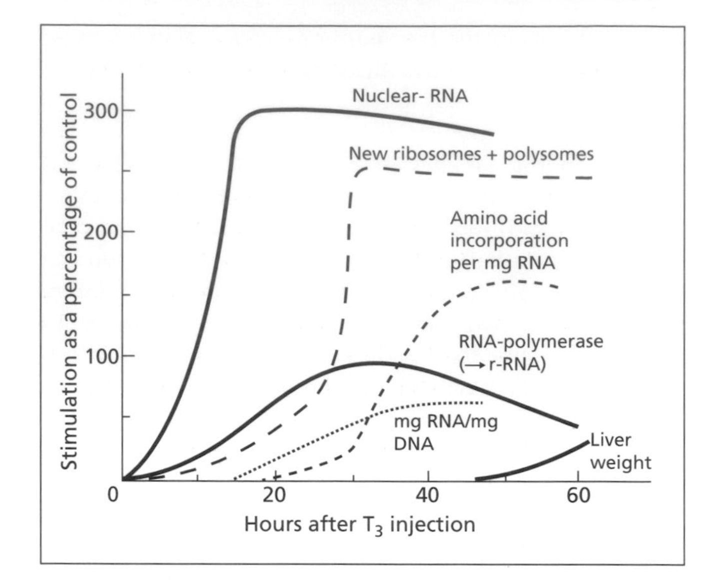

Figure 5.4 Effects of an injection of a relatively low dose of triiodothyronine (T_3) into a thyroidectomized rat. The time-course of synthesis of some intracellular nucleic acids and enzymes is shown as a percentage increase over the control with time after injection. An increase in nuclear ribonucleic acid (RNA) is the first significant event to be observed following the administration of thyroid hormone, and it results in increased ribosomal RNA and polysome formation. This produces increased protein (mainly catabolic enzyme) synthesis within the cell, shown as amino acid incorporation/mg of ribosomal RNA.

High-affinity mitochondrial receptors for thyroid hormones have been reported, but their full significance is at present unknown. They appear to be localized in tissues responsive to thyroid hormone, since they are not found in mitochondria from the spleen, testis, or adult brain, which are refractory to thyroid hormones.

Membrane transport of iodothyronines. Thyroid hormones are relatively hydrophobic, and hence may readily enter cells by diffusion through the lipid bilayers of the cell membrane. However, certain cells have been found to have a specific membrane transport mechanism for the iodothyronines, which facilitates the uptake of free thyroid hormones from the serum into the cells.

Deiodination of T_4

T_4 metabolism largely proceeds by progressive deiodination within the target cells. In a euthyroid individual, approximately 40% of T_4 is monodeiodinated at its outer ring to T_3 (Fig. 5.3). This requires one of two specific deiodinases that act at the outer ring. About 45% of T_4 is converted to rT_3 by an inner-ring monodeiodinase, which is also present in target cells. The remaining 15% of the T_4 is metabolized by minor pathways, such as deamination and cleavage of the ether link between the two substituted phenolic rings of the thyronine nucleus.

Peripheral regulation of iodothyronines. Peripheral monodeiodination is of crucial importance. In a euthyroid individual, up to 80% of T_3 in the circulation is obtained by this route, with only 20% being provided directly from the thyroid gland. It is suggested that, when a given cell has sufficient T_3 for its metabolic requirements, it switches to the alternative inner-ring monodeiodinase, which yields the biologically inactive rT_3, which is then rapidly cleared. T_4 may thus be a 'prohormone', its presence being required only to maintain a constant supply of T_3. However, it is possible that T_4 has other, as yet unidentified, actions (e.g. during fetal development) on thyrotrophs and neural tissues.

Two contrasting monodeiodinases are known to act at the outer ring of T_4 and thereby play a major role in T_3 supply. These are known as type I and type II iodothyronine deiodinase, respectively. They are tissue-specific, with type I predominating in liver, kidney and muscle, and type II in the brain and, notably, the pituitary. This tissue distribution is variable, and changes subtly with the thyroid status of an individual. The full significance of the two types is not yet clear. However, the kinetic characteristics and other properties of the two enzymes are strikingly different, suggesting an additional regulatory system for T_3 production by individual target tissues.

Type I is unusual in being inhibited by the antithyroid drug propylthiouracil (PTU). In addition, it is one of only two enzymes known to contain selenocysteine, which is essential for its full activity, and selenium deficiency may act as a contributing factor in the development of myxoedematous cretinism in iodine-deficient areas. Type I, being present in the parenchymatous tissue, is responsible for most of the peripheral conversion of T_4 to T_3. The hepatic and renal type I deiodinase provides the major source of T_3 in the circulation. Its activity is decreased in the 'sick euthyroid' syndrome (see p. 95). On the other hand, type II, which is confined largely to the central nervous system (CNS) and pituitary, must be key to the setting of the negative feedback at the thyrotroph and ultimately the provision of TSH. In addition, there is a type III deiodinase, which deiodinates at the inner ring exclusively and catalyses the conversion of T_4 to rT_3 (Fig. 5.3).

Modulation of actions of other hormones

Thyroid hormones influence the actions of several other hormones, but these effects are difficult to discriminate from the generalized increase in cell metabolism. Probably the most clinically important effect is the ability of T_3 to synergize with catecholamines to increase heart rate: combination of the two hormones produces a response that is greater than the sum of the effects that either exerts alone at the same concentrations. Most of the effects of other (nonthyroid) hormones are modified in conditions of underactivity or overactivity of the thyroid. However, with few exceptions, the changes can usually be attributed to the overall alterations in the metabolic states of the target cells, which are influenced by prevailing levels of iodothyronine hormones. Thus, insulin responses to intravenous glucose-tolerance tests are slightly exaggerated in hyperthyroidism and significantly depressed in hypothyroidism, when compared with the responses after corrective therapy. Note that comparison of intravenous rather than oral glucose-tolerance tests is necessary, since iodothyronine hormones can also alter the efficiency of carbohydrate absorption from the gastrointestinal tract.

SYNTHESIS OF THYROID HORMONES

Synthesis of thyroid hormones by the gland involves uptake of iodine from the blood and incorporation of iodine atoms into tyrosyl residues of thyroglobulin, the glycoprotein that is synthesized by follicular cells.

Iodide pump

The basal plasma membrane of the follicular cells contains a system for the active transport of iodide from the bloodstream into the cells against a steep iodide concentration gradient. While this iodide pump appears to be linked to the activity of the sodium/potassium (Na^+/K^+) pump in the basal state, a second pump is distinguishable in stimulated glands, leading to the suggestion that there might be two separate, but physically closely associated, systems in the basal cell membrane. The iodide pump shows all the characteristics of an energy-dependent and relatively specific transport system, as it requires adenosine 5′-triphosphate (ATP) and follows Michaelis–Menten kinetics. The iodide pump concentrates intrathyroidal iodide 20–100-fold above that of serum or the surrounding medium of cultivated thyroid cells.

Inhibitory anions

Several structurally related anions can competitively inhibit the iodide pump. For example, perchlorate (ClO_4^-) is employed clinically as a competitive inhibitor of the iodide pump, and large doses may be administered as a short-term measure to block iodide uptake by the gland. This is useful when studying the kinetics of thyroid-hormone secretion. It is also used as a prophylactic measure to inhibit the uptake of radioiodide by the thyroid if an individual has been contaminated by or has ingested radioactive iodine. The pertechnetate ion is also taken up by the iodide pump, and this is exploited by substituting a gamma radiation–emitting radioactive isotope of technetium in the anion, so that the thyroid gland can be imaged with a gamma camera.

Perchlorate is additionally used in the 'perchlorate-discharge test', in which the ability of the thyroid to synthesize iodothyronine hormones is assessed. The thyroid is first allowed to accumulate tracer doses of one of the short-lived radioisotopes, $^{131}I^-$ or $^{123}I^-$, and, following administration of ClO_4^- to block further radioiodine uptake, the rate of release of the radioisotope is followed over a period of time. The rate of radioiodine release is measured to assess whether the thyroid gland is normal, or whether there is reduced incorporation of iodine into thyroid protein, which occurs in some inherited enzyme deficiency diseases, when there is an exaggerated discharge of nonorganified radioiodine. The administration of high doses of radioiodine is used in the treatment of thyroid overactivity to ablate thyroid tissue.

Bromide (Br^-) and nitrite (NO_2^-) can competitively inhibit the iodide pump if their dietary intake is sufficiently high, as occurs in some regions of the world. Iodide itself does not inhibit the iodide pump, even at quite high circulating concentrations. Thiocyanate (SCN^-) and selenocyanate ($SeCN^-$) are two anions that are not transported into the gland, but they can inhibit the thyroidal iodide pump by a competitive mechanism.

Thyroglobulin synthesis

Follicular cells synthesize this large glycoprotein, which is unique to the thyroid gland and is iodinated after it is synthesized. T_4 and T_3 are subsequently made within this large precursor.

Structure

Thyroglobulin contains approximately 10% carbohydrate, composed of two major types of polysaccharide units, one of which terminates in sialic acid, which is responsible for the intense pink PAS staining reaction observed in the colloid. Thyroglobulin has a molecular weight of 660 000 and contains about 1% of iodine by weight. The molecule is composed of two apparently identical subunits, which can be dissociated under mild reducing conditions; this indicates that the subunits are either noncovalently associated or weakly attached through one or two disulphide bridges.

Synthesis and cytology

Messenger RNA (mRNA) is synthesized in the follicular cell nucleus, and the peptide chains of thyroglobulin are translated from specific mRNA on polysomes in the rough endoplasmic reticulum (Fig. 5.5). The exact number of peptide chains, and therefore the number of species of mRNA required to synthesize thyroglobulin, is still somewhat uncertain. However, a mRNA capable of yielding a peptide with a molecular weight of about 300 000 has been isolated and used to synthesize thyroglobulin in a cell-free system *in vitro*. Sugars such as galactose and sialic acid are added in the Golgi apparatus. Newly synthesized thyroglobulin is found in small vesicles, which are packaged in the Golgi. These vesicles move to the apical membrane, with which they fuse. They then release their contents into the lumen by exocytosis.

Iodination of thyroglobulin

Radioactive iodine has been used to locate iodide within the follicular cell after it has been transported across the basal membrane of the cell. Within 10 s of an injection of radioactive iodide, autoradiography shows high concentrations of iodine located over the apical cell membrane, with little radioisotope present elsewhere within the follicular cell. At longer time intervals, the band of radioiodine diffuses into the lumen of the colloid, and after some days the colloid becomes completely labelled with radioiodine.

The enzyme system carrying out the iodination of thyroglobulin is a peroxidase, which has now been cloned. This enzyme is synthesized and packaged in the Golgi complex into vesicles in an inactive form, probably along with thyroglobulin. At the apical cell membrane, the peroxidase enzyme is activated, either by changes that occur during membrane fusion or owing to the presence of iodide and cofactors required to activate the enzyme, such as a hydrogen peroxide (H_2O_2)-generating system. A thyroid peroxidase has been purified from thyroid tissue, and it requires an H_2O_2-generating system, which may be linked to a nicotinamide adenine dinucleotide phosphate (NADP)/glutathione redox cycle within the cell. The enzyme functions in a complex manner, in that it binds and oxidizes iodide to an active form, which is then transferred to the acceptor tyrosyl residue of thyroglobulin, which is itself bound at another site on the same enzyme:

$$\text{Enzyme} + I^- + \text{tyr-protein} \xrightarrow{H_2O_2 \;\rightarrow\; 2OH^-} \text{I. Enzyme. Tyr-protein} \rightarrow \text{Enzyme} + \text{I-tyr-protein}$$

This enzyme system has a particularly high efficiency for catalysing the iodination of thyroglobulin that has not previously been iodinated; this efficiency decreases somewhat when the thyroglobulin already contains some bound iodine.

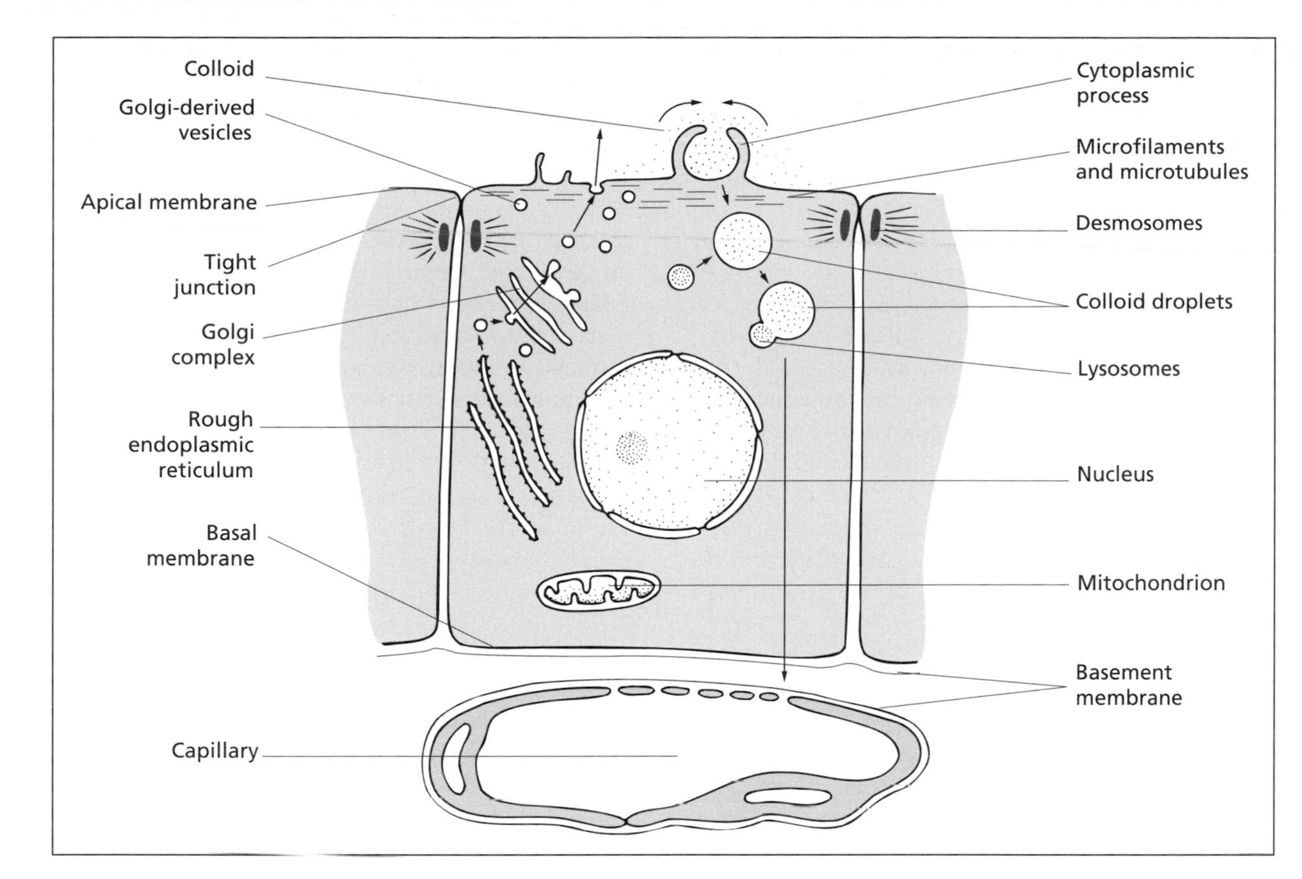

Figure 5.5 The intracellular organelles of a thyroid epithelial cell concerned in the synthesis, storage and degradation of thyroglobulin. Thyroglobulin is synthesized on the rough endoplasmic reticulum, packaged in the Golgi complex and released from small, Golgi-derived vesicles into the follicular lumen (shown at the top of the figure) to be stored as colloid. When stimulated by thyrotrophin, colloid is engulfed by cytoplasmic processes and reintroduced into the cell as colloid droplets. Lysosomes fuse with the colloid droplets and their acid hydrolases degrade the thyroglobulin, leading eventually to release of the thyroid hormones into local capillaries. Note also cytoplasmic microfilaments and microtubules under the apical surface of the cell, the nucleus and the mitochondrion. The capillaries are fenestrated and surrounded by a basement membrane. Desmosomes (which hold cells together) and tight junctions (which seal off the colloid) are also shown.

Drugs inhibiting iodination. The peroxidase enzyme, and hence the iodination reaction, is sensitive to inhibition by a number of antithyroid drugs, such as thiourea, propylthiouracil (PTU), or methimazole (methyl mercaptoimidazole (MMI)), all of which contain the N–C–SH grouping. These drugs, and particularly the mercaptoimidazoles, are employed to inhibit the iodination of thyroglobulin and hence stop or minimize production of thyroid hormones by an overactive thyroid gland. MMI is favoured in the USA, while carbimazole is the drug of choice in the UK, but since carbimazole is hydrolysed to MMI almost im-mediately after administration there is no advantage of one form of the drug over the other. This is an effective method of suppressing the synthesis and secretion of thyroid hormones.

Naturally occurring substances have occasionally been found to cause goitres in a local population, and these substances are therefore called goitrogens. Naturally occurring goitrogens have been isolated from drinking supplies (water wells), the milk of cows fed on certain green fodder and the brassicae (cabbages, etc.), which contain particularly high concentrations of goitrogens. These naturally occurring goitrogens act by inhibiting the iodination of thyroglobulin and hence the synthesis of thyroid hormones. Release of negative-feedback control at the pituitary results in increased TSH secretion and stimulation of the thyroid in an attempt to maintain circulating thyroid-hormone levels. The prolonged stimulation results in thyroid hyperplasia and a goitre.

Importance of the structure of thyroglobulin. In the iodination reaction, the tyrosyl residues of thyroglobulin that are exposed act as acceptor molecules. Thyroglobulin contains about 125 tyrosyl residues, but only about one-third are available for iodination, because they are situated at or near the surface of the glycoprotein; the other two-thirds are sequestered within the molecule. The iodination reaction not only results in the iodination of tyrosyl residues, but also initiates formation of the thyroid hormones within the structure of thyroglobulin.

T_3 and T_4 are derived from the coupling of iodotyrosines according to the following scheme:

$$\mathrm{MIT} + \mathrm{DIT} \rightarrow T_3$$

and

$$\mathrm{DIT} + \mathrm{DIT} \rightarrow T_4$$

where MIT and DIT are monoiodotyrosines and diiodotyrosines, respectively. The coupling reactions occur within the structure of the thyroglobulin molecule during the peroxidase-mediated iodination reaction; no coupling enzyme is therefore required (Fig. 5.6). The receiving DIT residue is linked to another part of either the same, or perhaps another, peptide chain as that of the transferred MIT or DIT residue, and either T_3 or T_4 is formed within the thyroglobulin structure, respectively. There is uncertainty as to whether the peptide chain is broken or whether an alanyl or seryl residue may be left as a remnant of the original iodotyrosyl residue, after coupling to form the iodothyronyl residue elsewhere in thyroglobulin. Thyroglobulin that has been iodinated contains a multitude of small peptide fragments, and these fragments are

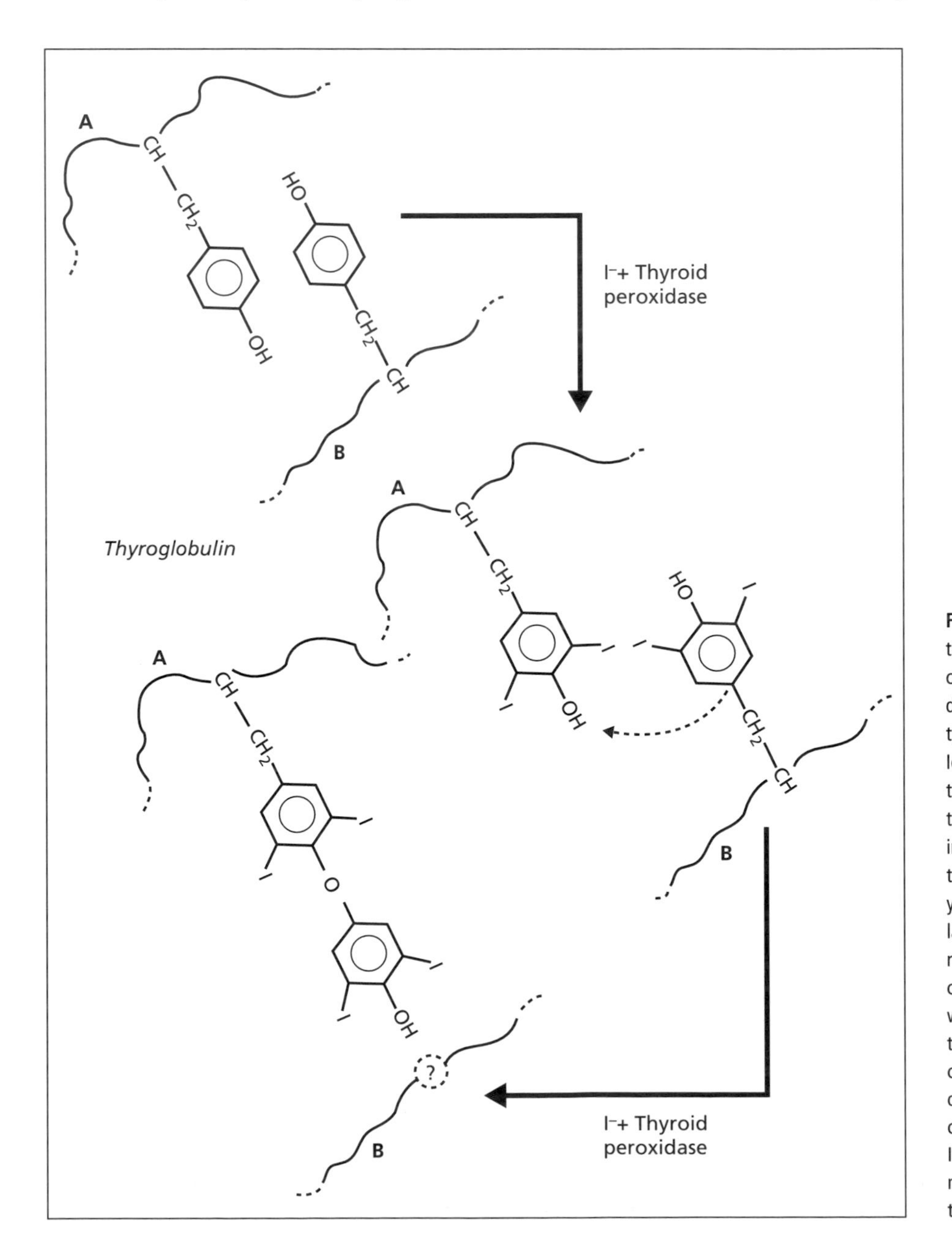

Figure 5.6 Synthesis of thyroid hormones within the structure of the thyroglobulin molecule. Two chains of thyroglobulin (labelled A and B to distinguish between them), each carrying a tyrosyl residue, are shown at the top left. Iodination by the thyroid peroxidase introduces two atoms of iodine into each tyrosyl residue in the ortho position relative to the hydroxyl group, in the central diagram. The dotted arrow indicates the molecular rearrangement which follows to yield the structure of T_4 linked to the chain labelled **A** at the lower left of the figure. This rearrangement requires the presence of oxidizing conditions, and may be spontaneously induced when particular key tyrosyl residues of thyroglobulin are iodinated. The fate of the B chain of the protein and the alanyl side-chain of the tyrosyl residue is uncertain: either the chain breaks or a seryl side-chain may form. If the tyrosyl residue on the B chain is only monoiodinated, triiodothyronine (T_3) is formed in the thyroglobulin molecule.

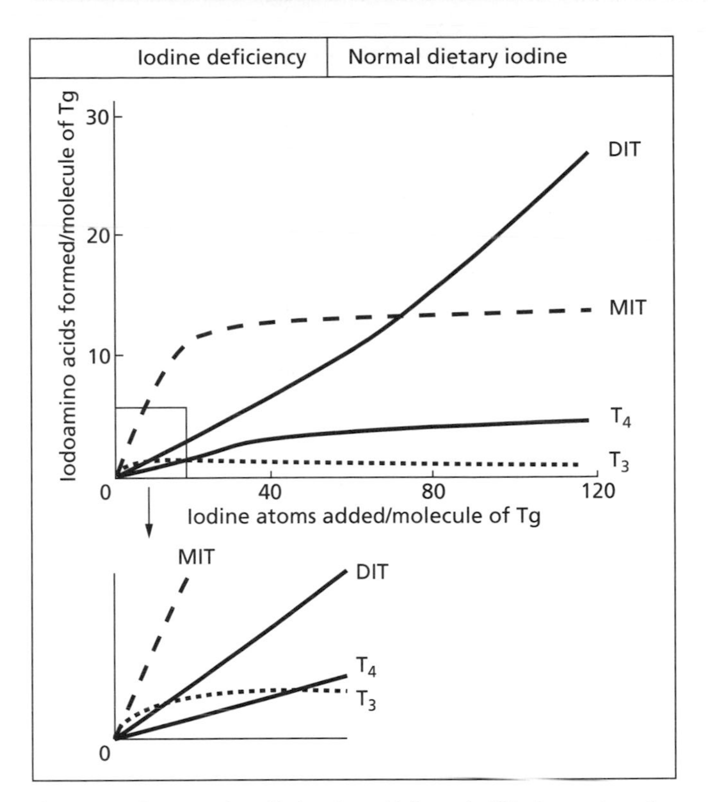

Figure 5.7 The proportion of iodoamino acids formed within the structure of thyroglobulin (Tg) as a function of the number of iodine atoms incorporated. MIT, monoiodotyrosine; DIT, diiodotyrosine; T_4, thyroxine; T_3, 3,5,3′-triiodothyronine. Initially, T_3 is synthesized in a relatively higher proportion than T_4 at very low levels of iodine incorporated (as shown in the inset to the figure), when the precursor MIT : DIT ratio is high. At higher levels of iodine, T_4 is formed preferentially, up to a maximum of about four molecules of thyroxine/molecule of thyroglobulin.

absent in iodine-deficient thyroglobulin. This observation suggests that the peptide chain is broken during the iodination and coupling reaction within thyroglobulin.

Iodination of thyroglobulin results in production of a maximum of four molecules of the two iodothyronine hormones linked within the structure of each protein molecule (Fig. 5.7): the small number of iodothyronines and the large size of thyroglobulin (molecular weight 660 000) suggest that specific active sites for iodothyronine synthesis occur in the thyroglobulin molecule. The iodinated protein is stored in the lumen of the thyroid follicle and some further iodination of the protein may take place within the lumen, presumably because some of the peroxidase-iodinating enzyme is released from membranes during the exocytotic process.

The effect of dietary iodide on hormone synthesis

The amount of iodine incorporated into thyroglobulin is directly related to the concentration of iodide reaching the thyroid gland from the circulation. Thus, when dietary iodide is limited or deficient, there will be little iodine incorporated into thyroglobulin. This will yield mainly MIT and only a few DIT residues in thyroglobulin (Fig. 5.7). An increase in the number of iodine atoms added yields progressively more diiodotyrosine. Under normal conditions of dietary iodide sufficiency, thyroglobulin will contain more DIT than MIT.

Under conditions of iodine sufficiency, when a lot of DIT is present, thyroglobulin will contain from two to four molecules of T_4; there will be relatively little T_3, because there is insufficient MIT to couple with DIT. Iodine sufficiency, which requires a dietary iodine intake of greater than 50 μg per day, corresponds to about 80 atoms of iodine per molecule of thyroglobulin on the *x*-axis of Fig. 5.7. It has been estimated that thyroglobulin in the normal human thyroid stores about a two-month supply of preformed T_4. This reserve is available to maintain the individual in the euthyroid state should conditions of iodine deficiency be encountered.

In iodine deficiency, thyroglobulin will contain relatively more MIT than DIT. In consequence, there will be smaller amounts of thyroid hormones. In addition, because of the higher ratio of MIT to DIT available to couple, the thyroglobulin will contain more T_3 than T_4 (see inset to Fig. 5.7).

Iodine deficiency and endemic goitre. Iodine deficiency is still a major problem in several areas of the world, especially in developing countries. In adults, a reduced iodine intake (below 50 μg per day) causes compensatory changes, so that the thyroid secretes T_3 in preference to T_4. Eventually, TSH secretion increases to maintain the concentrations of circulating thyroid hormones. The elevated TSH induces thyroid enlargement, and the rate of iodine uptake rises dramatically. This is due to activation of the iodine transport mechanism by TSH. Because dietary iodine deficiency is never absolute, the biochemical compensatory mechanism outlined above will usually ensure adequate production of thyroid hormones to meet the immediate needs of the individual. However, the supply of thyroid hormones will not be sufficient for a developing fetus.

Iodine deficiency during pregnancy is very serious, since the fetus is at risk from neurological damage. The syndrome of intellectual impairment, deafness and diplegia (bilateral paralysis) has been termed ‘cretinism’. This condition is different from ‘sporadic cretinism’, which results from an athyrotic fetus developing in an iodine-sufficient mother. Sporadic cretinism affects one child in 4000, and is at least partly preventable by treatment with T_4 immediately after birth. Many millions of infants world-wide are affected to a greater or lesser extent in terms of intellectual ability as a result of iodine deficiency.

Prophylaxis with iodine supplements has proved effective in reducing the incidence of cretinism in many areas of the world, although the effect of increased iodide on reducing well-established goitres in the adult is small. Supplementation of essential or common dietary constituents such as salt or bread is not always practicable, however, and in extremely isolated communities resort is then made to depot injections of iodized oils. These provide the thyroid with iodide supplies over periods of years.

Increase in dietary iodide intake may be associated with an increased incidence of hyperthyroidism; decreased intake with a marginal but chronic elevation of TSH may result in an increased incidence of thyroid cancer, especially if irradiation is involved, as it was in the Chernobyl accident. Iodine deficiency was prominent in eastern Germany, where iodine supplements to food or water supplies were forbidden. A sudden increase in dietary iodide can precipitate expression of autoimmune disease of the thyroid, but the incidence is related to other unknown factors that appear to affect a given community.

Iodine excess. Large doses of iodine, e.g. 5 mg/day, will initially inhibit the synthesis and release of thyroid hormones from the gland. This paradoxical effect arises from inhibition of two intrathyroidal reactions. Excess iodide inhibits the adenylate cyclase response to TSH, and it also inhibits iodine incorporation into thyroglobulin (sometimes called 'organification of iodide'). Thyroidal inhibition by excess iodine (the Wolff–Chaikoff effect) may sometimes be seen as a transitory thyroid enlargement when certain preparations, such as cough mixtures that contain high concentrations of iodide, are administered. The rapid and acute inhibitory effects of excess iodide can be used in the preparation of a thyrotoxic patient for thyroidectomy. The treatment is designed to restore the patient to a euthyroid state, and the excess iodide has an additional pharmacological effect that decreases the vascularity and increases the firmness of the gland. It also prevents the condition known as 'thyroid storm', which is a severe and acute escalation of hyperthyroidism which may occur during or after thyroid surgery, due to the release of excessive amounts of thyroid hormones.

After a few days of high iodide intake, thyroidal iodide transport diminishes to near zero, the intracellular iodide concentration falls, and the block of iodine incorporation into thyroglobulin is relieved—i.e. the Wolff–Chaikoff effect is reversed. In this way, humans can generally adapt to prolonged excesses of iodine intake and will eventually stabilize with normal circulating thyroid-hormone concentrations. These observations demonstrate the ability of the thyroid to maintain the euthyroid state in spite of wide fluctuations in dietary iodide intake.

REGULATION OF THE THYROID

The activity of the thyroid gland is controlled by TSH from the anterior pituitary gland: the secretion of this is controlled by thyrotrophin-releasing hormone (TRH) from the hypothalamus (see Chapter 3). TSH stimulates the secretion of thyroid hormones and these suppress TSH secretion by negative feedback (see Fig. 3.3).

Stimulation of the thyroid by TSH

TSH is bound to a specific receptor on the thyroid follicular-cell surface. This is a G-protein-linked receptor and leads to activation of both adenylate cyclase and phospholipase C (see Fig. 2.12). However, the former appears to be the dominant catalytic subunit and most of the actions of TSH are mediated by the second messenger cyclic adenosine 5′-monophosphate (cAMP) (see Fig. 2.13). This results in stimulation of cell metabolism and a tropic response in terms of cell size and activity.

After binding to its cell-surface receptor, TSH causes sequential increases in the following:

1 Intracellular cAMP concentration.

2 Transmembrane ion fluxes, with influx of Na^+ and an early efflux of iodide; translocation of calcium (Ca^{2+}) and activation of calmodulin also occurs (see Fig. 2.18).

3 Activation of various protein kinases (see Figs 2.3 and 2.4), which leads to protein or enzyme phosphorylation by phosphate transfer from ATP (see, for example, Figs 2.16 and 2.17).

4 Iodination of thyroglobulin due to increased H_2O_2 generation and also thyroid-hormone release.

5 Intracellular volume and number of colloid droplets, and the numbers, form and activity of microvilli at the apical cell surface (Fig. 5.5).

6 Cellular metabolism, including that of carbohydrate, which occurs principally via the pentose phosphate pathway, since the thyroid contains little glycogen; also phospholipid turnover.

7 Protein synthesis (including that of thyroglobulin) and also RNA turnover.

8 Iodide influx to the cell, which is a later response, because the iodide pump requires synthesis of a new protein for its activation.

9 DNA synthesis, although very limited mitosis and cell division occur in the adult thyroid *in vivo*.

The net result of TSH is to increase the synthesis of fresh thyroid-hormone stores, as well as increasing the release of the thyroid hormones within about 1 h. The most recently synthesized thyroglobulin is the first to be removed from the follicle, because it is nearer to the microvilli at the apical cell membrane than older thyroglobulin at the centre of the follicle. Because newly iodinated thyroglobulin around the edge of the follicle has a lower iodine content than the mature, centrally positioned thyroglobulin, this new glycoprotein has a relatively higher T_3 to T_4 ratio than that of the older thyroglobulin stores (Fig. 5.7). Hence a control mechanism exists within the gland, based on the turnover of thyroglobulin and its degree of iodination, which can not only produce more thyroid hormone, but also alter the amount of the more active T_3 that is secreted by the gland.

Thyroid-hormone secretion

In order to release thyroid hormones from the thyroglobulin stores in the follicle, the glycoprotein has first to be taken back into the thyroid cell, where lysosomal enzymes can release the iodothyronines for secretion into the circulation.

Colloid droplet formation. The apical cell membrane of thyroid follicles is covered by microvilli and pseudopods (Fig. 5.5). In stimulated thyroid glands, the number and length of the microvilli increase, and scanning electron micrographs show structures rather like individual rose petals. These cellular extensions envelop droplets of thyroglobulin, which then form vesicles within the cell, known as an intracellular 'colloid droplets'. This process is known as endocytosis. Colloid-droplet vesicles in activated thyroid cells may be seen under the light microscope after staining with PAS reagent. When viewed with the electron microscope, they may be distinguished from other vesicles, such as lysosomes, because they have the same electron density as the colloid, which is electron-opaque by virtue of the electron-absorbing mass of the large iodine atoms.

Microfilaments and microtubules. These cytoskeletal structures assist in the formation and directional movement of colloid droplets away from the apical membrane. With thyroid cells in culture, gross morphological changes are seen within minutes after the addition of TSH, and extensive reorganization of microfilaments and microtubules accompanies these events. Drugs such as cytochalasin and colchicine, which disrupt the cytoskeleton, inhibit thyroid-hormone secretion.

Lysosomal fusion and release of thyroid hormones. When thyroid cells are stimulated by TSH, lysosomes migrate towards the colloid droplets and fusion of the membranes of these two types of vesicle then occurs. The hydrolytic enzymes of the lysosome degrade thyroglobulin, releasing iodotyrosines and other amino acids and sugars. The latter are recycled within the gland, and MIT and DIT are relatively specifically deiodinated by microsomal enzymes (dehalogenases) to release iodide. This is recycled within the cell, and this 'scavenging' can be an important component of the iodine supply to the gland. The iodothyronine hormones are released from the gland by some mechanism which remains to be elucidated: they pass across the basement membrane of the follicle to gain access to the serum carrier proteins through the fenestrated capillary bed (Fig. 5.5) that surrounds the follicles.

INAPPROPRIATE SECRETION OF THYROID HORMONES

The effects of undersecretion and its treatment

Lack of thyroid hormones occurs either because of disease of the thyroid itself (primary hypothyroidism) or, less frequently, from lack of stimulation by TSH from the pituitary (secondary hypothyroidism). Tertiary hypothyroidism, due to hypothalamic dysfunction, is rare.

The effects of hypothyroidism in adults are the result of a lowered metabolic rate. The classic symptoms are listed in Table 5.1.

In children, thyroid hormones are necessary for normal growth, so short stature and obesity are the main features of hypothyroidism acquired during childhood (Fig. 5.8). Lack of thyroid hormone is particularly serious in the fetus, because it can cause irreversible brain damage (cretinism), which, as discussed above, is encountered in iodine-deficient areas of the world. The incidence of

Table 5.1 Principal clinical symptoms of hypothyroidism.

Appearance	Weight gain, coarse skin, dry hair, hoarse voice; puffy appearance due to deposition of glycosaminoglycans in skin and muscle; maybe a goitre
Disposition	Feels cold, particularly at the extremities; lethargic and depressed
Neuromuscular function	Changed tendon reflexes: muscles contract normally, but relax slowly; generalized muscle weakness and paraesthesias
Cardiac function	Reduced cardiac output: slow pulse
Others	Menstrual irregularities, due to altered gonadotrophin secretion associated with impaired oestrogen metabolism

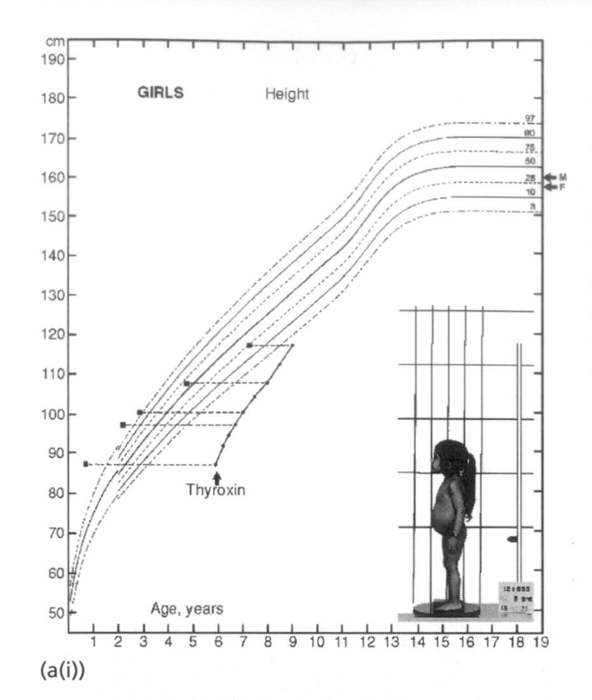

(a(i))

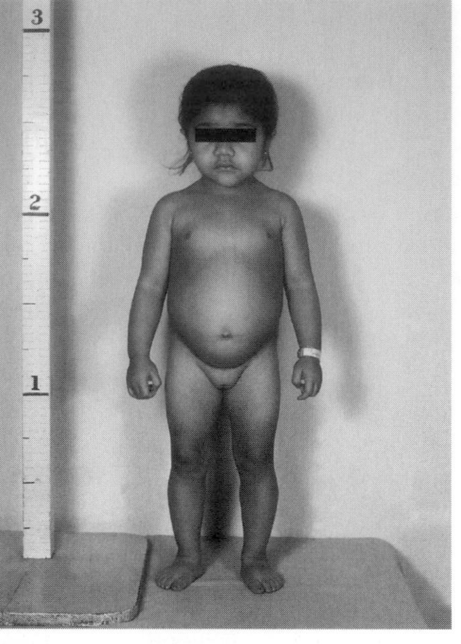

(a(ii))

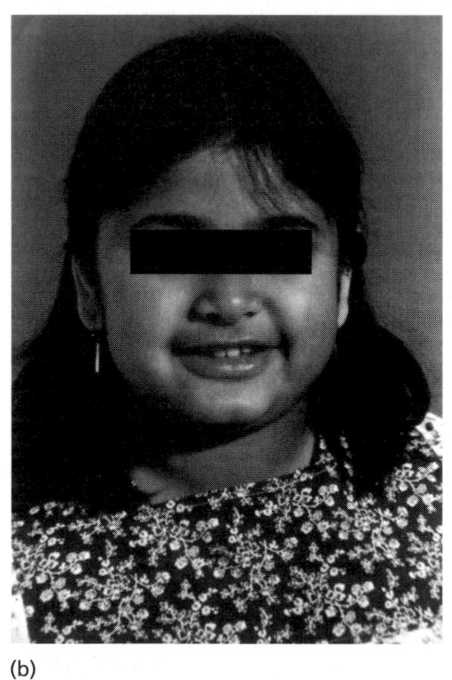
(b)

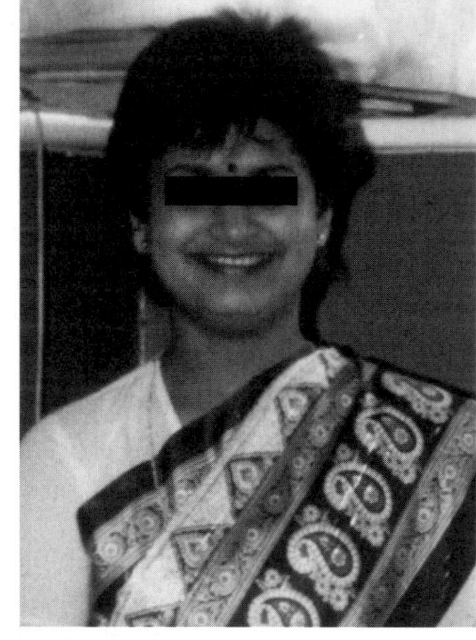
(c)

Figure 5.8 Effects of hypothyroidism. At the age of 6 years, this girl (upper panel, (a(i)) and (a(ii))) presented with short stature and extremely delayed skeletal maturation. Thyroxine concentration was very low and TSH grossly elevated, as were titres of thyroid antibodies. A diagnosis of autoimmune (Hashimoto) thyroiditis was made. The response to treatment is shown by rapid catch-up growth. Learning problems were not evident, as the condition was not congenital but acquired after the major development of the brain was complete. Three and eight years later, as a result of continued T_4 replacement (Fig. 5.8b, c), she has now gained a normal appearance.

neonatal hypothyroidism in Western society, which is referred to as 'sporadic cretinism' and is due to failure of the fetal thyroid to develop, is about one in 4000 births. It is most readily diagnosed by finding high circulating TSH. This is now part of routine neonatal screening, and is treatable with T_4 replacement.

Hypothyroidism can be treated by administration of T_4 by mouth at a dosage of about 100 μg/m^2 body surface area/day; 150 μg/day (slightly less than 100 μg/m^2) is usually sufficient for an adult. Replacement therapy will be for life.

The effects of overproduction and its treatment

Hyperthyroidism (thyrotoxicosis) is the result of overactivity of the thyroid gland. It often has an autoimmune origin (Graves disease, see below) and is only very rarely

Table 5.2 Principal clinical symptoms of hyperthyroidism.

General features	
Appearance	Weight loss, despite full appetite; sweating, tremor and maybe a goitre
Disposition	Agitated and nervous, easy fatigability, heat intolerance
Cardiac function	Tachycardia and atrial fibrillation
Neuromuscular function	Muscle weakness and loss of muscle mass
Others	Diarrhoea, shortness of breath, infertility and amenorrhea Rapid growth rate and accelerated bone maturation in children
Additional features associated with Graves disease	
Eye signs	Upper-lid retraction, stare, periorbital oedema, redness and swelling of the conjunctiva, exophthalmos (proptosis), impaired eye movement, inflammation of the cornea and, in most serious cases, optic-nerve compression, with loss of vision
Pretibial myxoedema	Thickening of the skin due to deposition of glycosaminoglycans over the lower tibia
Others	Patchy depigmentation of the skin (vitiligo), clubbing of the fingers (thyroid acropachy) and premature greying of the hair

due to overstimulation by excessive TSH from the pituitary. Many of the classic symptoms listed in Table 5.2 are due to the increase in BMR and enhanced β-adrenergic activity.

Hyperthyroidism of nonautoimmune origin is usually due to thyroid autonomy associated with either a toxic nodular goitre or a toxic adenoma (see below). Such patients will not have the diffuse and symmetrical goitre that is characteristic of Graves disease. However, eye signs of Graves disease (Fig. 5.9) will occasionally be present together with a nodular and asymmetrical goitre. It is possible that autoimmune Graves disease is then coexistent with hyperthyroidism of nonautoimmune origin. Eye signs may occur in a euthyroid patient; this condition is referred to as 'ophthalmic Graves disease'.

Hyperthyroidism may be treated by medical treatment in about 6 weeks. Since Graves disease is of autoimmune origin, the hyperthyroidism of a significant proportion of these patients may remit spontaneously. It is common to maintain patients on antithyroid drugs for a limited period (e.g. 1 year) and then to withdraw treatment to test for a spontaneous remission, but the repeated attendances at hospital to check that the patient is euthyroid may be problematic, particularly in puberty. One strategy is to use a high dose of an antithyroid drug, such as carbimazole, together with T_4 replacement. This is referred to as the 'block-replacement regimen', and may enhance the stability of the thyroid status of the patient while on treatment, as well as the chances of obtaining a spontaneous remission.

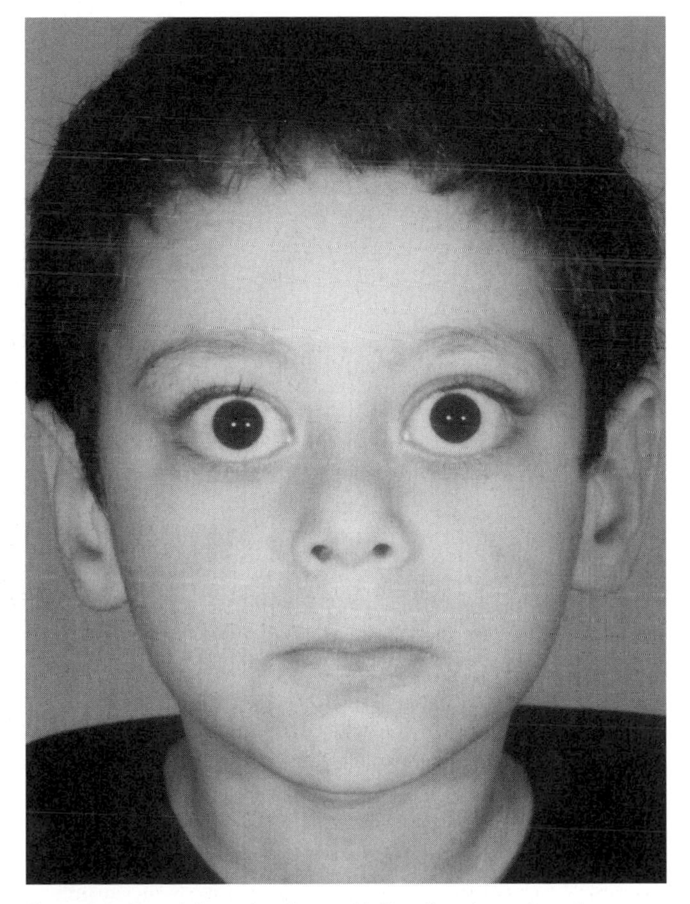

Figure 5.9 Graves' disease in a 4-year-old. Note the goitre and eye signs (exophthalmos).

The more radical treatments—surgery or radioiodine—are likely to be given earlier to non-Graves patients. Surgical treatment is often preferred for patients up to 45 years of age. About 15% of patients undergoing surgery (and most children) will be rendered hypothyroid, but this condition is relatively easily treated by replacement therapy with T_4. Because of the proximity of the parathyroid glands and the recurrent laryngeal nerves, hypoparathyroidism and vocal-cord palsies are hazards of thyroid surgery. Ablation with radioiodine is often preferred for the older patient.

Table 5.3 Examples of organ-specific autoimmune diseases.

Graves disease
Hashimoto disease
Pernicious anaemia
Addison disease
Autoimmune atrophic gastritis
Diabetes mellitus

The genesis of disordered function

Thyroid disease from autoimmune disorders

Disorders that affect the thyroid glands in areas of iodine sufficiency arise mainly from disorders of the immune system. In situations in which the immune system no longer treats tissues of the host as normal constituents of the body, but reacts against them as it would against a foreign tissue, the ensuing disease is known as an 'autoimmune disorder'. Thyroid autoimmune diseases are one of a group of organ-specific autoimmune diseases (Table 5.3), which are all characterized by circulating antibodies and lymphocytic infiltration of the tissue of a particular organ.

In contrast, other autoimmune conditions, such as rheumatoid arthritis and systemic lupus erythematosus (SLE), are not organ-specific. In these, the autoantibodies are directed against antigens that are widespread throughout the body and there are appropriately widespread manifestations of the disease.

The thyroid is particularly prone to autoimmune disease, which can result in either hypothyroidism, as in Hashimoto disease, or hyperthyroidism, as in Graves disease. The trigger that initiates an autoimmune response is not known. One hypothesis is that the thyroid cells begin to act as antigen-presenting cells. This followed the demonstration that major histocompatibility complex (MHC) class II antigen could be expressed by thyroid cells from both Hashimoto and Graves patients, but not from normal thyroid tissue. These aberrant cells may then present their cell components to T-lymphocytes, an activity usually undertaken by macrophages when they associate with an immunogen.

An alternative view is that the phenomenon of 'inappropriate MHC class II antigen expression' is secondary to lymphocyte infiltration of the thyroid and may be important as a means of perpetuating rather than originating the autoimmune process. The aetiology of the other facets of autoimmune thyroid disease, such as the eye signs and pretibial myxoedema of Graves disease, is unknown. It is possible that there is a cross-reactive antigen shared by the thyroid and a retro-orbital tissue such as the extraocular muscle.

In common with other autoimmune diseases, those of the thyroid often have a familial incidence. There is an association with human leucocyte antigen (HLA) haplotype, with, among Caucasians, HLA-DW3 and HLA-DR5 being associated with Graves and Hashimoto disease, respectively. As a group, thyroid autoimmune disorders comprise the commonest clinically significant autoimmune diseases in the community. Their incidence increases with age, and women are affected about 10 times more frequently than men.

Hyperthyroidism, Graves disease and thyrotoxicosis

Hyperthyroidism affects about 2% of women in the UK, and is about 10-fold less frequent for men. Approximately 50% of patients presenting with hyperthyroidism are suffering from the autoimmune condition referred to as Graves disease, although this percentage varies according to the past history of iodine intake by a community. Autoimmune hyperthyroidism is unusual in the sense that antibodies of the IgG1 subclass bind to the thyroid follicular-cell membrane either at or sufficiently close to the TSH receptor to cause stimulation of adenylate cyclase. This results in hypertrophy of the follicular cells (Fig. 5.2c), increased synthesis and secretion of thyroid hormones, and in some cases goitre formation.

These antibodies are called 'thyroid-stimulating antibodies' (TSAb). They were originally described by Adams and Purves in 1956, when they were named 'long-acting thyroid stimulators' (LATS), because of the slow onset and extended time-course of their stimulating activity when compared with stimulation by TSH in an *in vivo* bioassay. These stimulating antibodies are the only well-established example of autoantibodies that can mimic a stimulating hormone. In some mothers with high levels of TSAb, there is a risk of the fetus being affected by antibody crossing the placenta. This can cause fetal thyroid stimulation and hyperthyroidism, called 'neonatal thyrotoxicosis'. After birth, the symptoms due to the thyrotoxicosis need urgent treatment, but recede with a time-course that reflects the clearance of the maternal antibodies.

Primary hypothyroidism: Hashimoto thyroiditis and primary myxoedema

Hashimoto thyroiditis is characterized by a goitre, whereas there is little evidence for a preceding goitre for primary myxoedema. In Hashimoto thyroiditis, there is extensive lymphocytic infiltration, together with high concentrations of humoral antibodies, which are directed against thyroglobulin and thyroid peroxidase. The anti-peroxidase antibodies are often referred to as 'antimicrosomal antibodies'. The progressive destruction of thyroid follicular tissue results in hypothyroidism.

Primary hypothyroidism may also occur due to non-autoimmune conditions, such as inappropriate iodide intake. As discussed previously this may be due to limited availability of dietary iodide, which would be uncommon in Western countries and can usually be prevented by the biochemical compensation mechanism in the thyroid gland. It may also be due to excessive iodide intake, e.g. with the use of radiocontrast dyes, which may give rise to transient hypothyroidism. In addition, there are rare inborn errors of thyroid-hormone synthesis (thyroid dyshormonogenesis), which usually present with congenital hypothyroidism and a goitre.

Thyroid neoplasms: benign adenomas and thyroid carcinomas

The normal thyroid gland contains cells and follicles that are in different states of activity at any given time. Histological examination demonstrates that adjacent follicles, and even different cells within the same follicle, may be quiescent or active, which is described as follicular microheterogeneity. An exaggeration of follicular microheterogeneity can occur, and may lead to macroheterogeneity of the thyroid, with one or more nodules of stimulated thyroid follicular cells making a nontoxic nodular or multinodular goitre. A variety of toxic nodular goitres can be found. Some are benign adenomas and others are multinodular adenomas. They can produce sufficient thyroid hormone to result in thyrotoxicosis. The hormone production is autonomous, i.e. the cells do not require stimulation by either TSH or TSAb. The remainder of the thyroid is normal, and at time of presentation will be suppressed, due to low circulating TSH. The abnormality can be corrected either by surgical removal of the adenoma or by its destruction with radioactive iodine. Since only the autonomous tissue is hyperactive, selective destruction of this and not the surrounding normal tissue, which is suppressed, can be achieved.

There are a variety of neoplasms that can affect the thyroid gland, examples of which are the functioning benign thyroid adenomas discussed above and functioning thyroid carcinomas. The latter are a rare cause of fatal, malignant disease. Some malignant thyroid carcinomas retain a limited ability to take up iodine and synthesize thyroid hormone, but this is never sufficient to produce thyrotoxicosis. Carcinomas in the thyroid take up very little radioactive iodine during a diagnostic scan, and are therefore usually called 'cold' regions or nodules. In adults, approximately 12% of 'cold nodules' prove to be malignant. Following total thyroidectomy, the low level of cellular activity does, however, allow destructive treatment of tumour metastases, since they may take up radioactive iodine in the absence of competition from the thyroid, provided that they are stimulated by TSH.

There are two main classes of malignant tumours that arise from thyroid follicular cells. In iodine-replete areas of the world, papillary carcinomas are the most common. These are made up of varying quantities of neoplastic papillae and follicles. The other class is the follicular carcinoma, which consists of a mixture of neoplastic colloid-containing follicles, empty acini and alveoli of neoplastic cells. Intriguingly, follicular carcinomas predominate in geographical areas with low dietary iodine. Ionizing radiation to the thyroid gland of children has been established as an aetiological factor for thyroid carcinoma, but the treatment of thyrotoxic adults with radioiodine has not been associated with the induction of thyroid cancer.

CLINICAL BIOCHEMISTRY: AN OUTLINE OF THYROID-FUNCTION TESTS

A condition such as hypothyroidism is insidious in onset, and laboratory tests of thyroid function therefore play a key role in its diagnosis, particularly for the elderly. On the other hand, although thyrotoxicosis may have a more obvious clinical presentation, thyroid-function tests are still useful in the differential diagnosis of the condition and for subsequent monitoring of therapy. In addition, biochemical tests may reveal a subclinical condition and demonstrate a need for periodic testing of an individual in the future.

The measurement of both thyroid hormones and TSH is by immunoassay. These assays are now a matter of routine, and 'thyroid-function tests' form a large proportion, e.g. 40%, of the workload of an immunoassay service in a typical department of clinical chemistry. Frequently, 'testing strategies' are used, which often rely on a 'front-line' test for TSH (Fig. 5.10). A suppressed TSH would indicate either hyperthyroidism or secondary (or tertiary) hypothyroidism. Subsequent measurement of T_4 levels will usually distinguish between overactivity and underactivity of the thyroid. However, a further measurement of T_3 may be required, since occasionally T_3 but not T_4 is elevated in thyrotoxicosis. Because of compensating mechanisms discussed earlier, T_3 is not a reliable indicator of hypothyroidism. Alternatively, an initial finding of an elevated level of TSH in the 'front-line' test would almost always be due to hypothyroidism; elevated TSH as a cause of hyperthyroidism is extremely rare. The significance of equivocal TSH results, e.g. borderline raised levels, can be ascertained by a subsequent T_4 determination, which may indicate that an individual is approaching a hypothyroid state.

Pituitary malfunction, which may be causing secondary hypothyroidism, may be assessed by a TRH test. No increase in TSH secretion would then be observed in

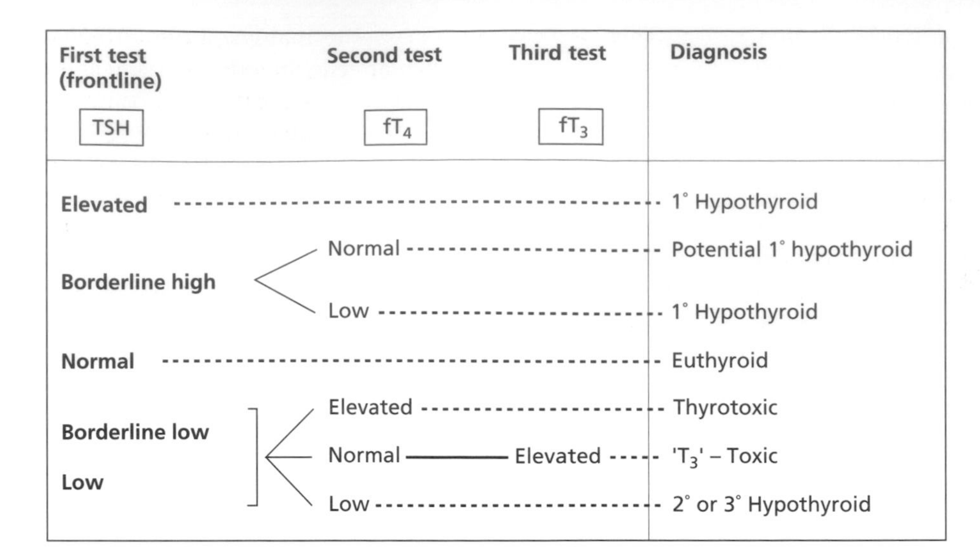

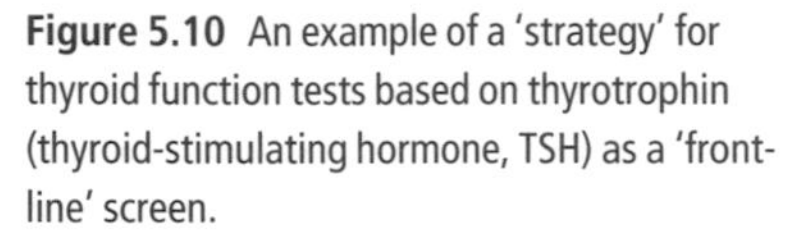
Figure 5.10 An example of a 'strategy' for thyroid function tests based on thyrotrophin (thyroid-stimulating hormone, TSH) as a 'front-line' screen.

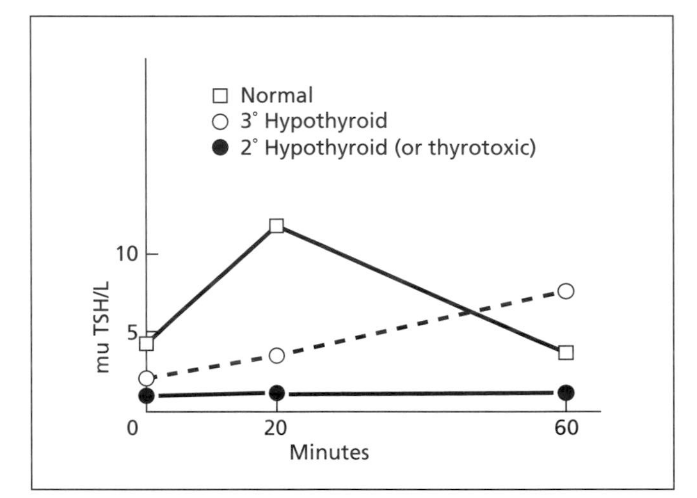

Figure 5.11 Typical responses to an intravenous thyrotrophin-releasing hormone (TRH) test used to test for pituitary or hypothalamic malfunction. Thyrotrophin (thyroid-stimulating hormone, TSH) is measured at 0, 20 and 60 min following the administration of TRH. Note the absent response for secondary hypothyroidism and the delayed response for tertiary hypothyroidism. The former indicates that the pituitary is incapable of responding to the TRH, while the latter indicates that the unstimulated thyrotroph requires time before it can respond to TRH.

this dynamic function test, whereas a delayed TSH response would be obtained for tertiary hypothyroidism (Fig. 5.11).

TSH measurements are made by immunometric assays, while immunoassays for thyroid hormones use the 'competitive' system (see Appendix 1). For thyroid hormones, there is an additional analytical complication due to the presence of thyroid hormone binding proteins. There is a choice between measuring the 'total' thyroid hormone concentration (TT_3 and TT_4) and measuring the free hormone or hormones (fT_3 and/or fT_4). There are a number of specially adapted immunoassays for free hormone measurement (see Appendix 1). Theoretically, the latter is the physiologically relevant parameter recognized by the target cells, and would therefore be the obvious choice. Levels of binding proteins may change, and the measurement of TT_4 or TT_3 might be dangerously misleading. For example, in a normal pregnancy, the levels of binding proteins rise. The concentration of total hormones rises in parallel, and can enter what would normally be considered the hyperthyroid range, but the concentration of the free hormones will remain in the euthyroid range. Consequently, greater reliance is often placed on the measurement of free as opposed to total thyroid hormones. There are, however, unusual situations in which some of the methods for free hormone determination are subject to artefacts and can give misleading results—for example, when grossly abnormal binding proteins or excessive free fatty acids are present. Such analytical uncertainties have increased reliance on the use of TSH measurements for establishing thyroid status.

Rare examples of peripheral resistance to the action of thyroid hormone are encountered. This is generally familial, and is regarded as being due to inherited defects of the intracellular thyroid-hormone receptor (see Figs 2.21–2.24 and Table 2.3). Such individuals may have elevated levels of both free and total thyroid hormones, but TSH levels will not be suppressed—i.e. there is a resetting of the hypothalamic–pituitary–thyroid axis.

Treatment for thyroid disorders requires prolonged monitoring, and thyroid-function tests play an important role in establishing the correct dosage of either replacement therapy or antithyroid drugs. In addition, they can also be used to check patient compliance. The pituitary responds rather sluggishly to acute changes in the circulating levels of thyroid hormones, an effect that is termed the 'pituitary lag'. Consequently, a noncompliant patient on replacement therapy who has, for example, taken T_4 just prior to clinic attendance, will be revealed by a raised TSH.

In some patients who suffer from physical (or in some instances psychiatric) illnesses that do not directly involve the thyroid gland, the level of total and free T_3 may fall below normal. In the most serious cases, total and free T_4 also falls. However, these changes are not accompanied by an increase in TSH. This condition is referred to as the 'sick euthyroid' syndrome, and should not be misinterpreted as thyroid-hormone deficiency. On recovery from the illness, T_3 and T_4 will return to normal of their own accord.

Additional tests

Investigating a patient by using a strategy such as that shown in Fig. 5.10 may lead to prolonged treatment, and, in the case of hypothyroidism, replacement therapy for life. Consequently, a frequent variant of this simple strategy is to use a measurement of one of the circulating thyroid hormones in addition to TSH, to act as confirmation. For example, a diagnosis of primary hypothyroidism would be confirmed with an fT_4 determination.

Additional tests may be used to establish a full diagnosis. For example, antithyroglobulin and/or antithyroid-peroxidase antibodies (anti-TPO) may be measured, since these will be elevated in conditions such as Hashimoto thyroiditis. Commercial kits are readily available to measure these antibodies.

Imaging of the thyroid is useful to establish whether thyrotoxicosis, in the absence of the obvious clinical signs of Graves disease listed in Table 5.2, is due to autoimmune (Graves) disease or is of nonautoimmune origin. Diffuse uptake on a radionuclide scan indicates Graves disease, while patchy uptake indicates toxic multinodular goitre; a single toxic nodule will show clearly as a 'hot nodule'. Should the scan prove equivocal, a measurement of TSAb should be useful, although assays for TSAb remain technically difficult and are not routinely available. Anti-TSH-receptor antibodies can be measured using a commercial kit. The latter relies on the inhibition of the binding of radiolabelled TSH to its receptor by the added antibody. However, interaction at the receptor level may not correlate with the potency of the antibody when stimulating the thyroid. For example, some antibodies that inhibit TSH binding do not stimulate and thereby 'block' the receptor *in vivo*, and are associated with hypothyroidism rather than hyperthyroidism.

Circulating thyroglobulin levels can be determined by immunoassay. Since the glycoprotein is sequestered, they are normally low. However, they can rise with hyperthyroidism, large multinodular goitres and certain forms of thyroid cancer. They are used to follow up a patient with papillary or follicular thyroid cancer. After total thyroidectomy, serum thyroglobulin levels should be low; any rise is indicative of metastases.

Finally, unexpected results from thyroid-function tests may be due to missing, excessive, or aberrant forms of thyroid hormone binding proteins. These can be investigated by electrophoretic separation of the serum proteins and measurement of the specific thyroid hormone binding proteins.

CHAPTER 6

Reproductive Endocrinology

SUMMARY

The maintenance of male reproductive capability depends on the secretion of testosterone from the testes. The male continuously produces a very large number of gametes (spermatozoa), whereas the female produces only one (or two) ova each month. The control of gametogenesis in the male depends on testicular stimulation by luteinizing hormone and follicle-stimulating hormone secretion, which is inhibited by a negative feedback of testosterone and a hormone produced by the seminiferous tubules, inhibin. The production of ova depends on a cycle of hormonal changes, involving follicle-stimulating hormone and luteinizing hormone, with negative feedback by ovarian hormones, oestrogens, progesterone and inhibin. Ovulation is initiated by a surge of luteinizing hormone at midcycle, resulting from a temporary switch from negative to positive feedback by oestrogens on the pituitary. The cycle of hormonal changes brings about follicular development, luteolysis and menstruation and, in so doing, maintains the female genital tract in a condition that allows fertilization and implantation to occur at the appropriate time. Oestrogens also maintain the secondary sexual characteristics.

In pregnancy, the fetoplacental unit acts as an endocrine organ, secreting human chorionic gonadotrophin, human placental lactogen, oestrogens and progesterone, and transferring fetal adrenocortical steroids into the maternal circulation, thus maintaining pregnancy and eventually initiating parturition.

Sexual differentiation and development over an extended period, from conception to puberty, depends on a complex interplay of genetic and hormonal factors. In the absence of a functioning testis, the female phenotype prevails, even if there is a 46XY chromosome karyotype.

Disorders of the reproductive system range from a common endocrine cause of infertility, such as a prolactinoma, to rare genetic disorders such as end-organ insensitivity.

INTRODUCTION

Reproductive endocrinology begins at conception, with the differentiation and determination of the sex of the baby. Fetal sexual development in the male, although not in the female, requires the integrity of the hypothalamo-pituitary–gonadal axis, and this axis becomes responsible in both sexes for the changes of puberty that culminate in reproductive capability. The sex hormones, augmented by those from the placenta, have a special role in the female during pregnancy and at parturition; they are also required for lactation. Later, the changes at the menopause are attributable to alterations in the hormones of reproductive endocrinology.

The study of gamete formation began with Leeuwenhoek's descriptions of human sperm, when they were first viewed under the microscope in the seventeenth century. Two hundred years elapsed before the development of the mammalian ovum in the ovarian Graafian follicle was also described. At this time, it began to be perceived that the gonads were not only responsible for gamete formation, but also produced humoral factors that regulated reproductive physiology. Berthold demonstrated that transplantation of a cock's testes into a capon induced normal development of a cockscomb in the castrated animal. The testicular androgen responsible for this, testosterone, was identified and crystallized in 1935. Shortly before this, ovarian oestrogens and progesterone had also been isolated and purified. Simultaneous progress was made in understanding the physiological regulation of the production of the gonadal steroids by the gonadotrophins secreted from the anterior pituitary, and eventually the higher regulation provided by the hypothalamus.

It was not until the 1950s that Jost demonstrated the crucial role of testosterone in determining phenotypic sex differentiation in the developing male fetus. The recent advances in molecular biology have elucidated the structures of the intracellular receptors for the steroid hormones and highlighted the importance of the enzymatic conversion of testosterone to dihydrotestosterone by some target cells, such that in some respects testosterone may be regarded as a prohormone.

SEX DETERMINATION AND SEXUAL DIFFERENTIATION

The genetic sex of an individual is determined at the time of fertilization when a spermatozoon bearing an X chromosome or a Y chromosome fuses with a normal X-chromosome–bearing ovum, which produces a female (XX) or a male (XY) zygote. Thus, the genetic sex of the male human subject is normally determined by the presence of a Y chromosome. However, the mechanism involved in the translation of the zygote's genetic sex into the sexual dimorphism of the adult male or female phenotype is dependent on a complex interplay of genetic, hormonal, psychological and social factors.

Genetic determinants

The X and Y chromosomes are called the sex chromosomes, and the remaining 44 are termed autosomes. In the male, the Y chromosome normally carries the genetic determinants essential for the development of masculine traits, while those for the female are on the autosomes or the X chromosomes, or both. The sex-determining region of the Y chromosome (SRY) is the chromosomal determinant that causes the undifferentiated, bipotential gonad to become a testis. Study of chromosomal disorders has shown that even with additional X chromosomes, as with an XXY male, the presence of the Y chromosome is decisive, so that testes will develop and phenotypically (i.e. anatomically) the individual will be male, whatever may happen later.

Hormonal determinants

The gonads initially appear as the two urogenital ridges, which are thickened areas of coelomic epithelial cells covering the mesonephros and associated underlying mesenchymal cells (Fig. 6.1). The germinal ridges are then progressively invaded by primordial germ cells, which have migrated from the endoderm of the yolk sac. By amoeboid movement, the primordial germ cells leave the endoderm, migrate dorsally in the mesentery, and enter the germinal epithelium. The thickened germinal epithelium containing the dividing germ cells, now called gonocytes, proliferates and sends cords of cells (the primary sex cords) into the underlying stroma. The establishment of these primitive gonads and the urogenital tract is indistinguishable in the two sexes up to about 6 weeks of development. The sex cords of the male then become separated from the germinal epithelium, and eventually develop into the seminiferous tubules. Leydig cells also begin to differentiate at this stage. In the female, the sex cords break up into clusters of cells, each containing a gonocyte, to form the primordial follicles. Indifferent gonocytes become spermatogonia in the testes and oocytes in the ovaries.

After 6 weeks' gestation, by which time the indifferent phase of differentiation should be complete, the urogenital tract consists of two components. First, there is a dual duct system—the mesonephric (or Wolffian) duct and the paramesonephric (or Müllerian) duct. These form the anlagen of the internal accessory reproductive organs (Fig. 6.2). The second component is made up of the urogenital sinus and tubercle, which differentiate to form the external genitalia, and in the male the terminal urethra (Fig. 6.3). The Müllerian duct develops later than the Wolffian duct. The cranial portion (mesonephric tubules) of the Wolffian duct connects to the gonad (i.e. the testis), but the cranial end of the Müllerian duct never does so. During differentiation of a male fetus, the Wolffian duct develops to form the rete testis, epididymis, vas deferens and seminal vesicles, while the urogenital sinus gives rise

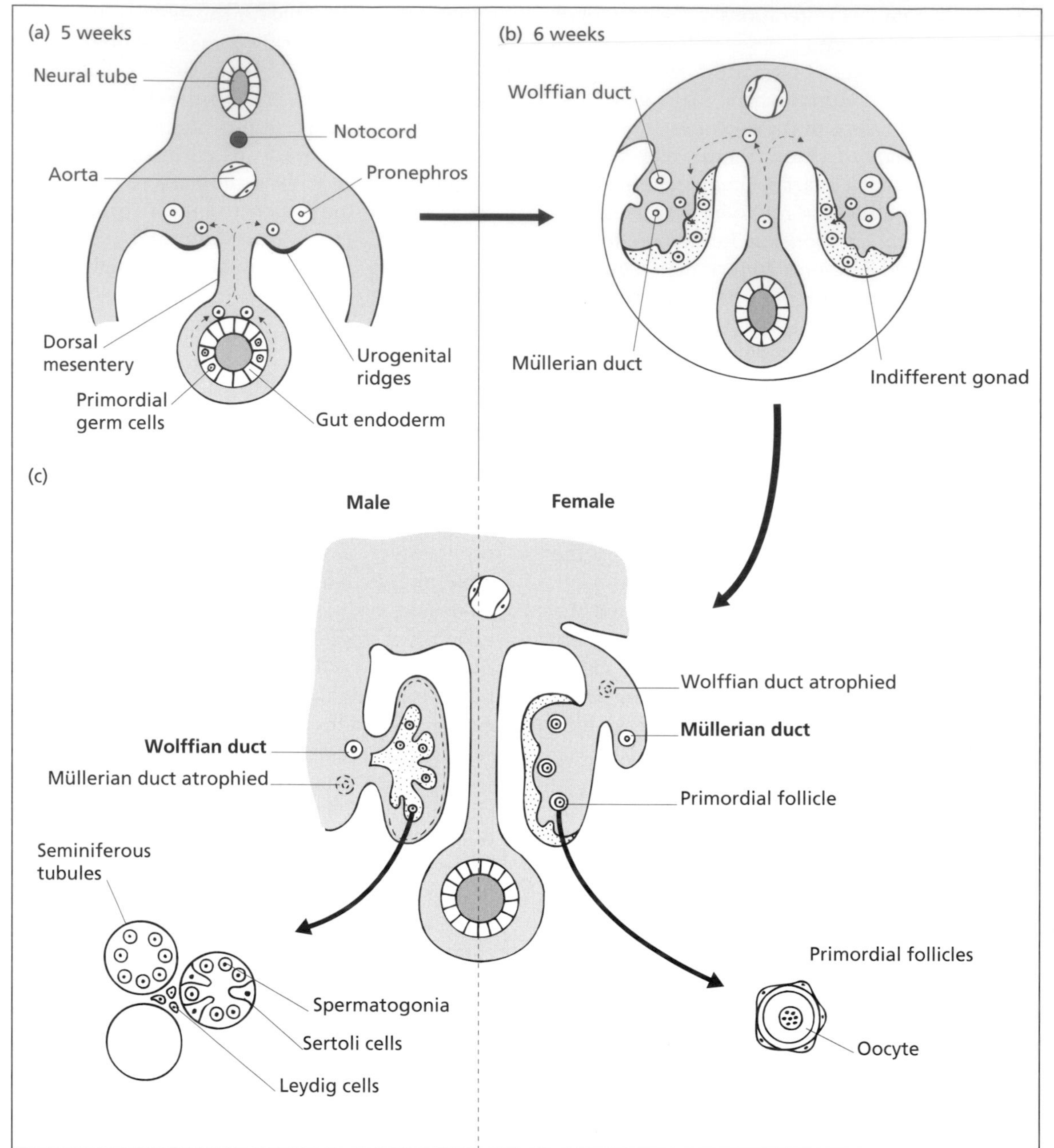

Figure 6.1 The early stages in the differentiation of the genital system. (a) A cross-section of a 5-week human embryo, showing the primordial germ cells migrating from the gut endoderm up the dorsal mesentery to the thickening urogenital ridges. The neural tube, notochord, pronephros and aorta are also shown. (b) A later stage (6 weeks) shows the invasion of the primordial germ cells into the urogenital ridges to form the indifferent gonads and the appearance of the Wolffian and Müllerian ducts. (c) In the male, seminiferous tubules differentiate and show spermatogonia and Sertoli cells. The steroidogenic Leydig cells appear between the tubules and the Müllerian duct regresses. In the female, primordial follicles consisting of an oocyte and flattened surrounding cells appear and the Wolffian duct regresses.

to the prostate (Fig. 6.2). In the differentiation of the female, the Fallopian tubes, the uterus and the upper half of the vagina develop from the Müllerian duct (Fig. 6.2).

During differentiation of the respective sexes, the duct that is not needed regresses. Regression of the Müllerian duct and virilization of the Wolffian duct in the male are an active process, dependent on the secretions of the fetal testis. In the absence of testicular secretion, the female form develops, even in the absence of the ovaries. The fetal testis secretes a Müllerian duct-regression factor

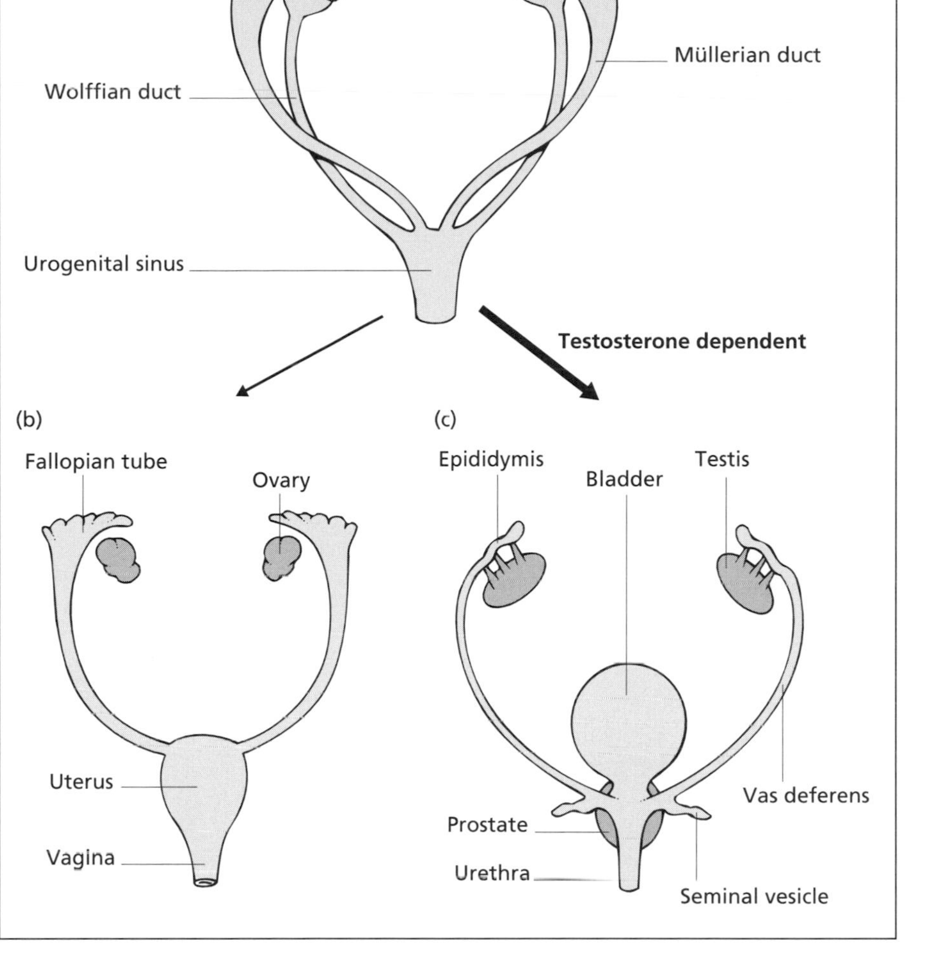

Figure 6.2 Embryonic differentiation of the male and female genital ducts and the formation of the internal genitalia. (a) The indifferent stage when both the Müllerian and Wolffian ducts are present. (b) The differentiation of the female genital ducts. In the absence of testicular hormones, the Müllerian ducts develop into the Fallopian tubes, the uterus and the upper section of the vagina. The Wolffian duct regresses. (c) The differentiation of the male genital ducts. Testosterone virilizes the Wolffian ducts to form the rete testis, epididymis, vas deferens and seminal vesicle. In addition, due to the secretion of anti-Müllerian hormone from the Sertoli cells, the Müllerian ducts regress.

called anti-Müllerian hormone (AMH), a glycoprotein that is initially synthesized by the Sertoli cells early in fetal life. It has a molecular weight of 145 000, with 13.5% of carbohydrates, and it is a homodimer, being made up of two identical chains. The Müllerian duct is sensitive to this hormone's action only for a short period, between the seventh and eighth week of intrauterine life. The action of the Müllerian regression hormone is ipsilateral. Failure of its synthesis or action results in the persistence of female structures into postnatal life.

The fetal testis also secretes testosterone, which is responsible for virilization of the Wolffian duct. Conversion of testosterone to 5α-dihydrotestosterone is necessary for virilization of the fetal external genitalia (Fig. 6.3) and the development of the prostate. This conversion is dependent on the action of the enzyme 5α-reductase in those fetal derivatives of the urogenital sinus.

Thus, a number of factors contribute to the development of the male reproductive system. The SRY is responsible for early testicular differentiation. AMH then induces regression of the ovarian duct, while testosterone virilizes the Wolffian duct. Differentiation of the external genitalia is dependent on 5α-reductase converting testosterone to 5α-dihydrotestosterone. The co-ordinated action of these factors is required to establish the gross anatomy of the phenotypic male by the end of the third month of pregnancy. Failure in one of these components, such as a deficiency of 5α-reductase, results in abnormal sexual differentiation, as is discussed later.

In the two latter trimesters of pregnancy, the testes descend from their position by the kidneys to the adult position in the scrotum. This process requires gonadotrophin from the developing pituitary, as well as testosterone and probably AMH. The descent is usually completed by birth, but is sometimes delayed: if descent does not occur, synthesis of testosterone in later life can occur, but

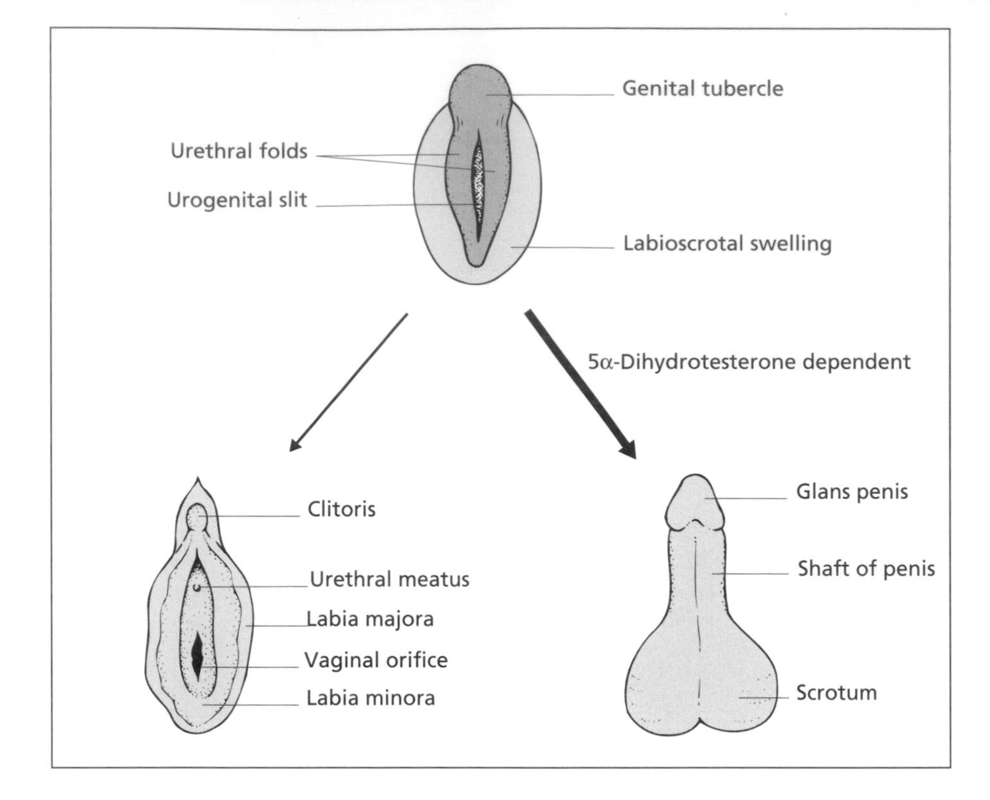

Figure 6.3 Embryonic development of the external genitalia. The genital tubercle is the bipotential primordium that forms in front of the urogenital slit. In the absence of 5α-dihydrotestosterone, a clitoris develops from the genital tubercle, and the labioscrotal swellings become the labia majora and labia minora. In the male, 5α-dihydrotestosterone is essential for the transformation of the genital tubercle into the penis and the fusion of the labioscrotal swellings to form the scrotum, into which the testes will descend.

spermatogenesis will fail, since this requires the lower temperature of the scrotum. However, this can be corrected effectively by surgery, provided this is done before the age of 6 years.

In the differentiation of the female, the Fallopian tubes, the uterus and the upper half of the vagina develop from the Müllerian duct. The development of the female lags behind that of the male. Regression of the Wolffian duct and the development of the female structure only commence towards the end of the first trimester, and the development of the gross anatomy of the female is not completed until the third trimester.

MALE REPRODUCTIVE SYSTEM

The male gonad has two important functions, the synthesis of the male sex hormones (androgens) and the production of gametes (spermatogenesis). Androgens are required for the differentiation of male characteristics in the fetus, for development at puberty and for the process of spermatogenesis.

Morphology of the gonads

In the testis, the seminiferous tubules, which make up the bulk of the tissues and produce sperm, are distinct from the lipid-laden, interstitial Leydig cells, which lie between the tubules and are the steroid-synthesizing cells (Fig. 6.4). Spermatozoa are produced in the seminiferous tubules, in which there are two types of cell, the germ cells and the Sertoli cells (Fig. 6.5). Tight junctions between adjacent Sertoli cells produce two compartments: a basal compartment, in which are found the spermatogonia, and an adluminal compartment, for the spermatocytes, spermatids and sperm. Each testis is attached to an epididymis, into which the tubules lead and in which maturation of the sperm occurs. The vas deferens leads from the epididymis to the urethra.

Androgen production

Synthesis and secretion

A number of androgenic hormones are secreted by the testes, including androstenedione, dehydroepiandrosterone (DHEA) and testosterone, which is the most powerful anabolic hormone. Synthesis of testosterone (Fig. 6.6.) takes place in the interstitial Leydig cells and proceeds, via cholesterol and pregnenolone, by the common pathway of steroidogenesis (see Fig. 4.4 and Appendix 3). In the normal male, the testis is the major site of androgen synthesis, with only a small contribution ($< 5\%$) from the adrenal. Apart from its action on the development of the internal genitalia and its action on muscle cells, testosterone

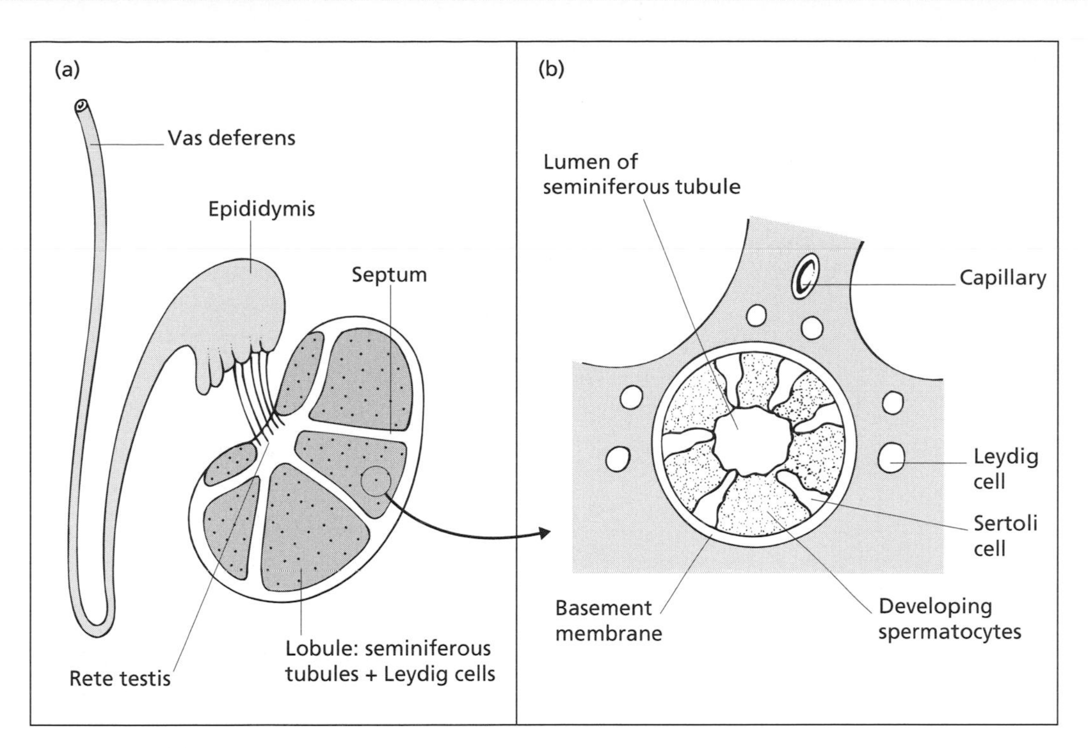

Figure 6.4 A testis in cross-section. (a) The testis is organized into lobules, in which lie the seminiferous tubules and the Leydig cells. Efferent ducts lead from the rete testis into the epididymis, which is eventually included in the spermatic cord together with the testicular blood vessels and lymphatics. (b) The organization of the seminiferous tubules and the interstitial Leydig cells, shown in cross-section.

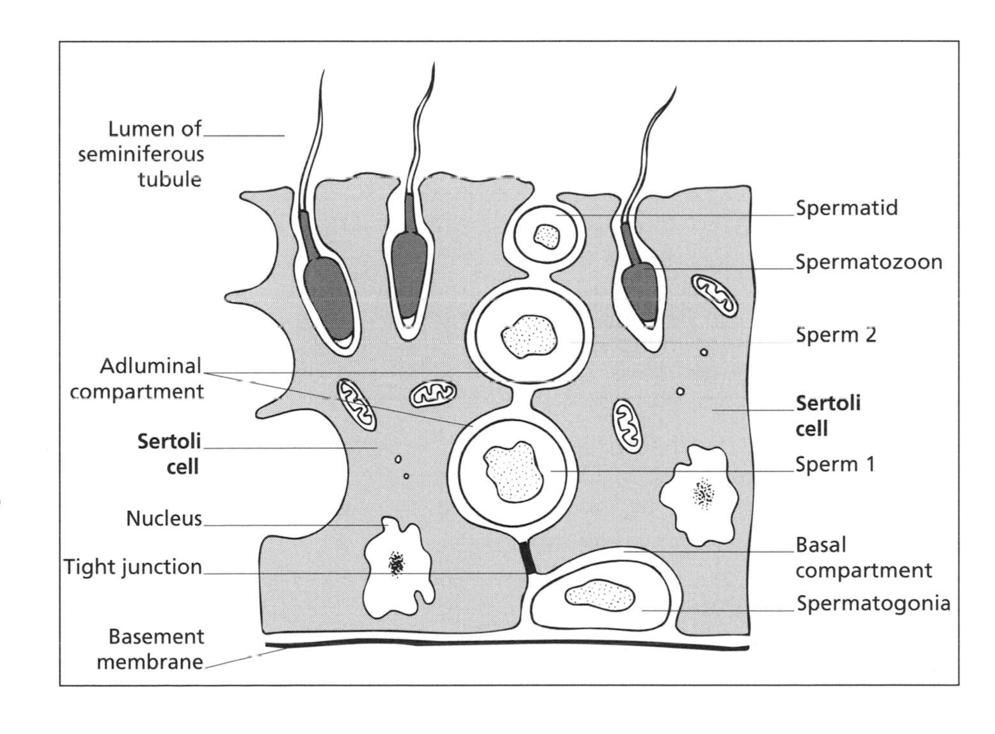

Figure 6.5 The structure of the wall of a seminiferous tubule. Sertoli cells span the thickness of the tubule from the surrounding basement membrane to its lumen. Two Sertoli cells are shown (shaded) in the figure. Tight junctions between adjacent Sertoli cells separate the spermatogonia in a basal compartment from the other stages in spermatogenesis in an adluminal compartment. The Sertoli cells closely surround the primary (sperm 1) and secondary (sperm 2) spermatocytes, the spermatids and sperm.

requires further metabolism by the microsomal enzyme 5α-reductase to dihydrotestosterone before it acts at its other target sites (Fig. 6.6). Because of this peripheral conversion, when acting on these specific tissues, testosterone may be thought of as a prohormone, and it is dihydrotestosterone that binds to the hormone-binding domain of the intranuclear receptors, which then activate deoxyribonucleic acid (DNA) transcription in some of its

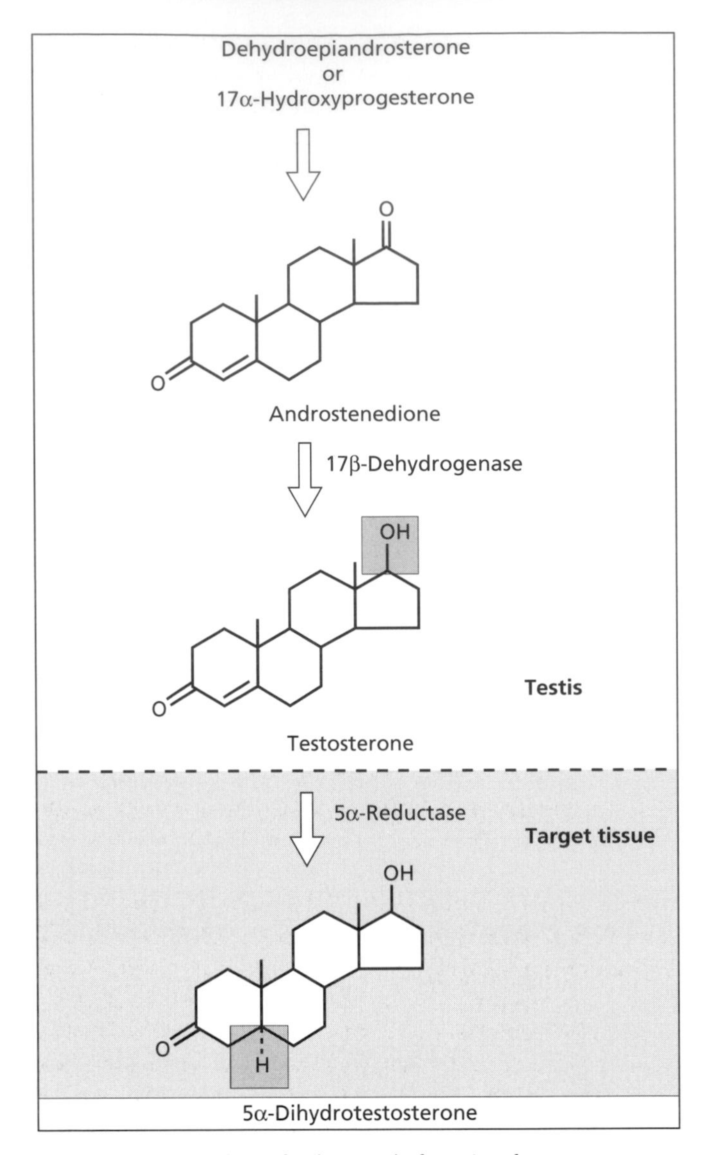

Figure 6.6 The biosynthesis of androgens. The formation of testosterone occurs in Leydig cells. Dehydroepiandrosterone is only a weak androgen, which can masculinize but does not affect secondary sex organs. Testosterone is secreted and is converted in some target issues to dihydrotestosterone.

target cells (see Figs 2.21–2.23). Testosterone may also be aromatized to oestradiol by its target cells, but dihydrotestosterone cannot be aromatized.

Actions of androgens

During childhood, gonadotrophin secretion is at a low level. There are occasional pulses of luteinizing hormone (LH) and follicle-stimulating hormone (FSH) in young children in the middle of the night, and the frequency and amplitude of these pulses gradually increase with the advancing years, so that by the age of 9–11 all children are experiencing regular nocturnal pulsatile gonadotrophin secretion. This results in sufficient sex steroid being present to produce the first external changes of the secondary sexual characteristics.

The onset of puberty in the male can be detected phenotypically by an increase in the size of the penis and testicular volume, the latter brought about by an increase in germ-cell layers and appearance of a lumen in each seminiferous tubule. The Leydig cells also increase in number and size, and are stimulated to synthesize and secrete testosterone. The increased testosterone concentration in the circulation stimulates skeletal muscle growth and development of the larynx, which results later in a deepening of the voice. Pubic hair and beard growth, together with sebaceous gland activity, is stimulated, and spermatogenesis commences. Rising testosterone levels promote epiphyseal fusion, which leads eventually to termination in the growth of the long bones.

Spermatogenesis

The primordial germ cells are laid down in the testes in the fetal period. Once they are committed to becoming spermatogonia, no further development to form spermatozoa takes place until puberty. In adolescent and adult life, spermatogonia continuously augment their numbers by mitotic division. They appear to be of two types: type A, which are reserve spermatogonia and which divide to give more of type A or, after several divisions, type B, which are destined to move from the basal compartment of the seminiferous tubule into the adluminal compartment, where they divide and form primary spermatocytes (Fig. 6.5). Primary spermatocytes then undergo the first meiotic division to form secondary spermatocytes, which have half the chromosomal number of the original spermatogonia. The second meiotic division produces spermatids; when first formed, the spermatid is a small rounded cell, which will gradually transform into a spermatozoon.

Their intimate association with the Sertoli cells is essential for these processes. Indeed, Sertoli cells are sometimes called 'nurse cells', and they secrete a steroidal, meiotic-stimulating factor. The spermatozoa are extruded by the Sertoli cells into the lumen of the tubule. Although apparently fully differentiated, the spermatozoa are not capable of independent motility or fertilization at this stage, and further maturation is required; this occurs during passage through the epididymis. The mature spermatozoa are fully mobile when they leave the epididymis, and they become mixed with the secretions of the seminal vesicle and prostate at the time of ejaculation. In many mammals, however, the freshly ejaculated spermatozoa are still incapable of fertilization until they have undergone a further process, called 'capacitation', in the female reproductive tract; this precedes the reactions brought about by the acrosome, and it is the latter changes that enable spermatozoa to penetrate the ovum. The acrosome is a large, specialized lysosome in the head of the sperm, and contains a number of acid hydrolases. During fertilization, the hydrolases are released and extracellular materials in the path of the sperm are digested, thus allowing it access to the ovum. Semen appears to contain a factor that inhibits capacitation; this is important, because capacitated sperm deteriorate very rapidly.

Control of testicular function

Testicular function is regulated by the two pituitary gonadotrophins, FSH and LH, both of which are glycoproteins (see Chapter 3). The initiation and maintenance of spermatogenesis normally requires the action of both FSH and LH. LH stimulates the synthesis of testosterone by the Leydig cells. Testosterone maintains spermatogenesis, although it cannot initiate it. Thus, if adult males are hypophysectomized, immediate administration of LH will maintain spermatogenesis. If, however, administration of LH is delayed or if the experiment is done in immature rats, spermatogenesis does not occur, since FSH is needed to initiate spermatogenesis.

The action of FSH and testosterone (and hence of LH) on the process of spermatogenesis is not thought to be directly on the germ cells, but via their action on Sertoli cells, which are triggered to produce several agents necessary for sperm maturation. One such substance, which has been identified in rat testicular fluid, is an androgen-binding protein which binds testosterone. This is secreted by Sertoli cells into the lumen of the seminiferous tubule and its production is stimulated by FSH and testosterone. In animals, it binds and hence provides a reserve of androgens in the testicular fluid, but its role in humans is still not certain; it probably mediates local concentrations of testosterone in the immediate environment of the developing spermatocytes.

The secretion of the two gonadotrophins controlling testicular function is regulated by a single gonadotrophin-releasing hormone (GnRH), a decapeptide produced in the hypothalamus. The secretions of the hypothalamo-pituitary unit are regulated by a negative-feedback mechanism involving steroid hormones, gonadotrophins and a gonadal peptide hormone, inhibin, from the Sertoli cells of the testis (Fig. 3.10). GnRH is released episodically, with pulses occurring every 90 min. Satisfactory gonadotrophin release only occurs in both males and females if this pulsatility is maintained.

LH controls the rate of testosterone synthesis in Leydig cells by regulating the enzymatic step involved in the conversion of cholesterol to pregnenolone, cholesterol side-chain cleavage. The action of LH on Leydig cells is mediated by a G-protein–linked receptor on the cell surface, which interacts in particular with the adenylate cyclase catalytic subunit (see Figs 2.11–2.13). The gonads, in their turn, exert an influence on the hypothalamic–pituitary system by a negative-feedback control whereby elevated concentrations of circulating testosterone inhibit the release of LH. Other steroids can also affect this feedback control, including oestradiol and 5α-dihydrotestosterone. At one time, it was thought that oestradiol was the important controlling compound, following the aromatization of testosterone in the brain. However, this cannot be the only mechanism operating, since 5α-dihydrotestosterone also suppresses LH secretion and yet cannot be converted to oestradiol. The secretion of LH is pulsatile, and seems to be much more sensitive to negative feedback by steroids than that of FSH.

Inhibin

A gonadal protein called inhibin selectively suppresses the secretion of FSH from the gonadotrophs. Originally detected in aqueous extracts of testis, inhibin has subsequently also been isolated from ovarian follicular fluid. It has a molecular weight of 32 000, and is made up of α- and β-peptide chains, which have molecular weights of 18 000 and 14 000, respectively, and are linked by disulphide bonds. There are two types of β-chains, which are referred to as β_A and β_B, and two forms of inhibin exist which have a common α-chain, these being either $\alpha\beta_A$- or $\alpha\beta_B$-dimers; these are also known as inhibin A and inhibin B, respectively. By using complementary DNA (cDNA) probes, it has been shown that the synthesis of the α- and β-chains occurs separately, with the genes for the relevant chains being present on different chromosomes. The situation is thus similar to the synthesis of the pituitary glycoprotein hormones, namely thyrotrophin and the gonadotrophins. It has been estimated that the messenger ribonucleic acid (mRNA) for the α-chain is present in the ovary in a 10- and 20-fold excess over that for the β_A- and β_B-chains, respectively. Inhibins A and B both circulate in women, but inhibin A is absent in men.

Dimers of β-chains have also been found in follicular fluid. They have different properties from inhibin, and although it is uncertain how or under what conditions the dimers are secreted, they are actually capable of increasing the secretion of FSH. Two dimers have been identified: one consisting of $\beta_A\beta_A$-subunits, called 'FSH-releasing protein', and the other consisting of $\beta_A\beta_B$-subunits, called 'activin'. Little is known about the control of either αβ or ββ dimerization.

The β-dimers have structural similarities to transforming growth factor β (TGF-β), which is a dimer of two subunits with a molecular weight of 12 500 linked by disulphide bonds. TGF-β acts as a local hormone in a variety of tissues, and can increase the secretion of FSH. It has been suggested that TGF-β, inhibin and activin may arise from a common gene family.

Male infertility

A defect of spermatogenesis, with reduced numbers or even total absence of sperm from the semen, is the cause of infertility in 10% of couples who find that they cannot conceive. The failure of spermatogenesis may be due to lack of LH and FSH secretion. Prolactin is important in the control of gonadotrophin release, and high concentrations of prolactin may cause testicular involution and impotence. Infertility, however, more commonly arises from primary failure of the testis itself, e.g. due to cryptorchidism (undescended testes) or damage to the testes by mumps. In some cases in which there has been testicular damage or the vas deferens has been resected, infertility may be due to the formation of antisperm antibody. Even if the sperm count is normal, there may be abnormal forms or reduced motility of the sperm; also, the sperm may have a low capacity for fertilization, although at present it is difficult to demonstrate this. Chromosomal abnormalities can also cause infertility, as in Klinefelter syndrome (47XXY karyotype). Investigation of infertility thus necessitates consideration of the endocrine, immunological and genetic mechanisms involved in reproduction, as well as psychological factors.

FEMALE REPRODUCTIVE SYSTEM

Mature germ cells are produced in females only intermittently, and usually only one germ cell reaches full maturity at a time, at intervals of approximately 28 days. Moreover, once production of mature germ cells has started at puberty, it continues for a limited time rather than for the rest of an individual's life. Thus, only about 400 germ cells reach full maturity to be released at ovulation. The cyclical production of mature oocytes in the ovary is associated with concordant changes in hormone production from the ovary and accompanying alterations in the uterus and the vagina.

Ovarian morphology and function: oogenesis

Oogenesis begins in the fetal ovary (Fig. 6.1) when the primordial germ cells proliferate to become oogonia. At week 11–12 of gestation, the oogonia enter the prophase of the first meiotic division, and then become arrested without completing the division. At this stage, they are called primary oocytes, and with the surrounding granulosa cells from the sex cords, they form the primordial follicles (Fig. 6.7). The primordial follicles reach a peak number of about 7×10^6 between week 20 and 28 of gestation, but from then on their number declines. At birth, there are only about 2×10^6, and by puberty only 300 000, each surrounded by a single layer of flattened follicular cells embedded in a cellular stroma. The centre or medulla of the ovary consists largely of blood vessels. The ovaries are sited close to the open ends of the Fallopian tubes, which pass to the body of the uterus, whose cervix opens into the vagina.

Formation of the Graafian follicle

At the beginning of a menstrual cycle, a group or cohort of 10–20 early follicles enlarge through the proliferation of the flattened follicular cells to form, in succession, primary and then liquid-filled secondary follicles (Fig. 6.7). These consist of several layers of membrana granulosa cells, surrounding an oocyte. In any one menstrual cycle, usually only one of the follicles matures fully. Stromal cells become arranged around the follicle to form the well-vascularized theca. Growth of the follicle proceeds, and a large cavity, the antrum, develops within the tertiary follicle, filled by the follicular fluid. In what is now termed a Graafian follicle, the oocyte is supported in the antrum by a stalk of granulosa cells, the cumulus oophorus. Up to this time, the granulosa cells are ionically coupled to one another and to the ovum by gap junctions. Then, in midcycle, ovulation occurs, whereby the ovum becomes uncoupled and the Graafian follicle ruptures, liberating the oocyte, which enters the fimbriated opening of the Fallopian tube. If the ovum is fertilized, development starts, and usually reaches the blastocyst stage before it enters the uterus to become implanted in the uterine endometrium. If the ovum is not fertilized, it dies.

Formation of the corpus luteum

The cells of the ruptured Graafian follicle proliferate, enlarge and fill the collapsed antrum of the follicle. This new structure becomes a solid, round mass of steroidogenic cells called the corpus luteum, which is initially red in colour, but then becomes yellowish. If fertilization and blastocyst implantation do not occur, the corpus luteum, having been active for most of the latter half of the menstrual cycle, begins to involute. The luteal cells then cease their synthetic activity and disappear, and the whole structure is replaced with scar tissue and becomes the corpus albicans. However, if implantation occurs, the corpus luteum increases in size and remains active during the early weeks of pregnancy until its function of steroidogen-

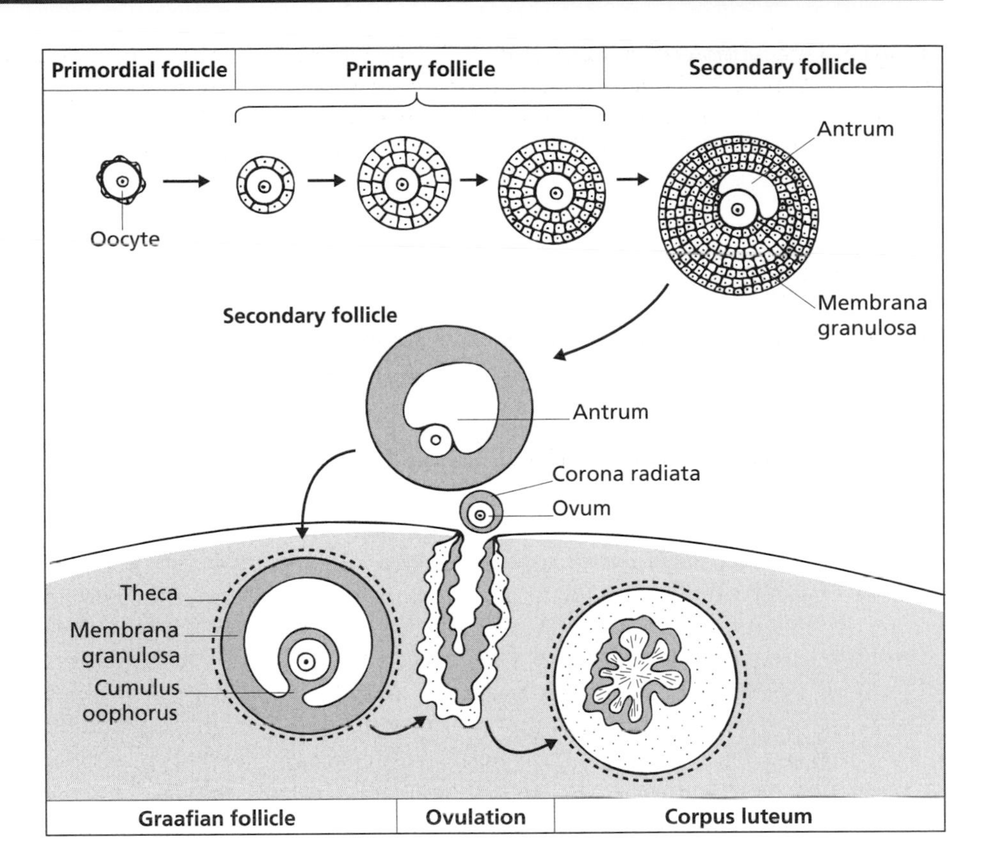

Figure 6.7 The growth, maturation and ovulation of a Graafian follicle, followed by the formation of a corpus luteum. To aid the clarity of presentation, the earlier stages are shown diagrammatically above and the later stages below in the shaded part representing the ovarian stroma, although the entire process takes place within this stroma. A primordial follicle consists of an oocyte surrounded by a layer of flattened cells. Growth of the primary follicle consists of multiplication and enlargement of the flattened cells to form a multilayered membrana granulosa. The appearance of a liquid-filled antrum indicates the formation of a secondary follicle. The antrum enlarges, and the oocyte remains attached to the membrana granulosa by a stalk of cells, the cumulus oophorus. Stromal cells become organized around the maturing Graafian follicle to form a steroidogenic layer of cells, the theca. When the follicle ruptures at ovulation, the ovum is expelled from the ovary surrounded by a layer of cells, the corona radiata. The granulosa cells of the collapsed follicle and the theca cells divide, enlarge and form a round, steroidogenic cellular mass, the corpus luteum.

esis is taken over by the placenta; thus, the corpus luteum maintains the uterine endometrium in early pregnancy.

Ovarian hormones

Control of ovarian hormone production

Hormone production in the ovary is cyclical. Two main steroid hormones are produced: oestradiol, which is an oestrogen, and progesterone, which possesses pregnancy-maintaining progestational activity (Table 6.1). The biosynthesis of oestradiol (Fig. 6.8 and Appendix 3) is remarkable in that its precursors (androstenedione and testosterone) are synthesized in the theca interna cells of the follicle and are then transported to the granulosa cells, where they are aromatized to yield oestrone and oestradiol (Fig. 6.9). Aromatization cleaves the carbon at position 19 (see Appendix 3), leaving the oestrogens with a phenolic A ring. Steroidogenesis is stimulated by LH, which activates the rate-limiting cholesterol side-chain cleavage enzyme (Appendix 3) by stimulating production of cyclic adenosine 5′-monophosphate (cAMP).

In the early follicular phase of the menstrual cycle, FSH initiates the further development of a number of primary follicles, and so increases the number of granulosa cells, while the number of theca cells increases under the influence of LH. This combination gives rise to an increased production of oestradiol between days 8 and 10 of the cycle. Just before ovulation, the granulosa cells of the follicle also develop receptors for LH, and these begin to synthesize progesterone.

When the empty follicle becomes a corpus luteum, the theca interna cells are trapped between granulosa cells, and both types of cells remain active, producing oestrogen and progesterone. The combination of the production of oestradiol and progesterone then has a negative-feedback effect, to suppress the production of LH and FSH (Fig. 6.10), although LH is needed to support the corpus luteum.

Effects of ovarian hormones on the uterus and vagina

The changing ovarian steroid output (Fig. 6.10) throughout the menstrual cycle is responsible for the alterations that are observed in the endometrium of the uterus and the rest of the female genital tract (Fig. 6.11). At the start of a new cycle, after menstruation is completed, the increased secretion of oestradiol stimulates the repair and proliferation of the endometrium and the synthesis of receptors for progesterone and oestradiol in its cells. The rise in progesterone that follows ovulation leads to changes in the secretion of the endometrium, which are

Table 6.1 The effects of female sex hormones.

Oestrogens	Progesterone
At puberty	
Stimulate the growth of the uterus and breast and determine the female figure by controlling the deposition of fat. They contribute to closure of the epiphyses. They have important effects on personality and sexual responsiveness	
During the menstrual cycle	
Cause endometrial proliferation and secretion of clear mucus from the cervix together with maturation of the vaginal epithelium. They have positive-feedback and negative-feedback effects on the hypothalamus and pituitary	Causes a rise in body temperature, the production of a secretory endometrium and secretion of thick cervical mucus with leucoctyes; this is inimical to sperm survival. It has a negative-feedback effect on the hypothalamus and pituitary
During pregnancy	
Cause growth of the breast duct system and myometrial hypertrophy together with fluid retention and increase in uterine blood flow	Causes a reduction of contractions and reduced smooth muscle tone. There is a rise in body temperature and growth of the alveoli of the breasts
Cellular effects	
Cause production of receptors for progesterone, and so the response to progesterone is dependent on oestrogenization	Stimulates the formation of 17-hydroxysteroid dehydrogenase, which leads to inactivation of oestradiol in target tissue by converting it to oestrone, which is only a weak oestrogen.

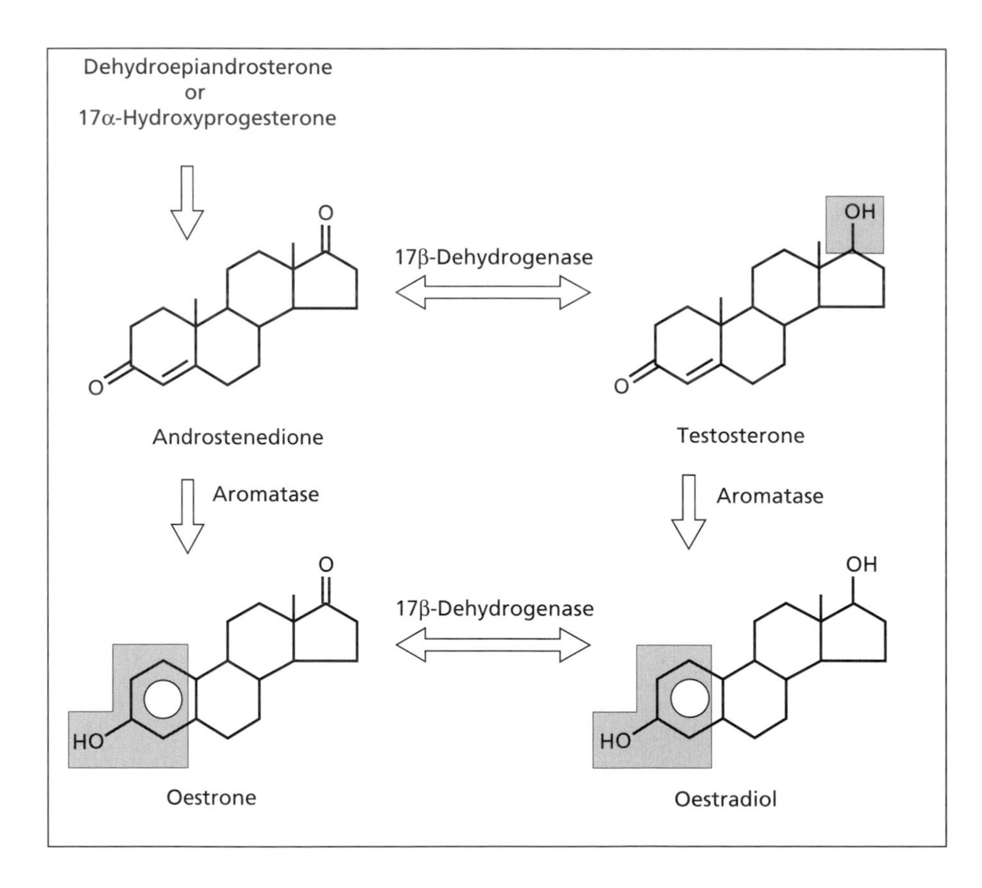

Figure 6.8 The biosynthesis of oestrogens. The precursors are formed in the theca interna and aromatized in the granulosa cells (see Fig. 6.9). Note that, after the menopause, oestrogen production is weak, and is solely due to the aromatization of androstenedione from the adrenal gland.

essential if implantation of a fertilized ovum is to occur. In the second half of the cycle, the endometrium doubles in thickness, and the simple tubular glands become tortuous and saccular. The maintenance of the secretory phase is dependent on the continued stimulus of oestrogen and the additional stimulus of progesterone from the corpus luteum, so that when luteolysis occurs, the endometrium breaks down, sloughs off, and menstrual bleeding occurs.

The cyclical hormonal changes also alter the consistency and pH of the cervical mucus. The changes in the

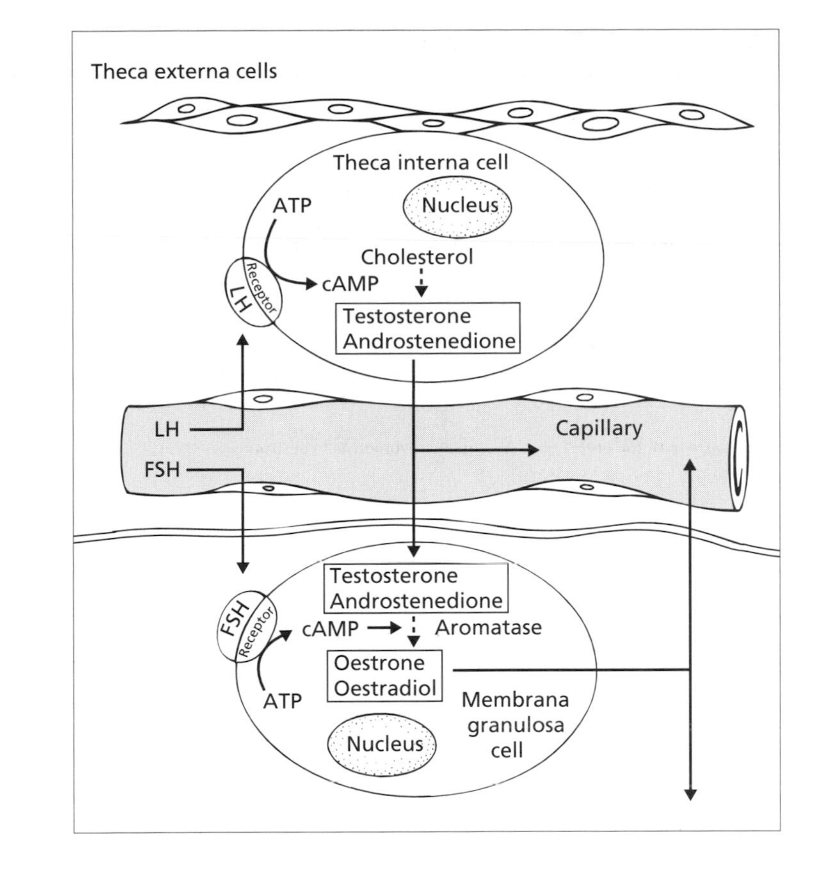

Figure 6.9 The structure of part of the wall of a Graafian follicle. Membrana granulosa cells are separated from the surrounding theca by a distinct basement membrane. The theca interna consists of androgen-synthesizing cells and capillaries; external to these are fibroblast-like cells of the theca externa. Luteinizing hormone (LH) stimulates receptors on the theca interna cells via cyclic adenosine 5′-monophosphate (cAMP) to synthesize testosterone and androstenedione. These either pass into the local capillaries or cross the basement membrane into the adjacent membrana granulosa cells. The latter are stimulated by follicle-stimulating hormone (FSH) to produce oestrogens by the aromatization of the testosterone and androstenedione (see Fig. 6.8). The oestrogens then enter the circulation or pass into the antrum of the follicle and act on the oocyte.

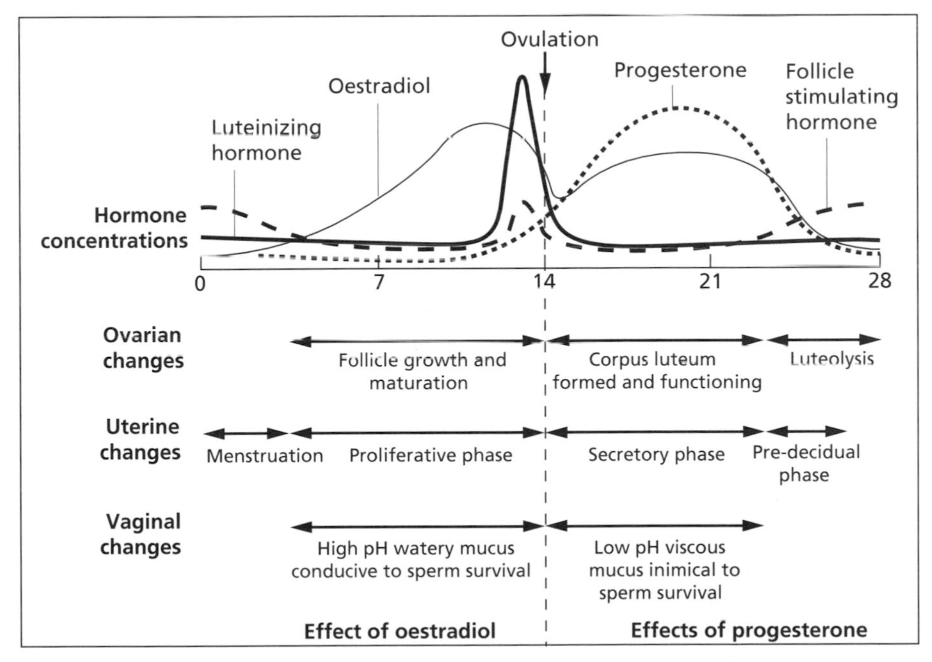

Figure 6.10 A schematic representation of the changes in the menstrual cycle shown as beginning with the start of menstruation on day 0 and lasting 28 days.

mucus are sufficient to render the entry of sperm into the uterus less likely during the luteal phase, when—because of high concentrations of progesterone—the mucus is viscous and of low pH, neither of which is conducive to survival of the sperm. In contrast, the mucus of the oestrogen-induced follicular phase is abundant, clear, watery and of higher pH, and consequently is more suitable for sperm transport and motility.

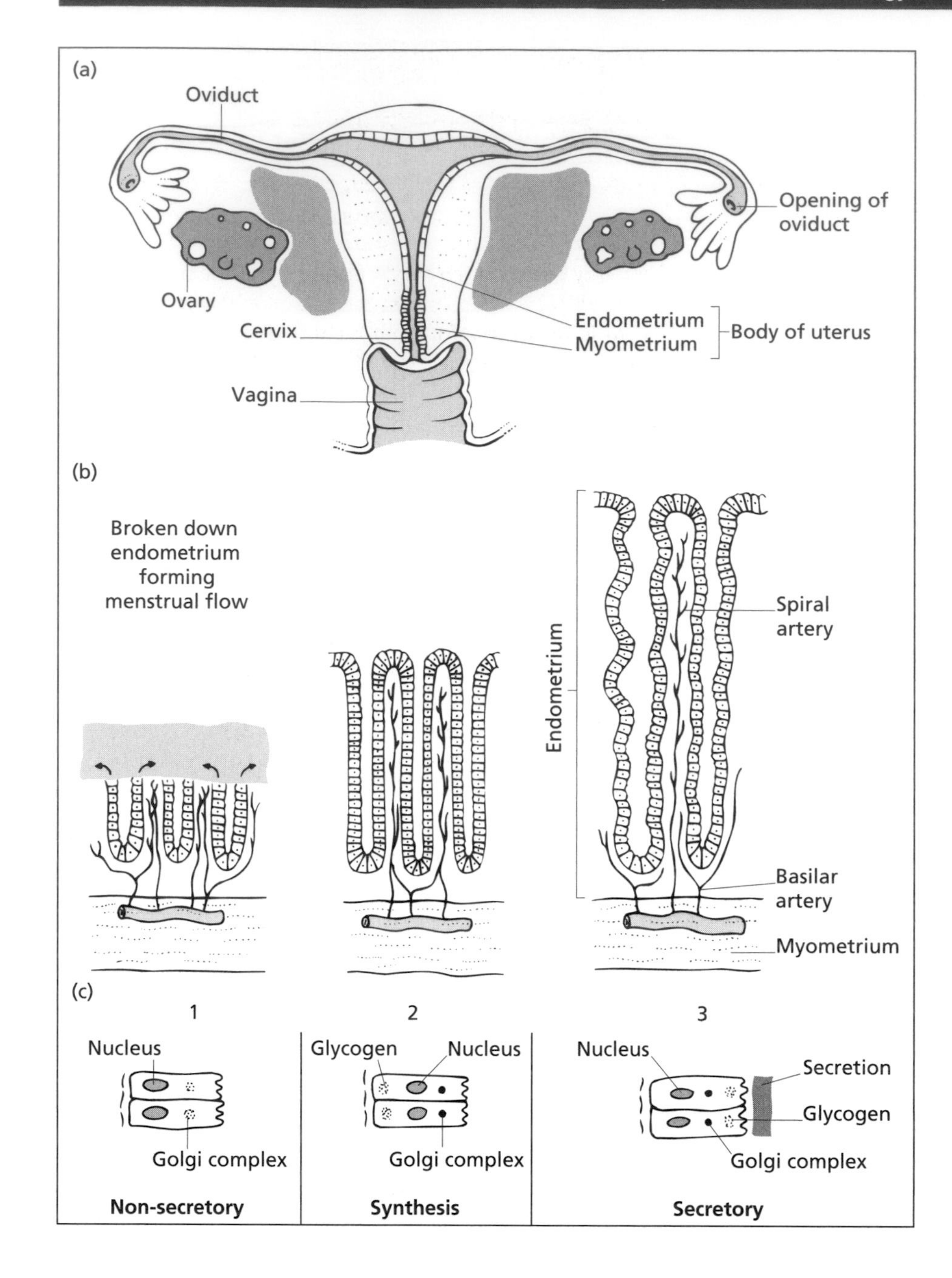

Figure 6.11 Changes in the uterine endometrium during the menstrual cycle (see also Fig. 6.10). (a) Section showing the body and cervix of the uterus and the vagina. The body of the uterus consists of an inner endometrial layer containing the uterine mucosa and a surrounding thick myometrium consisting largely of smooth muscle. (b and c) Changes in the uterine gland during the menstrual cycle. (1) Breakdown of the endometrium (days 1–3) occurs, in which the outer functional two-thirds is shed and the debris of the glands and endometrial stroma forms the menstrual flow. The basal third of the endometrium persists and its cells divide and grow over the exposed stromal tissue to repair the endometrium. The nucleus of the cells of the uterine gland shows a basal location. (2) During the oestrogenic, proliferative phase (days 3–14), the uterine glands grow in length as the endometrium thickens. Glycogen appears in the base of the glandular cells, pushing the nucleus towards the centre of the cell. (3) During the progestational, secretory phase (days 14–28), the uterine glands double in length and become tortuous and sacculated. Glycogen in the glandular cells migrates to the apex of the cell and, with other materials, is released to form the endometrial secretion, which reaches a maximum by day 20. Stromal oedema also increases to a maximum by day 21, approximately the time of normal blastocyst implantation. During the last 2–3 days of this phase, vascular changes occur in the spiral blood vessels, leading to their vasoconstriction. Blood-vessel rupture and extravasation then occurs, and lakes of blood form in the stromal tissue. Endometrial breakdown follows.

The actions of progesterone on the female reproductive tract, outlined above, have been exploited in the 'progesterone-only' contraceptive pill. Contraception is probably achieved through the effect of progesterone on cervical mucus and the endometrium.

Regulation of the menstrual cycle

In the UK, about 95% of girls have reached the menarche, i.e. started to menstruate, by the age of 15; 50% have done so by age of $12^1/_2$.

Control of follicle development. Regulation of the menstrual cycles occurs as a result of a number of interactions between the hormones of the hypothalamopituitary–gonadal axis, but the main regulation is intraovarian. Through the stimulus of FSH, a group of about 20 primary follicles begin to develop into secondary follicles, which produce oestradiol. Under the influence of increased concentrations of oestradiol, the follicles generate more receptors for FSH in the granulosa cells. Secretion of oestradiol and of inhibin by the follicles then begins to suppress the production of FSH from the anterior pituitary. When the concentration of FSH falls, only the ripening follicles with the highest concentration of receptors are able to sustain development, while the rest atrophy and regress. Thus, progressively, one follicle is selected to ovulate.

Initiation of ovulation. The occurrence of ovulation in the middle of the cycle is associated with a surge in the secretion of LH and, to a lesser extent, of FSH by the pituitary. The LH surge lasts for about 36 h, which is the time taken for the oocyte to mature. There is a local factor in the ovary that normally suppresses oocyte maturation, and this can be overcome by raised concentrations of LH. The midcycle rise in circulating gonadotrophins leads to increased synthesis of plasminogen activator in the follicle, and this aids ovulation, with concomitant follicle rupture and release of the ovum.

The principal cause of this surge in gonadotrophin secretion appears to be the action of oestradiol on the pituitary. Throughout the cycle, gonadotrophin output is stimulated by continuous pulsatile secretion of GnRH. In the early follicular phase of the cycle, the output of gonadotrophin is restricted by the negative feedback of inhibin and oestradiol on the pituitary. As the follicle ripens, oestradiol output increases and, by about day 12 of the cycle, a threshold concentration of oestradiol is exceeded. If this is maintained for about a further 36 h, there is a temporary switch from negative to positive feedback. Thus oestrogen-mediated positive feedback gives rise to a surge in release of gonadotrophins and so to ovulation. Gonadotrophin secretion is pulsatile, and varies according to a 24-h cycle, which is superimposed on the gross cyclical changes discussed above. One of the major causes of anovulatory infertility is an inability to progress from a nocturnal pulsatile gonadotrophin secretion, which is characteristic of early puberty, to the 24-h gonadotrophin pulsatility needed for reproductive capability.

Luteolysis. After ovulation, the collapsed follicle develops into the corpus luteum, and continues to produce oestradiol and progesterone under the stimulus of the low concentration of LH that remains after the midcycle surge. However, the output of LH continues to fall as the negative feedback of oestradiol on the pituitary is resumed.

The continued function of the corpus luteum depends on the stimulatory effect of LH, and so by about day 25, the falling output of this hormone results in failure of steroidogenesis. Menstruation follows, as there are no longer oestradiol and progesterone available to maintain the endometrium. This absence of oestradiol and progesterone removes the inhibition on the pituitary, which—under the stimulus of GnRH—resumes secretion of FSH and LH, and so the next cycle commences.

If implantation of a blastocyst occurs at about day 20 of the cycle, the resulting trophoblast begins to secrete human chorionic gonadotrophin (HCG), a glycoprotein hormone that has LH-like activity. This hormone maintains the corpus luteum, which continues its production of oestradiol and progesterone and so prevents menstruation.

Pregnancy

Conception and implantation

Normal conception requires that a spermatozoon should fertilize an ovum in the Fallopian tube. To achieve this, large numbers of sperm (approximately 25–30 million) have to be ejaculated into the vagina, whence they make their way through the cervix and body of the uterus to the Fallopian tube to encounter the ovum. Although only one sperm is necessary for final fertilization, the penetration of the ovum requires a sustained attack by many sperm, which release hydrolytic enzymes from their acrosomes. These loosen the corona radiata cells around the ovum and allow access for one sperm to penetrate. Once fertilized, the ovum is transported along the Fallopian tube by peristaltic contractions and the action of its ciliated epithelial cells. During this passage, it undergoes a series of cell divisions to reach the blastocyst stage of development, with about 16 cells. The secretion of a glycogen-rich mucus is necessary for nutrition of the blastocyst at this stage, and the uterine endometrium must be in a suitable secretory and receptive state for implantation to occur.

The life of sperm in the female genital tract is probably less than 72 h; there is a similarly short period during which the ovum is in the Fallopian tube and the cervical mucus is favourable for sperm survival. Thus, there is a relatively short period when coitus is likely to result in conception. This necessary coincidence of events provides the underlying rationale for the rhythm method of birth control, and is also of use in counselling couples who are attempting to achieve conception.

The fetoplacental endocrine unit (Fig. 6.12)

Successful implantation of the blastocyst in the endometrium is followed by its development into a trophoblast, which begins to secrete HCG into the maternal bloodstream; it is this glycoprotein hormone in maternal blood or urine that is the basis of most tests for the early detection of pregnancy. HCG maintains the oestradiol and progesterone secretion of the corpus luteum, and thus supports the fetoplacental unit. The increase in concentration of these steroids produced under the stimulus of HCG suppresses the pituitary production of FSH and so prevents further ovulation activity.

At about the ninth week of pregnancy, the fetoplacental unit expresses cholesterol side-chain cleavage activity, and so is able to synthesize both pregnenolone and progesterone (Fig. 4.4 and Appendix 3). Pregnenolone crosses to the fetus, and the developing fetal adrenal converts it to DHEA sulphate; this in turn is aromatized in the placenta, and is eventually excreted in maternal urine as oestriol (Fig. 6.12). Oestriol production begins from week 12, and with the onset of steroid production by the placenta, the corpus luteum of pregnancy gradually

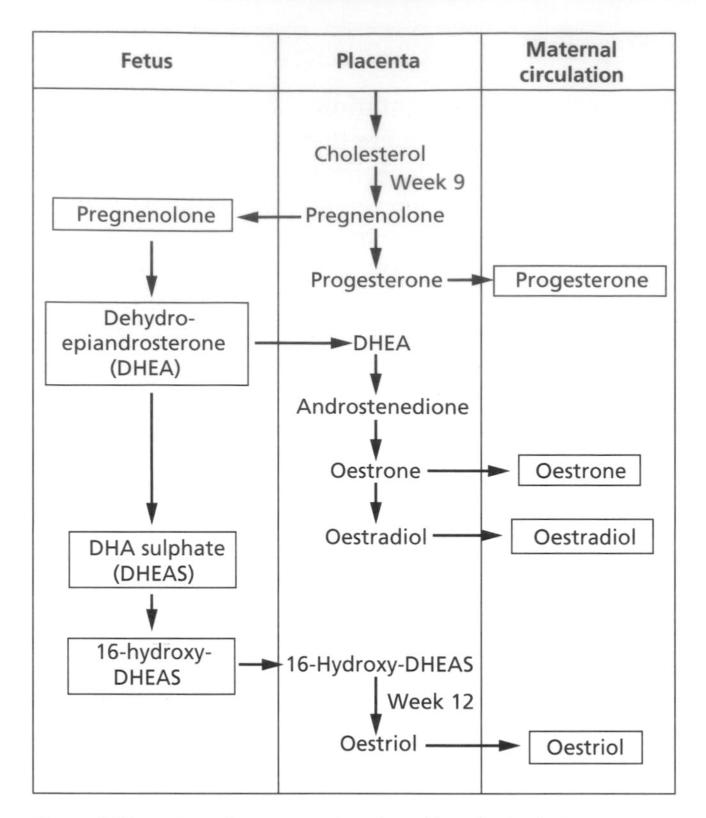

Figure 6.12 A schematic representation of steroid production in the fetoplacental unit. The placenta also produces protein hormones, particularly human chorionic gonadotrophin (HCG) and placental lactogen.

regresses. The fetoplacental unit provides a continuously rising output of progesterone and oestriol throughout pregnancy. This provides the rationale for measurement of maternal serum and urinary oestriol and urinary pregnanediol (which is a metabolite of progesterone), as indices of fetal well-being and placental function, although neither is a totally satisfactory index. Better information is obtained by serial ultrasound scans during pregnancy.

Changes in the breasts during pregnancy

Breast development in girls (thelarche) starts about 2 years before menarche, under the influence of ovarian oestrogens, which stimulate the proliferation of the duct system and the accumulation of fat in the breast. Further growth and development of the alveoli of the breast occur during pregnancy. In early pregnancy, the oestrogens stimulate further growth of the ducts. Later on, glucocorticoids from the adrenal, prolactin from the pituitary and placental lactogen, which is a prolactin-like hormone from the placenta, are required for the induction of the enzymes necessary for the production of milk (Fig. 3.7). However, the high oestrogen and progesterone concentrations prevent synthesis of milk proteins and lactation from starting until after delivery, even though the concentration of prolactin is high throughout pregnancy. The number of lactotrophs in the anterior pituitary increases, and prolactin is the only pituitary hormone to be present in sustained high concentrations in the circulation during pregnancy.

The role of the high prolactin concentration in pregnancy is not clear. It may, in part, be important to vitamin D synthesis through the stimulation of the 1α-hydroxylase in the kidney to increase the hydroxylation of 25-hydroxycholecalciferol (Fig. 7.14). Thus, the concentration of calcitriol increases to facilitate calcium absorption and maintain calcium balance during pregnancy and lactation. Prolactin may also be involved in the maintenance of osmolality of fetal fluids, and its concentration is high in amniotic fluid.

The onset of lactation after delivery is made possible by the fall in the circulating concentration of oestrogens and progesterone at parturition, and is dependent on the continued production of prolactin. The ejection of milk in response to suckling requires the action of oxytocin, secreted by the posterior pituitary in response to the suckling reflex. If lactation is maintained, due to the elevated prolactin concentration, the normal cycling of pituitary gonadotrophin release is delayed and fertility is reduced while breast-feeding is continued. Because of this action, prolactin has been referred to as 'Nature's contraceptive'. Even though on an individual basis it is not reliable, globally it forms an important negative regulator of fertility.

Parturition

The gestation of the human fetus is normally about 9 months. The nature of the signal for parturition is still not entirely clear (and may vary in different species), but glucocorticoids from the fetal adrenal gland probably play an important role. The concentration of progesterone falls, and there is an increase in circulating oxytocin (from the posterior pituitary) and of prostaglandins (from the uterus itself). Expulsion of the fetus is dependent on the production of prostaglandins (see Fig. 2.19), which stimulate the early uterine contractions, and on oxytocin (see Fig. 1.4), the release of which increases by positive feedback as the fetus moves down and distends the vagina.

The menopause

The menopause is defined as the time of the last menstrual period, which is usually around 50 years of age. The ovaries gradually cease to function cyclically; this is referred to as the climacteric. Ovarian failure results from exhaustion of primordial follicles, and causes low oestrogen and inhibin production and hence raised concentrations of LH and FSH. Because of the fall in oestradiol production, the vaginal mucosa and mammary glands become atrophic. Characteristic flushing attacks may occur, but the cause of this vasomotor instability is not known. After the menopause, for reasons that are not entirely clear, bone mass declines more rapidly than previously and osteoporosis may develop, due to the reduced production of oestradiol. After the menopause, oestrogen production depends entirely on peripheral aromatization of androstenedione from the adrenal gland to oestrone (Fig. 6.8), which is a weak oestrogen.

Hormone-replacement therapy in the menopausal period can therefore be used. If only oestrogen is given, it produces endometrial hyperplasia, and this increases the risk of a neoplasm developing. Consequently, progesterone should be given as well; this reduces the oestrogen receptors in the target-cell cytoplasm, and increases the activity of oestradiol 17β-dehydrogenase, which inactivates the oestradiol by converting it to oestrone (Fig. 6.8), which has a lower affinity for oestrogen receptors. This form of therapy is given intermittently and produces withdrawal bleeding.

Disturbances of the menstrual cycle

Primary amenorrhoea

If menstruation has not started by the age of 16, the condition of primary amenorrhoea may be said to exist. This may be of no significance, since periods may develop normally later. However, there are a number of other possible causes. For example, the ovaries may be absent, damaged, or rudimentary. If breast development has occurred, there must have been some production of oestrogen and therefore there must have been functional ovaries present; however, if breast development has not occurred, there may be a lack of active ovaries. Primary amenorrhoea can also be caused by depletion of oocytes and follicles because of chromosomal abnormalities, or by deficient functioning of the hypothalamus or pituitary. A defect of gonadotrophin production may be part of a generalized disturbance of the hypothalamus or pituitary, or due to an isolated deficiency of gonadotrophin secretion.

Secondary amenorrhoea

Menstruation usually occurs at intervals of 28–31 days. Pregnancy is, of course, the commonest cause of amenorrhoea but, apart from this, about 2% of women get bouts of amenorrhoea during their reproductive life. The term secondary amenorrhoea is used when an interval of 6 months or more occurs without a period in a girl or woman who has previously had normal periods. There are many causes for secondary amenorrhoea, including, for example, ovarian failure (i.e. a premature menopause), excessive androgen production, pituitary disease (including, particularly, prolonged overproduction of prolactin), disturbances in gonadotrophin production arising from a defect of negative feedback or a failure of initiation of a cyclical release of the gonadotrophins. Measurements of the concentrations of LH and FSH are useful, since if there is no feedback from ovarian secretions, the concentrations of gonadotrophin will be high. Psychiatric disturbance and abnormalities in nutrition can also cause amenorrhoea; these two occur together in bulimia (self-induced vomiting) and anorexia nervosa, of which amenorrhoea is an important feature.

Failure of ovulation. At the beginning and end of reproductive life, i.e. just after the menarche and just before the menopause, it is common for women to have menstrual cycles without ovulation. In some women, failure to ovulate also occurs during the reproductive period of life. In a few women, ovulation occurs rarely because of a lack of positive feedback by oestrogens. Lack of adequate pulsatile secretion of GnRH also causes failure of ovulation. Failure to ovulate may be associated with a short cycle, but is more often associated with irregular or long cycles. In a normal menstrual cycle, the endometrium is stimulated first by oestrogen and then by progesterone, and the breakdown of the endometrium occurs with the fall in the concentration of these steroids. If there is no ovulation, the only stimulus to proliferation of the endometrium is the secretion of oestrogen, and menstrual bleeding is due to oestrogen withdrawal after the nonovulatory follicles have atrophied. This leads to irregular periods. If the intervening time is long, the period may be heavy, particularly in the multiparous woman who is approaching the menopause, because of the relatively large uterus, but the mechanism is identical to the irregular periods of the postmenarcheal teenager.

Detection of ovulation. There are a number of indirect ways of inferring that ovulation has occurred; these depend on the assumption that a corpus luteum has been formed. For example, in the second half of a normal ovulatory cycle, there is a rise in the basal body temperature of about 0.5°C; if the temperature is taken daily before getting out of bed or eating or drinking, a rise in the basal temperature secondary to progesterone secretion (Table 6.1) indicates that ovulation has occurred. Similarly, examination of the vaginal epithelium may give an indication, since under the influence of both oestrogen and progesterone, the vaginal epithelium matures; if the vaginal smears are examined weekly, evidence of ovulation can be obtained. Likewise, if the endometrial mucosa is examined, the finding of a secretory endometrium in the second half of a cycle indicates that progesterone stimulation has occurred and that ovulation has preceded it. More direct evidence that a corpus luteum has formed may be obtained by measurement of progesterone in plasma obtained in the second half of the cycle; it is easier, however, to measure the excretion of a metabolite of progesterone, namely pregnanediol glucuronide, in urine. Easier still, and more direct, is to look at the ovaries, using ultrasound to see follicles and the development of a corpus luteum.

Artificial induction of ovulation. Before attempting to induce ovulation artificially, it is essential to know that the ovary contains ova (i.e. that the patient is not suffering from ovarian failure). If the pituitary is capable of secreting gonadotrophin and the ovary is capable of producing more than basal levels of oestrogen, it is feasible to treat the patient with the drug clomiphene, which acts as an 'antioestrogen' and stimulates the release of gonadotrophin. Clomiphene is in fact a nonsteroid compound that has only a very weak oestrogenic potency. It occupies oestrogen receptors in the hypothalamus, but does not activate the negative-feedback pathway. The net effect is that of an oestradiol deficiency, and GnRH will be secreted. The response to treatment with clomiphene can be followed directly by ultrasound, since before ovulation the diameter of the follicle is 8–10 mm and after treatment it should increase to 20–22 mm in diameter. The response can also be followed indirectly by monitoring body temperature or plasma progesterone.

It is also possible to induce ovulation by administration of gonadotrophins. Two preparations of these are available: human menopausal gonadotrophin, which is extracted from the urine of postmenopausal women and is a mixture of LH and FSH, and HCG, which is isolated from the urine of pregnant women and has predominantly the effects of LH. To induce ovulation, human menopausal gonadotrophin is first given to stimulate many follicles to develop, but caution is needed, since it may produce overstimulation and cyst formation. This is followed by administration of HCG, used to replace the normal midcycle surge in LH production and trigger ovulation. The dose of human menopausal gonadotrophin required to produce a satisfactory response varies from patient to patient, and the response must be monitored. The urinary total oestrogen, oestradiol, or oestrone excretion should be measured during treatment with human menopausal gonadotrophin, and the dose adjusted appropriately. If the response is too small, the dose should be increased, but, if the response is too great, HCG should be withheld because there is then a risk of over-stimulation, multiple ovulation and multiple pregnancy, with attendant dangers. The announcement of the successful delivery and survival of multiple babies usually indicates the outcome of such a medical mistake.

Once a satisfactory response to human menopausal gonadotrophin has been achieved, HCG can be given. Ultrasound scans or measurement of the plasma progesterone or urinary pregnanediol glucuronide excretion can be followed to establish whether ovulation has occurred. In judging the effectiveness of this type of therapy, it should be remembered that, in normal women who have regular intercourse, only 60% will become pregnant within 6 months and 85% within a year. It cannot be expected therefore that artificially induced ovulation will be successful immediately in all cases, and so repeated courses of treatment may be needed.

Administration of GnRH is obviously the treatment of choice in patients whose infertility arises from a hypothalamic defect causing secondary deficiency of pituitary gonadotrophins and consequent hypogonadism. The initial defect can be congenital, because there is a failure of hypothalamic development, which can be associated with a reduced sense of smell (Kallman syndrome). Pulsatile infusion of GnRH to induce ovulation can overcome this hypothalamic–hypopituitary hypogonadism. The object is to induce ovulation from a single follicle, as occurs normally. Pulsatile infusion of synthetic GnRH at a constant frequency (90 min) of a fixed amount of hormone is given to stimulate the pituitary. The ovary can then respond to the change in pituitary gonadotrophin secretions, and the feedback mechanisms will operate normally.

In vitro fertilization (IVF). It is possible to fertilize an oocyte *in vitro*, allow it to divide and then implant it in the uterus, after which pregnancy can follow a normal course. This method is useful when a woman has normal ovulatory cycles but is infertile because her Fallopian tubes are blocked. The likelihood of success is dependent on the number of fertilized ova that are implanted: with one or two, the success rate for a pregnancy concluding in normal delivery is 10–12%, while with implantation of three or four fertilized ova it is 15–20%. The rate of successful fertilization of ova *in vitro* is about 80%, so, to get three or four oocytes fertilized, it is necessary to have five or six available for fertilization. Thus, the immediate aim in inducing ovulation for IVF is different from that of *in vivo* fertilization.

In normal conception, one ovum is produced at a time and it leads to one baby; when ovulation is induced for IVF, again one ovum is all that is needed, although there is a risk of inducing maturation of multiple follicles during hormone therapy. For IVF, the aim is to induce maturation of multiple follicles, to be able to harvest six ova, if possible, in order to get one that matures to a full-term delivery of a single healthy baby. Thus, multiple ovulation has to be induced by high-dose gonadotrophin therapy. The response is followed by ultrasound scans of the ovaries and measurements of oestradiol. With six follicles maturing, there is a proportionately large increase in the amount of oestradiol in the circulation, and this may produce a premature rise in LH and cause premature ovulation. This can be prevented, however, by giving injections of a blocking analogue of GnRH to inhibit pituitary gonadotrophin release. The ova can be collected in a variety of ways, such as laparoscopy or by ultrasound-guided needle aspiration. A third approach is culdoscopy via the back of the vagina. Once the oocytes have been obtained, they are mixed with a washed suspension of sperm and incubated until cleavage is seen under the microscope. The embryos can then be introduced into the uterus through the vagina.

Endocrine regulation of fertility

The 'rhythm-control' or 'safe-period' method of contraception is based on the fact that the ovum, once released, is viable for only about 24 h, and that the sperm do not survive in a state in which they are able to achieve fertilization for more than 2 or 3 days. By avoiding intercourse for 7 days before the expected date of ovulation and 2 days after, there is a reduced prospect of pregnancy. The major difficulty in this method of control is in forecasting the exact time of ovulation, particularly in a woman with irregular menstrual cycles.

The most commonly used oral contraceptive pills contain a progestogen and an oestrogen. Commonly, a fixed daily dose of oestrogen and progestogen is taken for approximately 21 days, followed by a placebo or treatment-free period for 7 days. These preparations act by suppressing the hypothalamic–pituitary axis, depressing the gonadotrophin output and so preventing the maturation of follicles. In addition, the condition of the endometrium remains unsuitable for implantation, and the cervical mucus is not conducive to the passage of sperm, so that even if ovulation occurs, fertilization is less likely to follow. The failure rate of these mixed preparations is 0.08 per 100 woman-years.

These preparations may produce adverse reactions, such as depression, loss of libido, weight gain, mild hypertension and, less commonly, thrombosis, but probably only in women with a genetically determined predisposition to a clotting disorder, most commonly a partial (heterozygote) antithrombin III deficiency. They should not be taken by women who have themselves had thromboses or emboli, or, without careful thought, by women with a family history of such problems. They should be used with caution in patients with severe liver disease or malignant tumours, such as breast cancer, which may be sensitive to oestrogens, or where families have histories of such problems. It should also be noted that, if taken in combination with other drugs, either the contraceptive effect may be reduced or the action of the other drug may be modified.

Another form of oral contraceptive has only a progestogen in low dose to be taken daily. This is less effective, the failure rate being 1.1 per 100 woman-years. In many women, this 'minipill' causes irregular and frequent bleeding, and its mode of action is less certain. Ovulation is not inhibited in all cases, and the major contraceptive action is thought to be a consequence of the unsuitable conditions of the endometrium and cervical mucus.

ABNORMALITIES OF SEXUAL DIFFERENTIATION

With the extended and complex nature of the processes involved in the expression of the true phenotype, which were described previously (Figs 6.1–6.3), it is not surprising that disorders of sexual differentiation occur. Since normal development is a sequential process, failures in fetal life can be recognized in postnatal life by characteristic abnormalities. Some of these are detailed below.

Failure of anti-Müllerian hormone

If testosterone were the only hormone to be produced by the fetal testis, males would also have a vestigial uterus, with the upper two-thirds of the vagina and the Fallopian tubes (Fig. 6.2). A rare familial condition in which this occurs has been identified.

Inadequately masculinized males (male pseudohermaphroditism)

A male pseudohermaphrodite is an individual whose karyotype is XY and whose gonads are exclusively testes, but whose phenotypic characteristics are female to varying degrees. This condition may arise as a result of a number of abnormalities, some of which are described below.

Defects of testosterone biosynthesis

Deficiencies of all the enzymes in the pathway of biosynthesis of testosterone (Fig. 6.6) have been recognized clinically; a consequence can be that testosterone and hence dihydrotestosterone are not synthesized in normal amounts. Since their effects are not all-or-none, but are related to the circulating concentrations, ambiguity of the genitalia occurs.

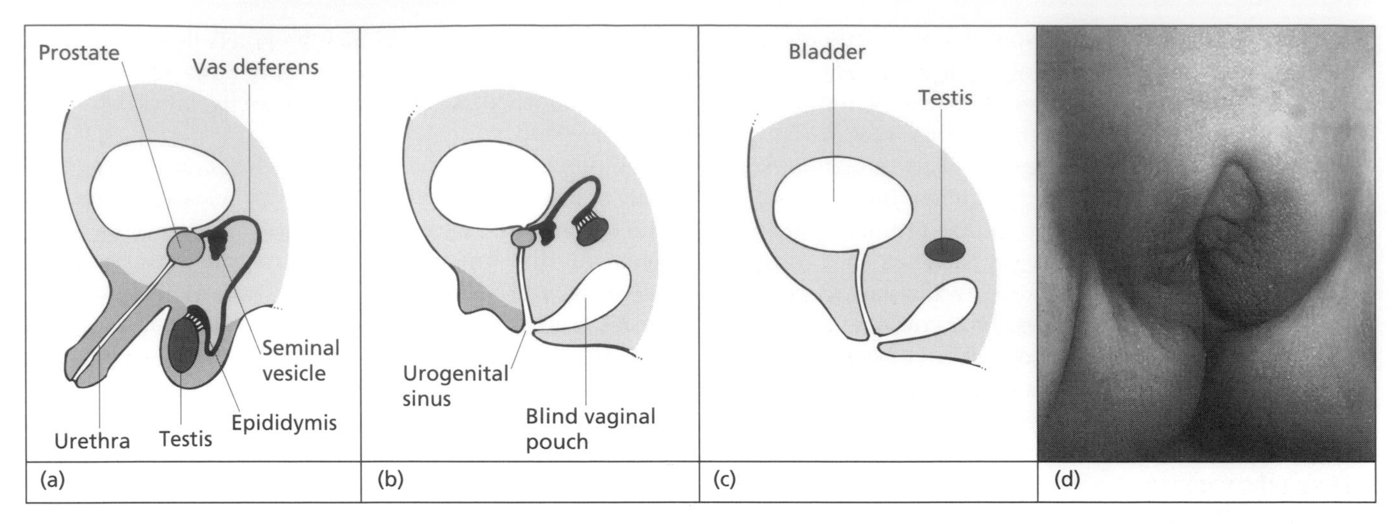

Figure 6.13 The normal male genital tract (a) and the changes that occur in (b) 5α-reductase deficiency and (c) androgen insensitivity. In the enzyme-deficient animal, structures arising from the genital tubercle (dark shading) are absent (e.g. penis), and a blind vaginal pouch is present. In androgen insensitivity syndrome, only the intra-abdominal testis is found. The epididymis, vas deferens, seminal vesicle, prostate and penis are all absent, so the external genitalia are female. (d) Genitalia of a 2-year-old male with 5α-reductase deficiency: note the genital ambiguity and swelling in the left labium due to a descended testis.

End-organ insensitivity

The underlying biochemical failures in two types of end-organ insensitivity have been recognized.

5α-reductase deficiency. These individuals cannot reduce testosterone to its active metabolite, 5α-dihydrotestosterone (Fig. 6.6). As a consequence, they can respond to the limited action of testosterone itself, but will exhibit defects due to the absence of 5α-dihydrotestosterone. Because of a lack of the latter *in utero*, there will be no development of the male external genitalia (Fig. 6.3), and these patients will have a small hypospadiac phallus, in which the urethra usually opens at the base of the phallus, at the junction of the penis and scrotum, and ambiguous female external genitalia (Fig. 6.13). A blind vaginal pouch is present, opening into the urogenital sinus. These patients will, however, develop male internal genitalia, since Wolffian duct development in the fetus is testosterone-dependent (Fig. 6.2). They will have labial testes and all the testosterone-dependent internal structures, but a reduced prostate (Fig. 6.13).

At puberty, there is a rise in testosterone production, and striking virilization occurs. The hypospadiac phallus enlarges as do the testes, which can descend into the labioscrotal folds, and this may be accompanied by spermatogenesis. There will also be increased muscular development and a deepening of the voice, but hair development and production of sebum are impaired. The reason for this virilization, which occurs when the levels of testosterone, but not 5α-dihydrotestosterone, are high, is not yet fully understood. It is possible that the elevated testosterone compensates for the relatively low affinity that this androgen has for the receptor, which would normally bind to, and be activated by, 5α-dihydrotestosterone. Because of the high testosterone, breast development does not occur at puberty in these patients, who appear to change sex at the age of puberty.

The deficiency in 5α-reductase is an autosomally recessive inherited condition. It has been particularly studied by behavioural endocrinologists in rural communities in the Dominican Republic, where the change in gender identity from female to male at puberty appears to be accepted with remarkable equanimity. Patients with this condition need surgery to correct their anatomy early in life, depending on whether or not an adequate phallus is present, and be raised unambiguously either as males or females.

Failure to respond to testosterone (androgen insensitivity). In androgen-insensitive individuals (Table 2.3), the androgen receptor (see Figs 2.21–2.23) is either absent or has an altered amino acid sequence such that it can no longer bind androgens. Defects of the receptors for either testosterone itself or 5α-dihydrotestosterone, or both, can occur and give rise to a spectrum of clinical abnormalities. Despite the defective androgen receptors, AMH will express its local action. An individual who is insensitive to both testosterone and 5α-dihydrotestosterone will thus be born with nonvirilized, female external genitalia (Fig. 6.3). However, due to regression of the Müllerian duct, the upper two-thirds of the vagina will have been obliterated (Fig. 6.2). There will be no uterus or Fallopian tubes. In addition, due to lack of supportive action of testosterone, the Wolffian ducts will also have failed to develop. There will as a consequence be no epididymis, seminal vesicles, or vas deferens (Fig. 6.13c).

These individuals are reared as females, and breasts develop normally at puberty, because there is effectively no testosterone to oppose the oestrogen that is circulating in normal pubertal boys, and which is derived from aromatization of testosterone. This is why the condition used to be called 'testicular feminization'. Pubic and axillary hair is absent because of androgen insensitivity. The patients are tall, because they are genotypically male.

Masculinized females (female pseudohermaphroditism)

A female pseudohermaphrodite has an XX karyotype, and ovaries are present, but there are varying degrees of phenotypic masculinization. There is no abnormality of the ovary or its functional capacity and no abnormality of internal genital development, so reproductive function is often possible after appropriate treatment. Females usually become virilized, as a result of enzyme abnormalities involved in adrenal steroid biosynthesis. In some of the varieties of congenital adrenal hyperplasia, there is excess production of androgens (see Chapter 4), which results in the masculinization of the genitalia of the female fetus.

True hermaphroditism

Only when both female and male gonadal elements can be definitely demonstrated in the same individual can true hermaphroditism be said to exist. The chromosomal pattern may be XX, XY, or a mosaic. There may be a testis on one side of the body and an ovary on the other; more commonly, there is an 'ovotestis' present on one or both sides. The phenotype depends on the number of Leydig cells; the amount of testosterone such gonads produce at puberty is inadequate for a male but excessive for a female. Thus, at puberty, a 'male' patient may develop gynaecomastia, or a 'female' may develop excessive body hair.

Effect of abnormal exposure to hormones *in utero*

Exposure to androgens before week 12 of pregnancy leads to fusion of the labia (scrotalization) of a female fetus. This occurs classically in congenital adrenal hyperplasia, but it can also result from secretion of androgens from a maternal (usually adrenal) tumour or through ingestion of androgenic (anabolic) steroids. Oestrogen administration can also have serious effects. In the late 1950s, diethylstilboestrol (a synthetic compound that has oestrogenic activity, even though it does not have a steroid nucleus) was used in an attempt to improve the prognosis of pregnancy in diabetic patients, because the morbidity and mortality in infants of diabetic mothers are considerable. This treatment had no effect on the outcome of pregnancy, but it became apparent that some of the daughters of mothers who had been treated in this way developed a carcinoma of the vagina when they were about 20 years old. Similar changes could be reproduced in rats treated with diethylstilboestrol early in pregnancy; neoplastic change subsequently developed at the time of puberty. In other words, there were two endocrine events in the development of this tumour, the first *in utero* and the second at the time of puberty, and if puberty was prevented in the rats, neoplasms did not develop.

OUTLINE OF BIOCHEMICAL TESTS OF THE HYPOTHALAMIC–PITUITARY–GONADAL AXIS

Immunoassays are routinely used on a large scale to measure both gonadal steroids and also the glycoprotein gonadotrophins secreted from the anterior pituitary. As discussed in Appendix 1, 'competitive' ligand-binding assays are used for the steroids, whereas immunometric, 'sandwich' assays are used for the glycoproteins. Immunometric assays are also used to measure serum prolactin levels. This can be highly relevant, since hyperprolactinaemia is both a common endocrine abnormality and an important cause of infertility in both sexes, due to its perturbation of the pulsatility of GnRH.

Both androgens and oestrogens bind to binding proteins in the circulation: 97% of testosterone and oestradiol are normally protein-bound. For testosterone, the principal binding protein is sex-hormone–binding globulin (SHBG), but SHBG has a lower affinity for oestradiol. One consequence of the difference in the affinities is that a decrease in SHBG preferentially increases free testosterone more than free oestradiol, and thus is androgenic. Conversely a rise in SHBG, which may occur because of apparently unrelated conditions such as hyperthyroidism or liver cirrhosis, causes a lack of androgen effect. This can account for breast development (gynaecomastia) in males with these conditions. Although in most circumstances we rely on measurements of total steroid levels (i.e. free and bound), which can be obtained by chemical dissociation of the steroids from their binding proteins prior to their immunoassay, it can be important to monitor binding-protein concentrations.

Disorders in the male

It is clearly important to distinguish between primary hypogonadism, which may be due to malfunction of either Leydig cells or seminiferous tubules or both, from secondary hypogonadism. The latter may be due to pituitary or hypothalamic disease. Primary hypogonadism would typically be indicated by decreased levels in testosterone and increases in circulating LH and/or FSH, whereas decreases in the gonadotrophins together with testosterone would be indicative of secondary hypogonadism. With the gonadotrophins, a rise in only LH concentrations may be associated with impaired Leydig-cell function, whereas a rise in only FSH could indicate seminiferous-tubule defects.

Clear discrimination may be obtained by dynamic function tests. For example, intramuscular HCG, which has actions that are similar to LH, should stimulate testosterone levels in a normal male but will not do so in a patient with primary hypogonadism due to Leydig-cell failure. Subcutaneous GnRH will stimulate LH and FSH production from a patient with a hypothalamic lesion, while a diminished or absent response is seen with a pituitary lesion.

Disorders in the female

In females, the measurement of oestradiol and gonadotrophin concentrations differentiates primary hypogonadism, due to ovarian failure, from secondary hypogonadism, due to either pituitary or hypothalamic dysfunction. The natural fluctuation in oestrogen secretion makes measurements of oestradiol less useful than those of gonadotrophins. Ovarian failure is indicated when raised LH and particularly FSH are detected, whereas decreased levels are seen with a pituitary or hypothalamic lesion. Dynamic function tests, testing the capability of the pituitary or hypothalamus to respond to provocation, play an important role in differential diagnosis.

Hormone measurements are also valuable for the investigation of hirsutism and virilization in women. For example, one of the commonest causes of hirsutism, namely the polycystic ovary syndrome, will be associated with a marginal elevation in testosterone and a low FSH but an increased LH. A ratio of LH : FSH of 3 or greater during the early follicular phase of the menstrual cycle is particularly characteristic of this condition, which is the commonest reproductive disorder in women. Genetic studies suggest that premature baldness is the male phenotype. Substantial elevation of testosterone levels, together with the adrenal androgens DHEA sulphate and androstenedione, with additional features of virilization, such as clitoromegaly, suggests the presence of an adrenal tumour. High levels of 17α-hydroxyprogesterone are characteristic of congenital adrenal hyperplasia (Chapter 4).

The early rise in circulating HCG and its detection in urine forms the basis for pregnancy testing. These tests rely on antibodies that are directed against the hormonally specific β-subunit of HCG and may be either in the form of highly quantitative immunometric assays (see Appendix 1) or adapted as slide or tube tests based on the inhibition of the adhesion of coated latex particles. A significant rise in β-HCG can be detected as early as 6 days after conception if measured in blood, and after 14 days in urine.

CHAPTER 7

Calcium Regulation

SUMMARY

Maintenance of calcium homoeostasis is important for all cells, not merely for the skeleton. During growth, calcium balance is positive. In adult life, there is an equilibrium between absorption from the gut and loss through urine. This is regulated by parathyroid hormone, vitamin D and possibly calcitonin. Parathyroid hormone acts primarily on bone and kidney. Vitamin D is also a hormone, the active form of which is calcitriol (1,25-dihydroxycholecalciferol), which is produced in the kidney and acts largely on the gut to increase absorption of calcium.

INTRODUCTION

Rickets, a childhood bone disease that causes softening and bending of the bones, was clearly described in the seventeenth century. It was subsequently found that fish-liver oil, exposure of patients to sunlight, or even irradiation of certain foods prior to their consumption could cure both rickets in children and the corresponding adult condition, osteomalacia. This was explained by the realization that the irradiation could yield vitamin D, in skin and also in food, and that this vitamin is present in fish-liver oil. Vitamin D, which is a collective term for a group of related compounds, is important for maintaining the absorption of calcium from the gut.

Two other factors, parathyroid hormone (PTH) and calcitonin, also control serum calcium. PTH, which raises serum calcium, is produced from the parathyroid glands, which are attached to, but separate from, the thyroid. Calcitonin, which lowers serum calcium, is secreted by specialized cells located within the thyroid gland. These cells, the C-cells, are functionally and morphologically distinct from the thyroid follicular cells, which secrete thyroid hormones.

CALCIUM IN THE BODY

Calcium is an important intracellular and extracellular ion, which makes up a major component of the skeleton and is needed for blood clotting and for the activity of many enzyme systems. Within the cell, calcium varies from 0.1 to 1 μM, although there can be sudden pulses of an impressive magnitude, as for example pass across the oocyte after it has been penetrated by a sperm. In interstitial fluid, calcium is much higher, e.g. 1.5 mM, and in blood is higher still, e.g. 2.5 mM. Movement of calcium across cell membranes occurs all the time, and change in flux is an important event, with physiological consequences. The importance of changes in calcium within the cell, acting as a 'messenger', for hormones was described in Chapter 2. Release of calcium within the cell can be an important intracellular signal—leading, for example, to activation of secretion processes or to muscular contraction. Even small alterations in extracellular calcium concentration affect the excitability of cells, and a low serum calcium concentration—hypocalcaemia—can lead to epilepsy or tetany.

The concentration of calcium in extracellular fluid is closely controlled. In human serum, it is normally 2.2–2.6 mmol/L. This calcium exists in three forms: approximately 44% is bound to albumin and so is not readily diffusible, about 9% is complexed to citrate and the remainder (≈1.3 mmol/L), the most important fraction, is uncomplexed ionized calcium. The importance of ionized calcium in the circulation can be illustrated by considering the effects of overbreathing. This can cause tetany because of a fall in the ionized calcium concentration in serum. This results from the disturbance of the following equilibria:

$$CO_2 + H_2O \rightleftharpoons H_2CO_3^-$$
$$H_2CO_3 \rightleftharpoons H^+ + HCO_3^-$$
$$\text{Protein} - H \rightleftharpoons \text{Protein}^- + H^+$$
$$\text{Protein}^- + Ca^{2+} \rightleftharpoons \text{Protein} - Ca$$

With a fall in the partial pressure of carbon dioxide ($P\text{co}_2$), there is alkalosis, due to a decrease in H^+ production from H_2CO_3. Hydrogen ions consequently dissociate from albumin to compensate. This leads to increased binding of calcium ions to the protein, so that the ionized calcium concentration is decreased. This can be sufficient to induce clinical features of hypocalcaemia, such as tetany. Initially, there will be no change in the total calcium concentration, but in chronic alkalosis ionized calcium levels may be restored to normal by homeostatic mechanisms, and under these circumstances, total calcium concentration will rise. Despite the physiological importance of ionized calcium, it is total serum calcium that is generally measured, since measurement of ionized calcium is difficult.

Calcium balance

There is continuous exchange of calcium between different sites in the body (sometimes called 'calcium pools'), and a balance between these various sites is usually maintained. There is a total of about 1 kg of calcium in the adult body, and about 99% of it is in bone, in the form of hydroxyapatite, $3Ca_3(PO_4)_2 \cdot Ca(OH)_2$. Thus, outside bone, there is only about 10 g of calcium available for other cellular processes in the body.

In the adult, an equilibrium is reached between absorption and excretion (Fig. 7.1). Dietary intake provides about 25 mmol (that is, 1 g) of calcium; intestinal secretions add another 7 mmol of calcium to the contents of the intestinal lumen, and only part of the calcium in the lumen is absorbed into the bloodstream. Absorption is balanced by the renal loss of calcium, which ranges between 3 and 7 mmol in 24 h. Calcium excreted in the urine is only a small proportion (about 2 or 3%) of the calcium that is filtered through the glomeruli, since the majority is absorbed by the renal tubules. In growing children, there is calcium retention, and intestinal absorption of calcium exceeds renal excretion by about 10 mmol/day to provide for the needs of the skeleton.

Regulation of calcium balance within the body is closely associated with that of phosphate, although regulation of the latter is rather less precise. The normal range of serum phosphate in adults lies between 0.6 and 1.3 mmol/L, but it is higher in children. A higher proportion of dietary phosphate is absorbed than is the case for calcium, and so urinary excretion, which depends on the phosphate intake, can vary from 15 to 50 mmol/24 h, varying especially with meat intake. A gene on the short arm of the X chromosome is important in the renal regulation of phosphate excretion.

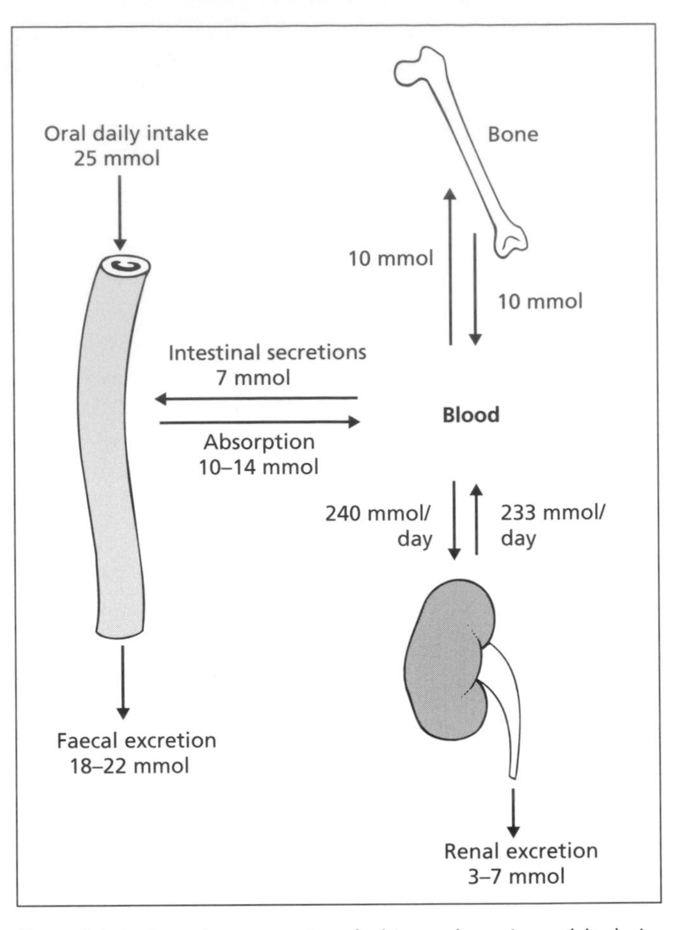

Figure 7.1 A schematic representation of calcium exchange in an adult who is in calcium balance. The daily net absorption from the gut (total absorption less intestinal secretion) equals urinary loss. In contrast, in a growing child, net absorption exceeds renal excretions, to allow for retention of calcium in the skeleton, and so the child is in positive calcium balance.

REGULATION OF CALCIUM

Mineral metabolism can be regulated by alteration in bone turnover, by changes in absorption from the diet and by alteration of renal excretion. These homeostatic mechanisms are controlled by PTH and vitamin D.

Bone

Function, composition and morphology

Bone supports the body and protects vital organs, including brain and bone marrow. It also acts as a reservoir of calcium and phosphate, and can contribute towards acid–base regulation (through phosphate and carbonate). In childhood and early adult life, the skeleton is growing, but in later life, and especially after the menopause, there is an overall loss of bone.

Apart from calcium, the skeleton contains about 90% of the body's phosphate, 50% of its magnesium and 33% of its sodium. It is a hard, calcified connective tissue consisting of cells (osteoprogenitor cells, osteoblasts, osteocytes and osteoclasts) and a calcified extracellular matrix. The constituents of the matrix will vary in relative amounts according to the particular bone type and the age, sex and species from which it has come. In general, the inorganic or mineral component accounts for 65% of the bone's weight, while the organic constituents, such as collagen fibres, make up the rest. As there are relatively few cells per unit mass of bone, they make a negligible contribution to bone mass. Collagen accounts for 90–95% of the organic matrix of bone; the rest is made up of proteoglycans, glycoproteins, sialoproteins and a small amount of lipid. Osteocalcin accounts for 1–2% of the protein in bone; it is also called 'bone Gla-protein' because it contains γ-carboxyglutamic acid. This can bind hydroxyapatite with high affinity (1 mg of osteocalcin binds 17 mg of hydroxyapatite). Osteocalcin is also found in plasma, and since this osteocalcin is derived from newly formed bone, it can be used as an index of osteoblast activity. Osteonectin is a glycoprotein found in the bone matrix. It can bind collagen and hydroxyapatite, and *in vitro* it can facilitate calcification of type 1 collagen, so it may be important *in vivo* as a mineral nucleator.

Osteoblasts. Osteoblasts play an important role in calcium homeostasis. They are cells with the ultrastructural features of active protein-synthesizing cells (i.e. numerous polyribosomes, an extensive rough endoplasmic reticulum and a large Golgi complex). Osteoblasts synthesize the organic constituents of bone (osteoid), and are subsequently involved in the mineralization (i.e. calcification) of the newly secreted osteoid. The precursors of osteoblasts are fibroblast-like cells. These proliferating osteoprogenitor cells appear on bone surfaces and differentiate into osteoblasts. Mineralization of osteoid initially occurs rapidly (60–70% is completed within 6–12 h of initiation), but secondary mineralization takes 1–2 months.

Once osteoblasts have completed their function in matrix formation, they become surrounded by the new matrix, and change into relatively inactive cells called osteocytes. These make contact with their neighbours by means of cytoplasmic processes, which lie in tiny channels within the matrix called canaliculi. The canaliculi are in continuity with the extracellular spaces of the Haversian canals, in which lies the blood supply of the bone. Thus, the canaliculi provide the means by which osteocytes get their nutrients, eliminate their unwanted products of metabolism and receive hormonal stimulation. Osteoblasts play an important role in calcium homoeostasis.

Collagen. Collagen synthesis occurs on the rough endoplasmic reticulum of osteoblasts (Fig. 7.2), where a large molecule, procollagen, is assembled. This consists of three polypeptide chains organized in an ahelical conformation. Once translocated into the lumen of the rough endoplasmic reticulum, post-translational modifications to this larger molecule occur to yield the final smaller molecule of collagen in the extracellular space, after the procollagen has been extruded into it by exocytosis.

Collagen is rich in the amino acids glycine, proline and hydroxyproline, and has the general formula (glycine–proline.X)$_{333}$, where X is another amino acid. Extracellular collagen has a molecular weight of about 300 000. It is a semirigid, rod-like molecule approximately 300 nm long and 1.5 nm in diameter. These rod-like collagen molecules polymerize in a highly specific manner extracellularly, with like ends orientated in the same direction. Adjoining linear aggregates of collagen molecules are staggered with respect to one another, at positions that are approximately one-fourth to one-fifth of their length (Fig. 7.2), and are held firmly together by intermolecular cross-linkages. Linear arrays or bundles of collagen molecules form a microfibril, and several microfibrils aggregate to form a collagen fibril. The 'hole zone' between the end of one tropocollagen molecule and the next becomes filled with calcium salts during the process of calcification, as do the spaces between the microfibrils. Both collagen and its associated proteoglycans probably contribute to the initiation of hydroxyapatite crystallization by epitaxy, holding the components of the apatite in position so that the process of 'seeding' can start.

During bone formation, the calcified matrix and especially the collagen fibres are laid down as either compact or woven bone.

1 In compact bone, a series of concentric lamellae with a central blood vessel form a Haversian system or osteone. This lamellar bone is found in the cortex of adult long bones, and it is relatively inert metabolically.

2 In woven bone, the collagen fibres are in the form of loosely woven bundles. Spongy (cancellous) and trabecular bones are made up of woven bone, and are found, for example, in young subjects and at fracture sites. Loosely woven bundles also occur on the endosteal surfaces of

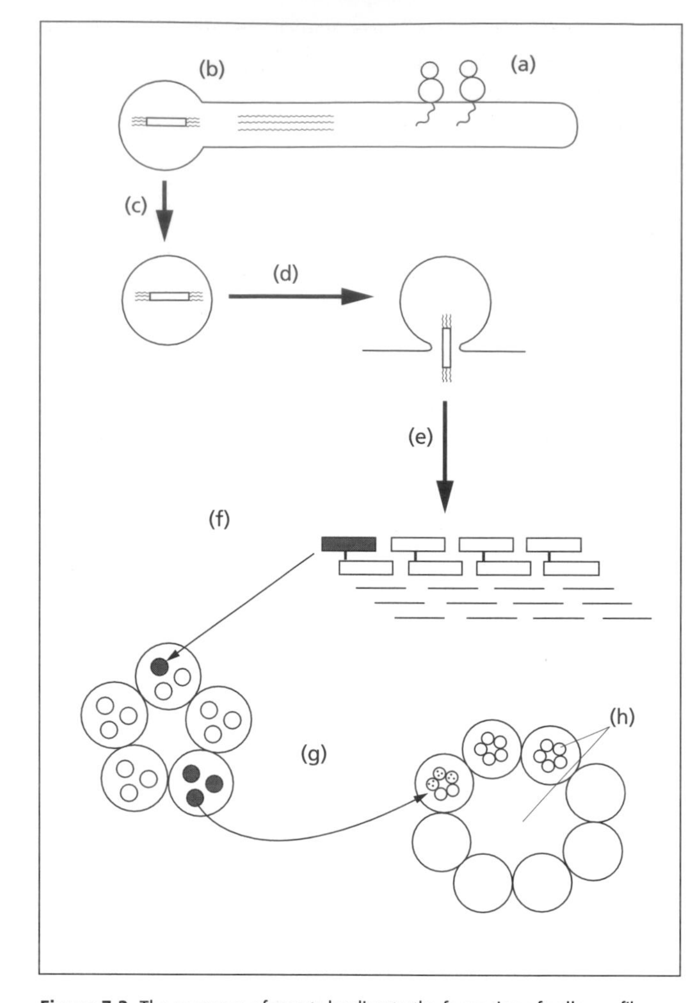

Figure 7.2 The sequence of events leading to the formation of collagen fibres in a fibroblast and the process of osteoid mineralization. (a) Ribosomes attached to the endoplasmic reticulum translate messenger ribonucleic acid (mRNA) for collagen, and polypeptide chains are translocated into the lumen of the endoplasmic reticulum. (b) Three polypeptide chains align and then helically coil, except for the extension peptides, to form procollagen. (c) The procollagen molecule is processed into a secretory vesicle, probably through the Golgi complex. (d) Procollagen is released from the osteoblast by exocytosis, and the collagen molecule is formed after scission of the extension peptides. (e) Linear and side-to-side alignment of collagen molecules by cross-bridges results in the formation of microfibrils. Hole zones are found between the ends of a linear array of collagen molecules. (f) Cross-section of five linear aggregates of collagen, forming a microfibril. (g) Several microfibrils align to form a collagen fibril. (h) During mineralization of osteoid, the hole zones and the spaces between the collagen microfibrils and fibrils become filled with calcium hydroxyapatite crystals. Alkaline phosphatase secreted by the osteoblasts causes calcium phosphate complexes to precipitate, leading to the formation of the hydroxyapatite.

medullary long bones and in some bone disorders, e.g. hyperparathyroidism. Usually large numbers of osteocytes are present, which is indicative of high rates of bone turnover.

Osteoclasts. The other main cell type in bone is the osteoclast. These are large multinucleated cells formed by fusion of mononuclear phagocytes from bone marrow. Osteoclasts appear on the surfaces of bone which is subsequently resorbed, especially under the stimulation of PTH. The role of the osteoclast in the resorption and remodelling of bone is well established: they appear to break down bone components through the action of lysosomal enzymes, which they release extracellularly.

PTH controls calcium levels of the body fluid, principally by regulating the removal of calcium from bone. In mammals, elevations of plasma calcium levels occur several hours after PTH administration. PTH also increases osteoclast numbers and activity both *in vivo* and *in vitro*. However, these effects are usually noted long after the changes in plasma calcium levels have occurred, leading to the belief that, in mammals at least, osteoclasts are not rapidly responsive to PTH and perhaps are not involved in the acute regulation of calcium metabolism. The situation appears to be different in birds, where, during egg-laying, administration of PTH induces functionally active osteoclasts within 20 min and at the same time causes a marked increase in the plasma concentration of calcium. Calcitonin reduces osteoclast activity.

Interference with any of the above processes (the synthesis and secretion of osteoid constituents, eventual mineralization or resorption and remodelling) can lead to profound changes in bone structure and growth.

Bone growth and remodelling

In the young, bone is growing—i.e. it increases in size, particularly in length. Apart from formation of new bone, there is remodelling of existing bone, so that its formation and reabsorption are coupled (Fig. 7.3). In the adult, bone remodelling and turnover continue, but at a slower rate. In females, particularly after the menopause, resorption can exceed formation, so that bone mass then becomes reduced.

A number of factors interact to regulate the balance of bone turnover. These include local factors (both chemical and mechanical) and hormonal factors. For example, PTH stimulates the production of growth factors, such as insulin-like growth factor II (IGF-II), from human osteoblasts. These can act immediately as paracrine stimulators of neighbouring osteoblasts. In addition, they can be stored in the bone matrix and released later by bone resorption. The finding that bone is a storehouse for growth factors suggests that they are important determinants of local bone formation. Osteoblasts also produce osteoclast-activating factors, which act locally.

The early action of PTH in stimulating bone resorption is thus indirect, through activation of osteoblasts (Fig. 7.3). There are probably several osteoclast-activating factors,

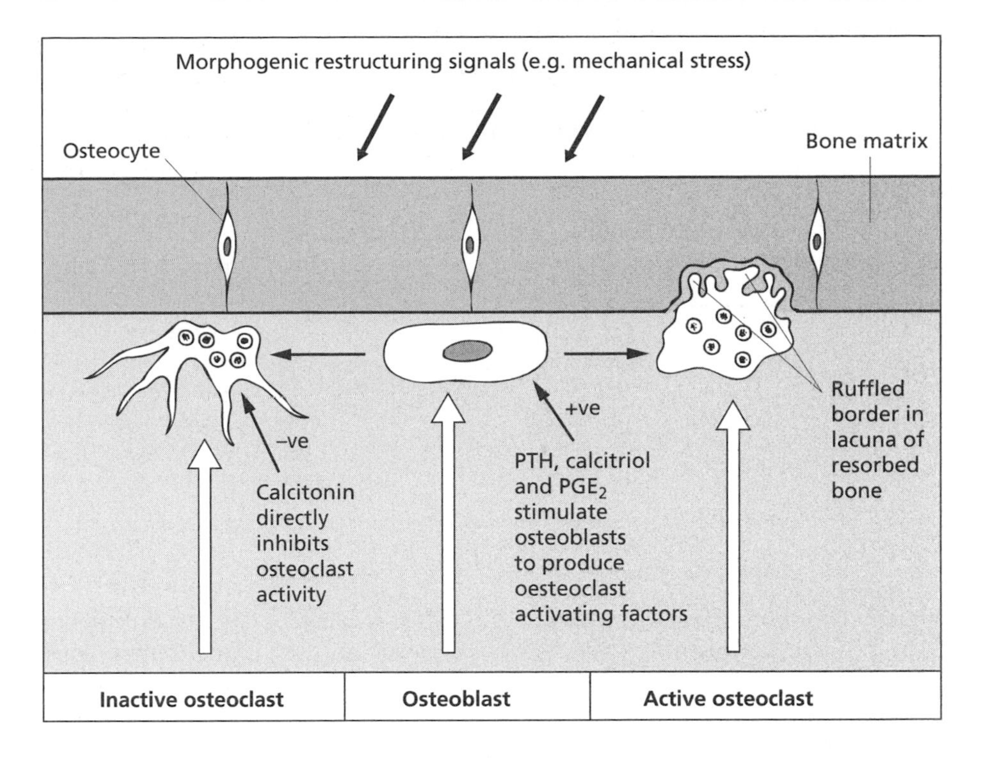

Figure 7.3 Factors that affect the remodelling of bone. Morphogenic restructuring signals such as mechanical stress can influence bone remodelling, while hormone factors control osteoblast activity. Calcitonin has an inhibitory action, with formation of an inactive osteoclast. Parathyroid hormone (PTH), calcitriol and prostaglandin E_2 (PGE_2) act on the osteoblast to produce osteoclast-activating factors that stimulate bone-matrix resorption by osteoclasts. Other hormones, such as thyroid hormones, can increase osteoclast activity.

including interleukin-1, the production of which is stimulated by PTH. The turnover of bone and its regulation are important to calcium homoeostasis at all ages. Thus, if the parathyroid gland is removed in adult humans, serum calcium falls within 48 h. This is because the return of calcium to the circulation is reduced, since there is a reduction in bone resorption.

The parathyroid glands

Development and morphology

In the human, there are usually four parathyroid glands, but there may be additional accessory glands. They are small, lentil-sized glands, and each weighs 40–60 mg; they are usually larger in women than in men. They lie on the posterior surface of the thyroid, between its capsule and the surrounding cervical sheath. An important point to be noted is that variations in number, size and location of the parathyroids are common; this is a consequence of the embryological development of the parathyroids (see Chapter 5). Both the regularly occurring and accessory glands may be situated at some distance from the gland's normal location. It has been estimated that in humans about one in 10 glands is aberrant; they may be found down in the mediastinum or high up in the neck, but can also be found in the thyroid itself or, sometimes, posterior to the oesophagus. This is relevant to a surgeon seeking to remove overactive parathyroid tissue.

There is a rich blood supply to the glands, derived mainly from the inferior thyroid arteries, but also occasionally from the superior thyroid vessels. The venous drainage is via the superior, middle and inferior thyroid veins. Numerous lymphatics are present in the gland, and although the sympathetic innervation derives from the superior and middle cervical ganglia, there is no secretomotor supply to the glandular tissue.

In humans, each gland is surrounded by a thin connective-tissue capsule, from which septa pass into its substance. The principal cell type is the 'chief', which is responsible for the synthesis and secretion of PTH. The cells are arranged in irregular, anastomosing cords and sheets or occasional acini, separated by vascular channels. After puberty, fat cells appear within the parenchyma, and in older people they may make up 60–70% of the volume of the gland.

Parathyroid hormone

This is made up of a single chain of 84 amino acids. The whole sequence of the molecule is not necessary for expression of full biological activity. The amino-terminal portion is the important part. A synthetic peptide has been made which comprises the first 34 residues of the intact molecule. This one-third fragment of PTH has full biological activity, and can increase not only serum calcium concentrations, but also urinary excretion of phosphate—that is, produce phosphaturia.

PTH is synthesized as a larger molecule, and two

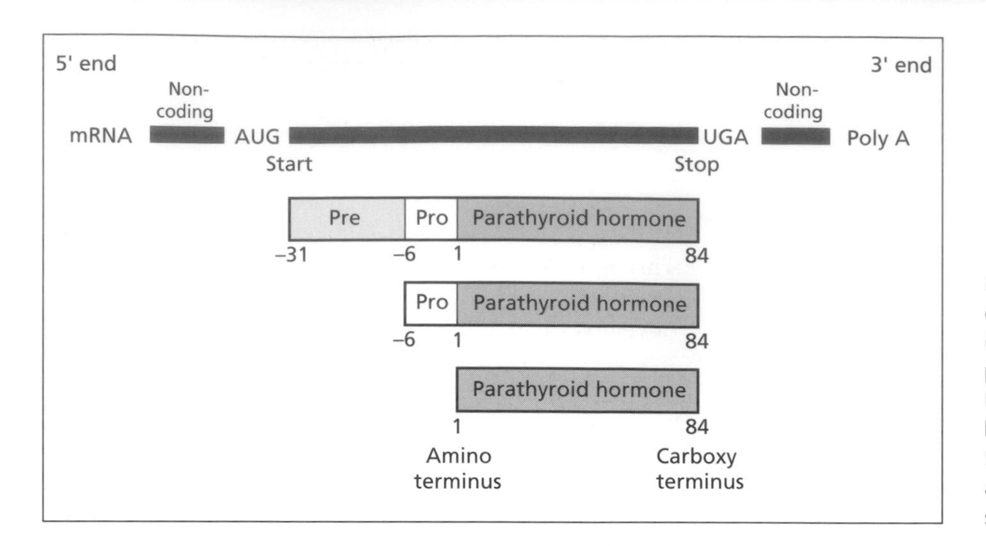

Figure 7.4 Messenger ribonucleic acid (mRNA) codes for the synthesis of parathyroid hormone (PTH), which begins with creation of a signal peptide with 25 amino acids, –31 to –6, of prepro-PTH. The signal peptide is normally removed before synthesis of the hormone is completed. Pro-PTH has 90 amino acids, the first six of which are removed before the 1–84 hormone is secreted.

precursor forms have been identified (Fig. 7.4). The smaller of these is called pro-PTH, and has been identified in extracts of parathyroid glands, although it is probably not secreted. Its existence illustrates the general phenomenon (see Chapter 1) that secreted proteins (including hormones) are synthesized in larger precursor forms. PTH is routinely measured in blood by immunoassay.

Rapid changes in the secretion of PTH can occur, indicating that it is not dependent on *de novo* synthesis, but relies on the release of stored hormone, or possibly changes in the metabolism of the hormone within the parathyroid cell, which can break down the peptide hormone that it has synthesized. Accelerated or slowed breakdown of PTH would alter the amount available for secretion.

Actions of PTH. PTH regulates the concentration of both calcium and phosphate in blood. The rise in serum calcium concentration after administration of PTH is due in part to the direct effect of the hormone on bone, where it increases resorption. PTH also has a direct effect on the renal excretion of calcium, the net effect on the kidneys being a composite one. On the one hand, there may be a rise in renal excretion because of a greater filtered load induced by hypercalcaemia itself. On the other, PTH stimulates the reabsorption of calcium in the tubules and this will reduce excretion. The overall effect of the PTH on urinary excretion of calcium is thus variable, depending upon the relative magnitude of the two effects. PTH also causes phosphaturia, leading to a lowering of serum phosphate and a consequent rise in serum calcium.

In both bone and kidney, the effects of PTH are the result of hormone binding to G-protein–linked cell-surface receptors (see Figs 2.1 and 2.12). Activation of adenylate cyclase follows (see Fig. 2.13), and cyclic adenosine 5′-monophosphate (cAMP) appears to be the dominant intracellular second messenger (see Fig. 2.12). In bone, the hormone binds to osteoblasts, whereas in contrast, calcitonin binds to osteoclasts (Fig. 7.3). Calcitriol probably has a permissive effect on PTH actions on osteoblasts. In the kidney, binding of PTH occurs to multiple cell types, but specific competitive binding occurs at the cell membrane of the primary foot processes of glomerular podocytes and at the antiluminal surface of all three segments of the proximal tubule. The effect of PTH on adenylate cyclase in the renal tubules can be used as the basis of an *in vitro* bioassay; for this, isolated cell membranes from the renal cortex are used.

When cAMP production is stimulated by PTH *in vivo*, some of it escapes from the cell and the concentration of cAMP in blood and urine rises. This elevation of cAMP in blood arises largely from an action of the hormone on the kidney; this can be shown by following the appearance of cAMP in the renal vein, where its concentration rises more rapidly and to a higher value than elsewhere. The increase in renal excretion of cAMP is due to a direct excretion into the renal tubules, although a small part may also be due to the increased filtered load attributable to the rise in circulating cAMP. It should be noted that there is no known biological role for the cAMP that appears in blood and in urine, its principal function being as an intracellular messenger. The extracellular changes in cAMP serve, however, as a marker of the intracellular events. The changes in cAMP precede all other responses that follow the administration of PTH. In humans, the changes in cAMP in plasma and urine occur within minutes, while phosphate excretion does not alter for a few hours (Fig. 7.5), and repeated injections of PTH may be needed over 2–3 days before there are significant shifts in serum calcium concentrations.

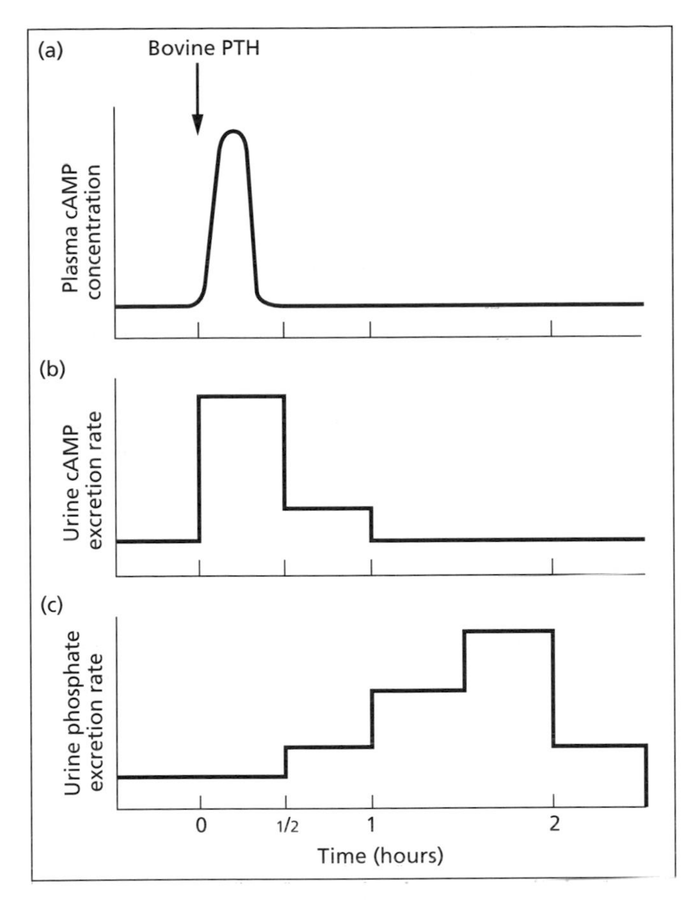

Figure 7.5 Injection of parathyroid hormone (PTH) intravenously in humans increases the activity of renal adenylate cyclase. Some of the cyclic adenosine 5′-monophosphate (cAMP) produced appears in blood (a) and urine (b). The phosphaturic response (c) then follows.

Control of the secretion of PTH. Secretion of PTH occurs continuously to maintain its concentration in the circulation, from which it is cleared rapidly, with a half-life of about 5 min. Since PTH is important in the regulation of calcium and phosphate metabolism, it might be expected that both of these would affect the activity of the parathyroid glands, possibly through feedback mechanisms. The most important regulator in the secretion of PTH is the serum calcium concentration (Fig. 7.6). The calcium receptor is also a G-protein-linked, 7-pass receptor on the surface of the chief cells in the parathyroid gland. It is linked to phospholipase C (see Fig. 2.1). It has an exceptionally long ectodomain (see Chapter 2). Hypercalcaemia suppresses secretion, while hypocalcaemia (which can be produced by administration of an agent such as ethylenediamine tetra-acetic acid (EDTA), which complexes calcium ions) stimulates secretion. The secretion of PTH is proportional to the degree of hypocalcaemia (Fig. 7.7). Magnesium is important for the release of PTH, and this is one of the reasons why the premature baby, who often has hypomagnesaemia, becomes hypocalcaemic.

Effects of oversecretion of PTH. Excessive PTH causes hypercalcaemia and phosphaturia. This is most commonly due to a benign tumour of one of the four parathyroid glands, although sometimes it is due to hyperplasia of all four. This is called primary hyperparathyroidism, to distinguish it from the secondary overactivity of the glands that develops in an attempt to compensate for long-standing hypocalcaemia, which can occur, for example, because of malabsorption of calcium. Secondary hyperparathyroidism can also be caused by chronic renal failure, when there will be a decreased synthesis of calcitriol. In addition, tertiary hyperparathyroidism can develop in a patient given a renal transplant. Patients with end-stage renal failure can occasionally become hypercalcaemic due to the development of autonomous PTH secretion, which is associated with prolonged hypocalcaemia. In such a patient, PTH secretion will remain elevated even after renal transplantation and restoration of renal calcitriol metabolism.

Primary hyperparathyroidism causes subperiosteal resorption of bone. Sometimes this is so extensive that it leads to cyst formation, with development of a so-called 'brown tumour', for example in the skull or pelvis. Bone disease, causing bone pain and difficulty in walking is the major feature in only about 15% of patients with primary hyperparathyroidism. However, abnormal bone histology can be found in most cases of primary hyperparathyroidism.

Renal calculi are much more common than bone disease, occurring in half of the patients with hyperparathyroidism. The renal stones are made of calcium and phosphate and hence are radiopaque. The stone formation is presumably due to long-standing hypercalcaemia and hypercalciuria (increased urinary excretion of calcium), although the latter feature does not occur in all patients. The stones develop in the calyces of the kidney and may move down the ureter, thereby causing renal colic; blood in the urine (haematuria) and recurrent infections of the renal tract (pyelonephritis) are consequences of the presence of stones. The kidneys may be damaged by the presence of renal calculi, which may even lead to renal failure if untreated. Hypercalcaemia *per se* can also impair renal function, leading to thirst and polyuria.

Treatment of primary hyperparathyroidism is by surgery, with removal of the overactive parathyroid. However, patients whose calcium is only mildly elevated and who are devoid of symptoms of hypercalcaemia and suffer no renal impairment may remain healthy for many years without treatment. A high fluid intake should be maintained to discourage kidney stone formation.

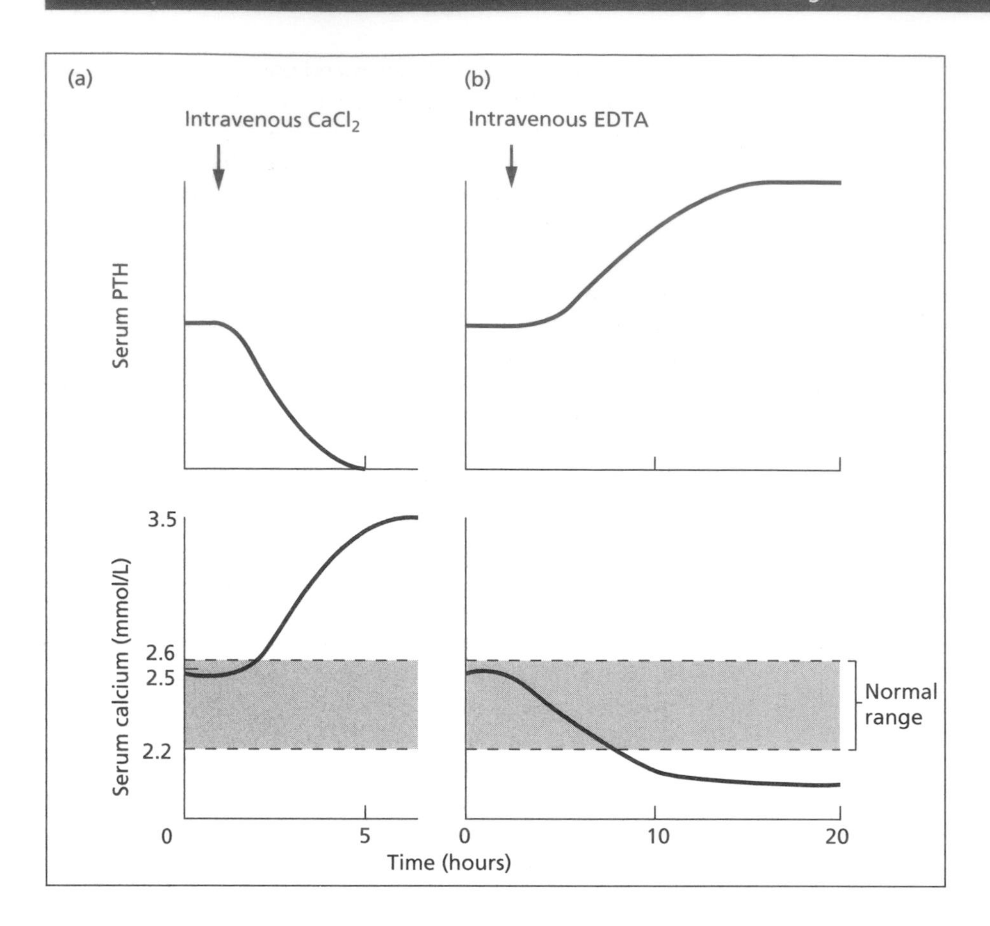

Figure 7.6 Changes in parathyroid hormone (PTH) secretion in response to alterations in serum calcium. (a) Rise in serum calcium reduces the secretion of PTH; this can be produced by infusion of calcium. (b) Conversely, a fall in serum calcium, produced by infusing ethylenediamine tetra-acetic acid (EDTA), which complexes calcium, stimulates PTH secretion.

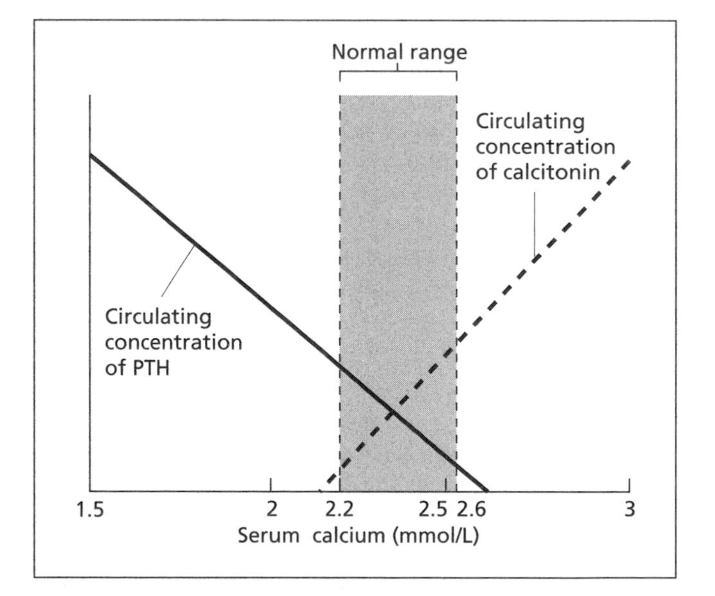

Figure 7.7 Calcitonin secretion is stimulated by a rise in serum calcium, which suppresses secretion of parathyroid hormone (PTH). Conversely, hypocalcaemia stimulates PTH release and reduces calcitonin.

Because the parathyroid tumour may be embedded within the thyroid, tucked away behind the oesophagus or down in the mediastinum within the thymus, it is desirable to locate the overactive parathyroid gland pre-operatively. Isotopic imaging with ^{201}Tl, which is avidly concentrated in parathyroid tissue, may help locate the tumour, but the best means of doing this is by parathyroid venous sampling. In this technique, blood is taken from different points in the venous tree by cannulation of veins in the neck, and the hormone content is measured (Fig. 7.8). The pattern of distribution of the hormone from different positions in the neck can indicate the probable location of the tumour, especially if samples have been taken from the superior, middle and inferior thyroid veins into which the parathyroid venous effluent drains.

Effects of undersecretion of PTH. Lack of PTH causes hypocalcaemia and hyperphosphataemia. The clinical effects are an increased excitability of nervous tissue, causing paraesthesia (pins and needles) or attacks of tetany and even of epilepsy. Surgical removal of parathyroid glands causes hypocalcaemia, and symptoms appear within 24–48 h. The glands may be removed accidentally during an operation for thyroid disease, because of the close physical relationship between the two glands. Frequently,

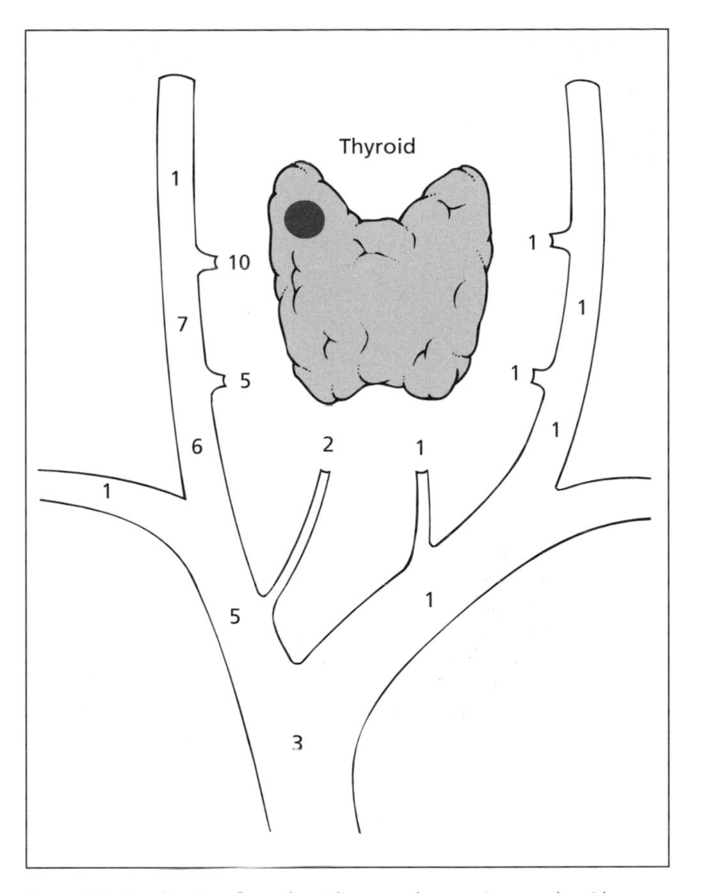

Figure 7.8 Localization of parathyroid tumours by assaying parathyroid hormone. Blood samples are taken after cannulation of the great veins of the neck and also the small thyroid veins. The numbers indicate the relative concentration of hormone in a patient with a tumour of the right upper parathyroid gland. The peak concentrations are in the right superior thyroid vein and the right internal jugular vein. The concentrations (shown in arbitrary numbers) are lower in the other veins such as the inferior thyroid veins and superior vena cava, thus pointing to the probable location of the tumour in the upper right parathyroid.

however, there is no known cause for failure of the parathyroids, and the condition is therefore called 'idiopathic hypoparathyroidism'. Other causes of hypocalcaemia, and the biochemical tests used for differential diagnosis of the condition, are discussed later.

Resistance to the actions of PTH. Failure of the tissues to respond to PTH also leads to the development of hypocalcaemia. This occurs in a condition that mimics the effect of idiopathic hypoparathyroidism and is therefore called 'pseudohypoparathyroidism'. In this condition, the serum phosphate concentration is high and the serum calcium is low, and there is secondary hyperparathyroidism with high (rather than low) concentrations of circulating PTH. The patients may have mental deficiency and other stigmata that may suggest the diagnosis: these include shortness of some of the metacarpals, particularly the fourth and fifth, giving rise to short fourth and fifth fingers, and a characteristic roundness of the face (Fig. 7.9). Paradoxically, in patients with pseudohypoparathyroidism, there may be ectopic calcification, with deposition of calcium salts subcutaneously, in muscle and in brain; the cause for this is not clear. The diagnosis can be established by showing that, when PTH is given, there is a lack of the normal response (Fig. 7.10). In pseudohypoparathyroidism, administration of PTH does not cause a rise in plasma or urinary cAMP, although it will produce a normal response in patients with idiopathic hypoparathyroidism or surgically induced hypoparathyroidism.

The resistance to the action of PTH in pseudohypoparathyroidism is due to a defect in bone and kidney. In some patients, this is due to decreased G-proteins, which couple the hormone-occupied cell-surface receptor to the adenylate cyclase catalytic subunit (see Fig. 2.13 and Chapter 2).

Both hypoparathyroidism and pseudohypoparathyroidism are usually treated with oral calcium, in combination with calcitriol (see Fig. 7.13). Care must be exercised to avoid vitamin D intoxication, which could irreversibly impair renal function.

Calcitonin

This is the only hypocalcaemic hormone. In mammals, calcitonin is secreted from the parafollicular or C-cells in the thyroid gland. In the embryonic development of the thyroid (see Chapter 5), the C-cells, which are originally derived from the neural-crest cells, become dispersed among the thyroid follicles. There is a common blood supply to C-cells and thyroid follicular cells. C-cells in mammals are not innervated.

The C-cells possess a number of cytochemical characteristics that are used as a paradigm for the class of cells known as the APUD system. The acronym APUD is derived from the words *a*mine, *p*recursor *u*ptake and *d*ecarboxylase—their significance being that the cells contain amines, they can take up amine precursors, and they contain a decarboxylase. The amine is fluorogenic (such as catecholamine or 5-hydroxytryptamine), and the amine precursor can be 5-hydroxytryptophan (5-HTP) or 3,4-dihydroxyphenylalanine (dopa). Thus, the characterization of the APUD cells is based on cytochemical characteristics.

Apart from the C-cells of the thyroid gland, which secrete calcitonin, the APUD system includes the chromaffin cells of the adrenal medulla, and also some other cells, which secrete peptide hormones. The latter include those of the anterior pituitary, the cells of the islets of Langerhans in the pancreas and the cells that secrete

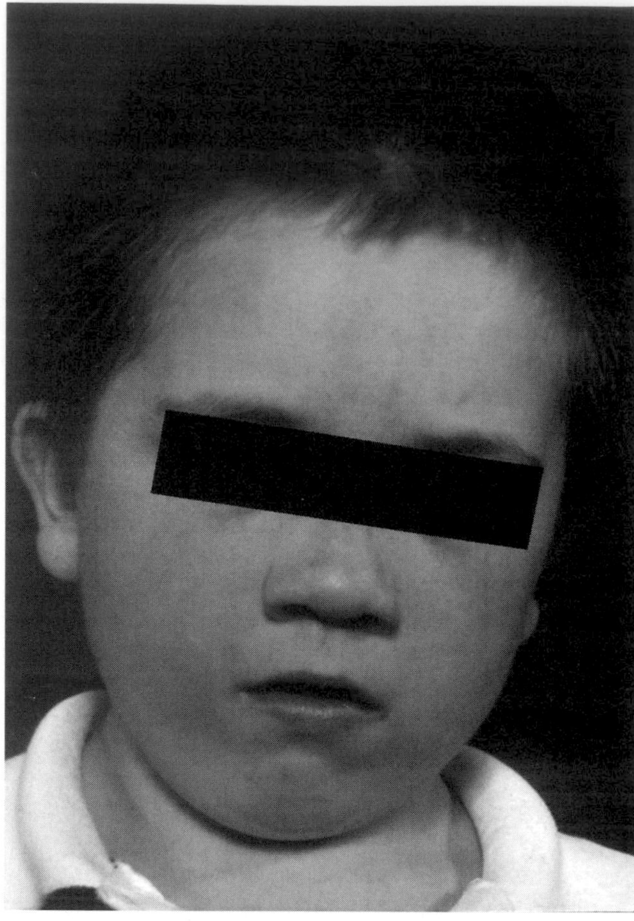

(a)

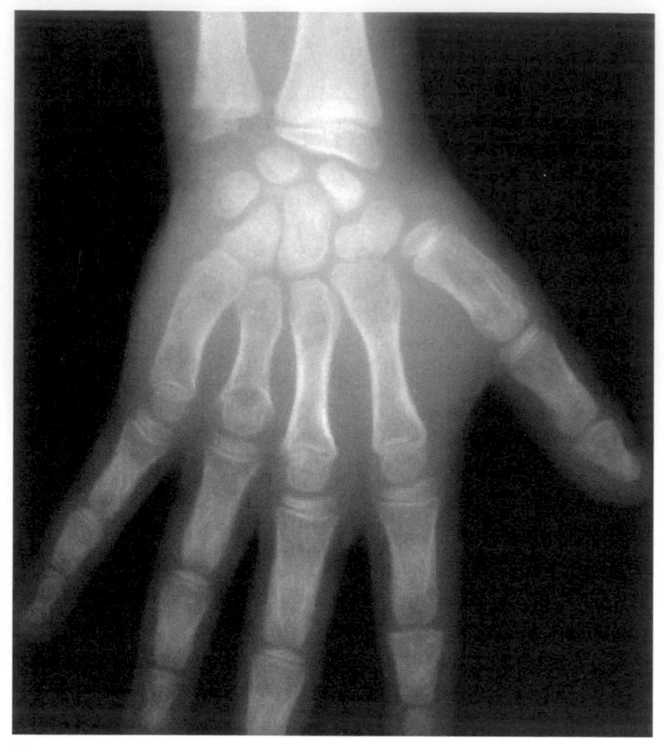

(c)

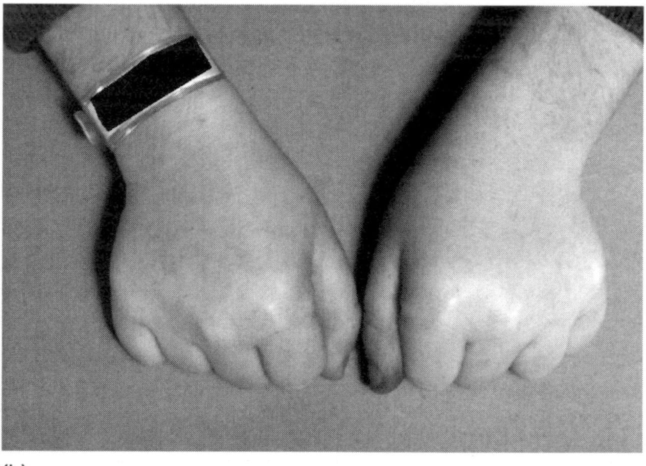

(b)

Figure 7.9 Clinical features of pseudohypoparathyroidism: (a) round face; (b) and (c) short fourth metacarpals.

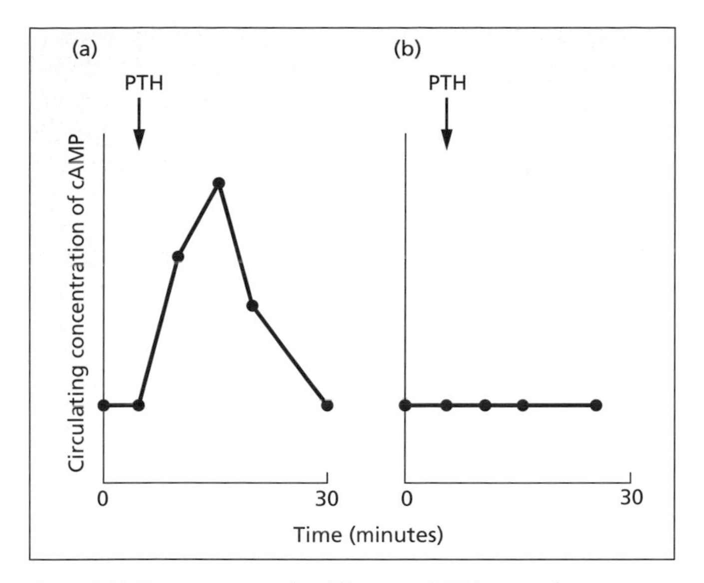

Figure 7.10 Responses to parathyroid hormone (PTH) in terms of circulating concentrations of cyclic adenosine 5′-monophosphate (cAMP) in hypoparathyroidism and pseudohypoparathyroidism. (a) In hypoparathyroidism, the response to injected PTH is normal, as shown by the rise in circulating cAMP. (b) In contrast, in a patient with pseudohypoparathyroidism, there is no response because of resistance in the target cells.

hormones from the gastrointestinal tract. However, apart from the adrenal medulla and C-cells, the origin of the other cells does not seem to be from the neural crest. The pathological importance of the APUD system is that this group of cells may give rise to a wide spectrum of neoplasias that maintain many of the phenotypic characteristics of their normal progenitor cells. In a patient, more than one endocrine tumour may be produced, and so they are called multiple endocrine neoplasias (MEN). They have been grouped into two classes. MEN-I lesions arise from those APUD cells that do not appear to originate from the neural crest (e.g. parathyroid, anterior pituitary, pancreatic islet and gastrointestinal endocrine cells) while MEN-II lesions arise from APUD cells of neural-crest origin (e.g. thyroid C-cells and adrenal medullary cells). Tumours of the parathyroid glands can arise in patients with MEN-I or MEN-II.

Calcitonin is a peptide containing 32 amino acids with a disulphide bridge, yielding an amino-terminal circle of amino acids between residues 1 and 7; there is a proline amide group at the carboxy terminus.

The calcitonin gene lies on the short arm of chromosome 11 in humans. It has six exons and five introns (Fig. 7.11), and the gene encodes for a much larger peptide than calcitonin, with 136 amino acid residues rather than the 32 amino acids of calcitonin. The calcitonin gene is also transcribed in tissues other than the parafollicular cells of the thyroid, and differential splicing of the exons can occur, so that different peptides are made in diverse tissues (Fig. 7.11). One of these is a 'calcitonin gene-related peptide' (CGRP) that consists of 37 amino acids. Like calcitonin, it can be synthesized and secreted by the thyroid, but more is made in the nervous system, particularly in

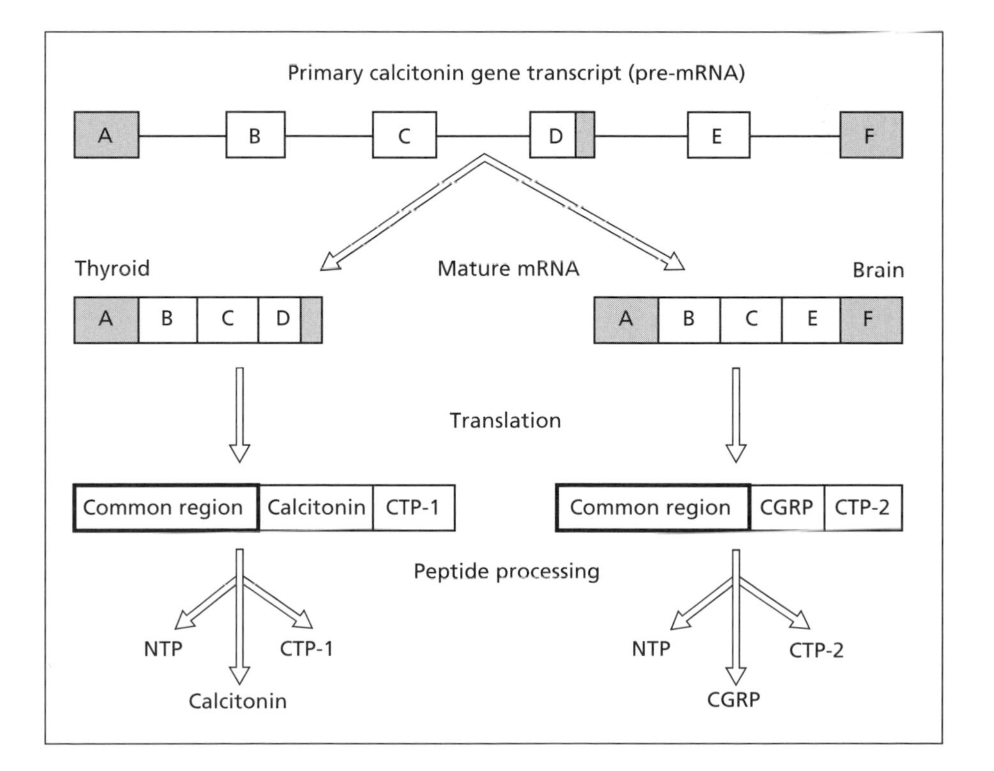

Figure 7.11 Peptides arising from the calcitonin gene. The calcitonin gene consists of six exons, shown here as A–F. These can be differentially spliced after transcription to give different forms of mature messenger ribonucleic acid (mRNA). The sequence of calcitonin is encoded in exon D; splicing of exons A, B, C and D gives an mRNA which, when it is translated, yields preprocalcitonin. From this, an amino-terminal peptide (NTP), calcitonin and a carboxy-terminal peptide (CTP-1) are produced by post-translational processing. An alternative splicing process, using exons A, B, C, E and F, yields a different mRNA. The product of this has a common amino-terminal region, the 'calcitonin gene-related peptide' (CGRP) and a different carboxy-terminal peptide (CTP-2). The left-hand pathway in the diagram predominates in parafollicular cells of the thyroid to yield calcitonin, while the CGRP pathway predominates in the brain.

the hypothalamus and pituitary. CGRP may be important as a neurotransmitter, and it also has very powerful vasodilator properties.

The hypocalcaemic effect of calcitonin depends primarily on its ability to inhibit the mobilization of calcium from bone. This it does by suppressing the activity of the osteoclasts. It may also have some stimulatory effect on bone formation, and thus increase calcium uptake, although this is probably less significant. Secretion of calcitonin is stimulated by hypercalcaemia (Fig. 7.7), which at the same time suppresses secretion of PTH.

Thus, calcitonin is capable of counteracting the effects of PTH. It has been postulated that it is important in protecting the body from the effects of a sudden influx of calcium, such as would be produced by drinking a pint of milk, which contains 25 mmol (1 g) of calcium. In patients who have undergone thyroidectomy, intravenous infusion of calcium causes a greater rise in serum than it does in normal subjects. Nevertheless, the physiological role of calcitonin remains uncertain, although increased concentrations of calcitonin are found in pregnant and lactating women, and so it may be more important under these conditions. It has been suggested that calcitonin is a 'vestigial' hormone that is important for vertebrates living in calcium-rich sea water.

Effects of overproduction of calcitonin. Overproduction of calcitonin occurs in patients who have tumours of the parafollicular cells of the thyroid; this is called medullary carcinoma of the thyroid. This tumour can be a familial, inherited condition. However, it can also occur without there being any family history of such a tumour. Sometimes the presence of a medullary carcinoma of the thyroid is associated with the presence of another tumour, of the adrenal medulla, called a phaeochromocytoma (Chapter 4), so that—as discussed previously—the patients have tumours of two groups of APUD cells (MEN-II). Patients with a medullary carcinoma of the thyroid usually present with a goitre in the neck, owing to enlargement of the thyroid gland. The concentration of calcitonin is very high in the circulation of these patients. Despite this, the serum calcium is entirely normal, and there is no demonstrable abnormality of calcium homoeostasis or bone architecture. The reason for this is not clear, but, because of it, there is doubt as to whether calcitonin has a significant role to play in calcium homoeostasis, at least in humans. It may be more important in growing children and in pregnant women, contributing to growth or preservation of the skeleton. In nonmammalian species, its role may be more significant, and in birds it can modulate eggshell formation.

Vitamin D

Structure and metabolism of vitamin D

Although known as a vitamin, and thus regarded as a compound that has to be provided in the diet, vitamin D can be formed in the skin. Exposure to ultraviolet light in sunshine converts 7-dehydrocholesterol to vitamin D_3 (cholecalciferol). Figure 7.12 shows how irradiation with

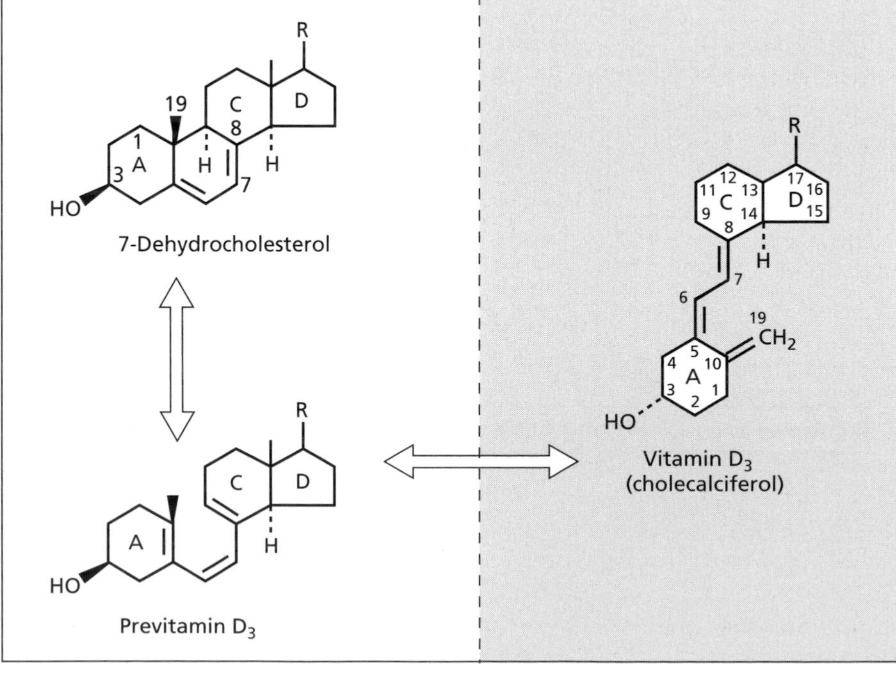

Figure 7.12 The formation of vitamin D_3. Ultraviolet irradiation, for example on skin, opens the B ring of 7-dehydrocholesterol to give previtamin D_3; rotation of the A ring then gives vitamin D_3 (cholecalciferol). In this illustration, R is the side-chain of cholesterol, 7-dehydrocholesterol and vitamin D_3 (see Fig. 7.13). Projection of groups relative to the plane of the rings: ◢, forwards; ⋰, backwards.

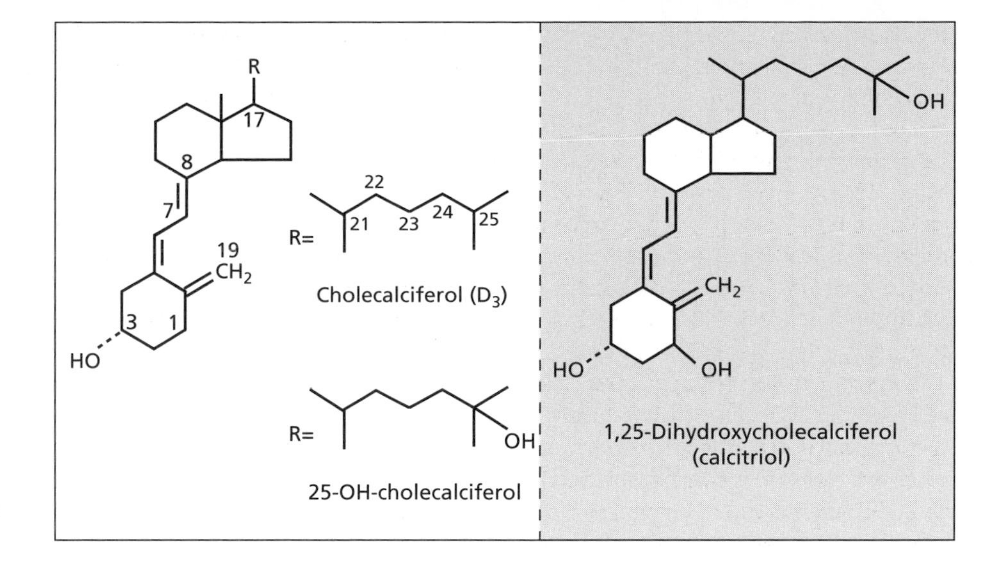

Figure 7.13 The formation of calcitriol. Cholecalciferol (vitamin D_3) is first hydroxylated in the liver to 25-OH-cholecalciferol. The latter is then hydroxylated at C-1 to 1,25-dihydroxycholecalciferol, which is also known as calcitriol. The hydroxyl group is in the alpha orientation, and so the renal enzyme responsible is known as 1α-hydroxylase.

ultraviolet light opens the B ring of the steroid nucleus (Fig. 1.5 and Appendix 3) to give previtamin D_3; then there is rotation of the A ring to give vitamin D_3. This can be absorbed into the circulation, and is the natural form of vitamin D. Formation of vitamin D_3 in the skin is important, since the natural sources of vitamin D in the diet are limited to fish and eggs. Vitamin D_2 (ergocalciferol) is a pharmaceutical product of plant origin made by irradiation of ergosterol, which is found in extracts of wheat germ, for example. Vitamin D_2 is used in food fortification, e.g. in margarine. In some countries, it is added to milk. Its structure is identical to that of vitamin D_3, except for a double bond between C22 and C23 in the side chain.

By 1965, because of the work of Kodicek in Cambridge and DeLuca in America, it was realized that vitamin D had to be further metabolized before it was capable of exerting its biological activity (Figs 7.13 and 7.14). This involves the addition of hydroxyl groups. The first step occurs in the liver, in which a hydroxyl group is added to the side-chain, converting cholecalciferol to 25-hydroxycholecalciferol (i.e. 25-hydroxyvitamin D_3), which is the major form of vitamin D in the circulation (unless the patient ingests ergocalciferol, which is converted to 25-hydroxyergocalciferol, i.e. 25-hydroxyvitamin D_2). Further metabolism of 25-hydroxycholecalciferol is necessary; this occurs in the kidney, which adds an additional hydroxyl group in the A ring to give 1,25-dihydroxycholecalciferol (Fig. 7.13). In view of the three hydroxyl groups in this structure, this is referred to as calcitriol; this is the most potent form of vitamin D. Other circulating metabolites of vitamin D formed from 25-hydroxycholecalciferol include 24,25-dihydroxycholecalciferol, made by 24-hydroxylation in the kidney. The concentration of

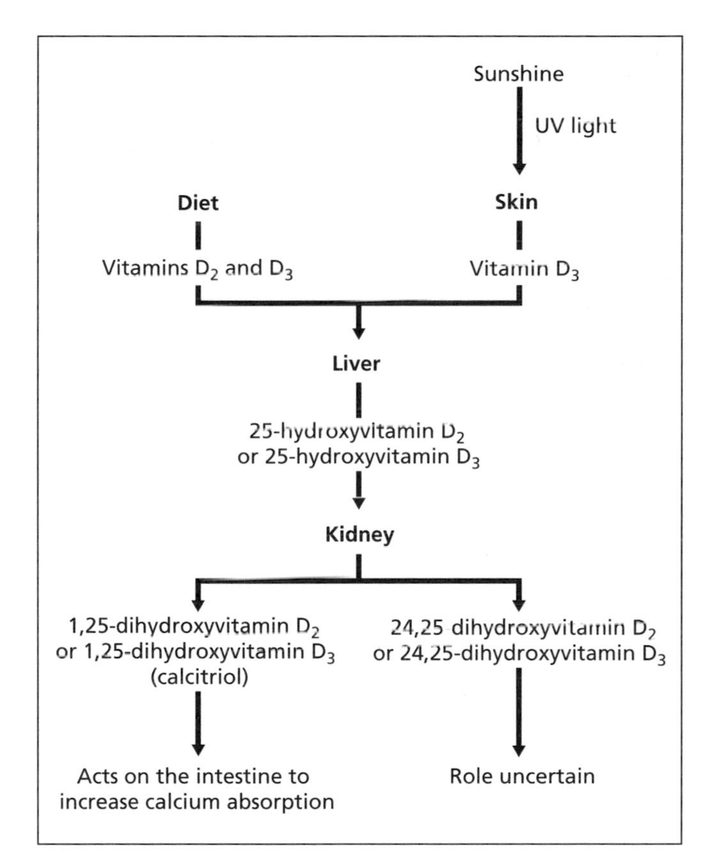

Figure 7.14 The sources and metabolism of vitamin D. The term vitamin D is used when it is not necessary to differentiate between vitamin D_2 and D_3.

25-hydroxycholecalciferol in the circulation is quite high (3–30 ng/mL), but the concentration of calcitriol is very low (20–60 pg/mL). There is a circulating vitamin D-binding protein that has high affinity for 25-hydroxy-

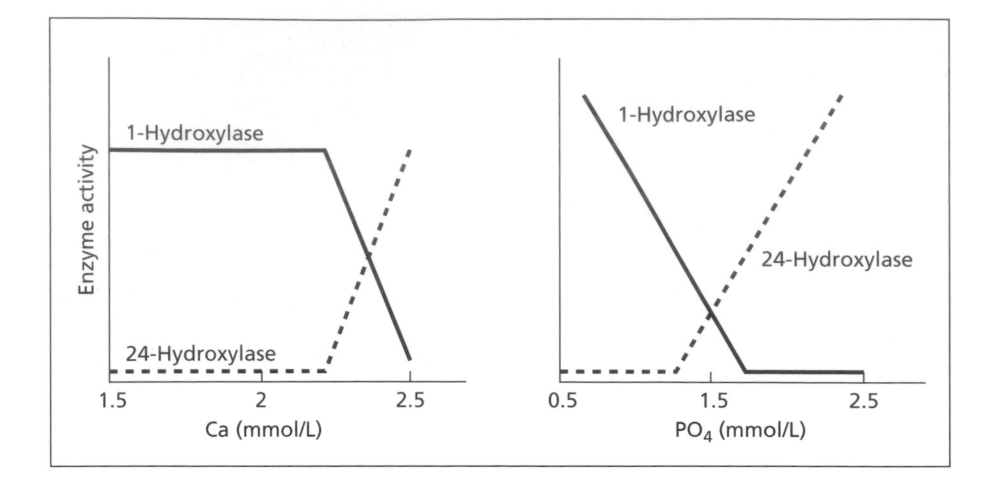

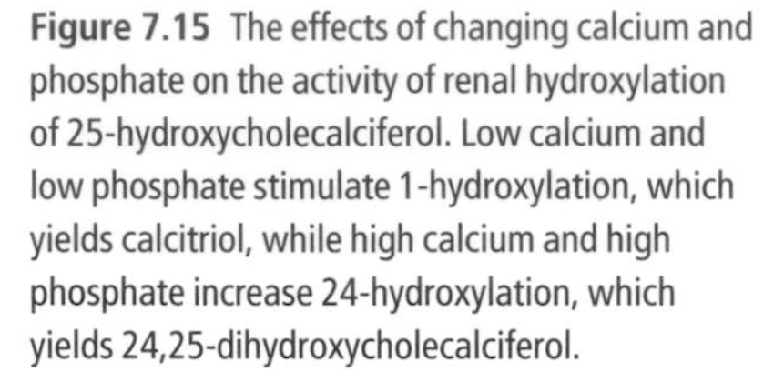
Figure 7.15 The effects of changing calcium and phosphate on the activity of renal hydroxylation of 25-hydroxycholecalciferol. Low calcium and low phosphate stimulate 1-hydroxylation, which yields calcitriol, while high calcium and high phosphate increase 24-hydroxylation, which yields 24,25-dihydroxycholecalciferol.

vitamin D and 24,25-dihydroxyvitamin D but low affinity for calcitriol.

Effects of vitamin D. Under normal circumstances, probably all the effects of vitamin D are due to calcitriol. It remains to be established whether any of the other metabolites of vitamin D have a physiological role or whether they are breakdown products. The main action of calcitriol is to stimulate calcium absorption. This occurs by a direct action on the intestinal mucosa, where it acts on nuclear receptors. These are a subgroup of the steroid–thyroid-hormone nuclear receptor superfamily (see Figs 2.1 and 2.21). The effect of calcitriol on the nucleus leads to an increase in the synthesis of messenger ribonucleic acid (mRNA), which in turn leads to increased protein synthesis. Among the proteins formed in the intestinal cell is a calcium-binding protein believed to be important in transporting calcium across the intestinal cell. Calcitriol also increases the secretion of osteoclast-activating factors by osteoblasts (Fig. 7.3).

Vitamin D as a hormone—the regulation of the metabolism of vitamin D. Since calcitriol is synthesized in the kidney and is secreted in the bloodstream to act on a distant tissue (the intestine), it can be regarded as a hormone. In this sense (and others), the kidney is therefore an endocrine gland. This endocrine system is subject to feedback control. The activity of the 1α-hydroxylase system in the mitochondria of the renal tubule is dependent on the serum calcium and phosphate concentrations (Fig. 7.15). Low calcium stimulates the 1α-hydroxylase system, while high calcium activates 24-hydroxylase, which can convert 25-hydroxycholecalciferol to 24,25-dihydroxycholecalciferol. The latter is probably biologically inert, and the formation of 24,25-dihydroxycholecalciferol is reciprocally related to the production of calcitriol. A low serum phosphate also activates the 1α-hydroxylase system. In addition, PTH stimulates and calcitonin suppresses the 1α-hydroxylase. There may be other interactions between the parathyroid glands and vitamin D endocrine systems, and it appears that derivatives of vitamin D can modulate the secretion of PTH, so as to maintain calcium homoeostasis.

Effects of deficiency of vitamin D

Deficiency of vitamin D causes rickets in children; in adults the corresponding condition is osteomalacia. Both conditions are characterized by failure of calcification of osteoid, which is the matrix of bone, and the manifestations depend on whether or not the bone is growing.

In children, there is a failure of remodelling, so that the growing ends are swollen (Fig. 7.16). This can be seen at the wrists and at the costochondral junctions, the swelling of which leads to the development of what is called a rickety rosary. Endochondral ossification fails, and this leads to excessively thick plates of epiphyseal disc cartilage, which is soft and poorly calcified. In addition, both the primary and secondary spongiosa are inadequately calcified, so that the bone bends. This results in deformity, with bow-legs or knock-knees. Radiologically, it can be shown that the changes are greatest at the growing ends of bones. The X-ray appearance of rachitic bones is characterized by classical changes at the distal ends of long bones, including cupping, fraying, widening and generally decreased bone density.

In the adult, the main feature is pain. The bone may partially fracture to give what is called a 'Looser zone' or pseudofracture. In addition, there may be profound muscle weakness, affecting particularly the hip and shoulder muscles, due to an associated proximal myopathy. Osteomalacic bones have generally decreased density, but since the epiphyses are closed in adulthood, rickets is not present. In the mature skeleton, osteomalacia leads to the

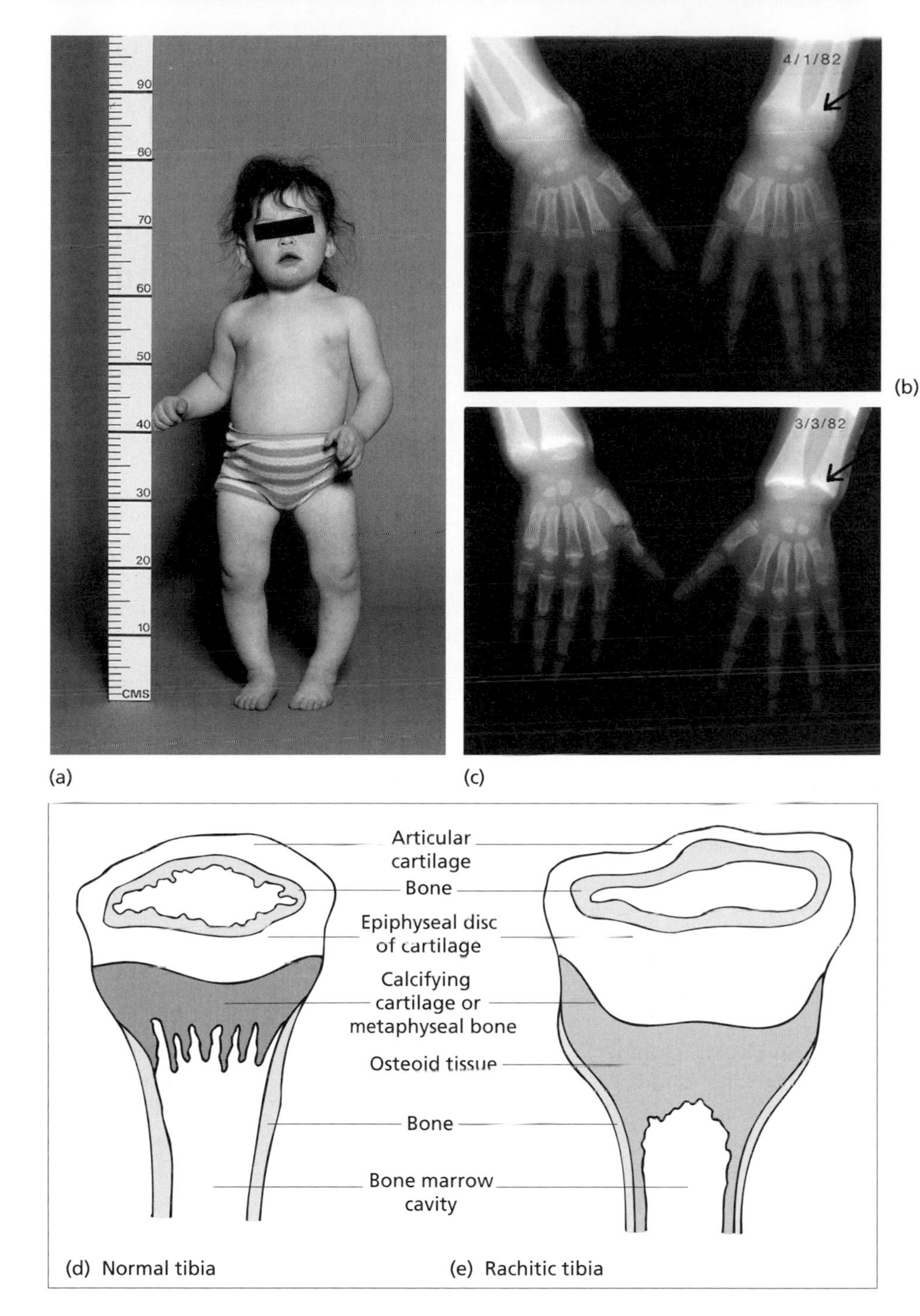

Figure 7.16 Rickets. (a) Clinical appearance in a 3-year-old. Note the bowing of the tibiae. (b) Radiological features showing expansion, irregularity and 'cupping' of the metaphyses (arrow). (c) Radiological features of healing rickets: note the increased density and definition of the same metaphysis (arrow). Note also the reduction in the radial epiphyseal cartilage thickness from (b) to (c). The growing tibial head in (d) is normal and that in (e) is rachitic. (d) A normally growing epiphyseal disc of cartilage is seen, with the underlying zone of calcifying cartilage. (e) The epiphyseal disc of cartilage is greatly enlarged, and underneath it there is a thick zone of osteoid tissue, i.e. uncalcified bone matrix. Note also the generally thickened epiphyseal region in the rachitic bone, as shown in (b).

production of wide layers of osteoid, which eventually come to cover the vast majority of available bone surfaces.

In vitamin D deficiency, the serum calcium may be low. This can cause tetany, and it increases parathyroid activity. Hypocalcaemia does not always occur, however, and so this cannot be the main cause for the failure of calcification of the osteoid in bone. It is therefore likely that vitamin D derivatives have a direct action on bone to induce mineralization, although it has been difficult to prove this *in vitro*.

The normal daily requirement in humans is 100–400 U (2.5–10 μg) of vitamin D daily. Deficiency can be treated with small doses, although the amount given is often rather greater than the normal requirement, e.g. 3000 U/day. Improvement occurs within weeks, but it takes a much longer time, perhaps a year, before the skeleton is entirely normal. The condition can be treated with a smaller amount of calcitriol, e.g. 0.5 μg/day. When vitamin D_3 is given orally to a vitamin D-deficient patient, it is rapidly hydroxylated to 25-hydroxycholecalciferol and then to calcitriol. The doses of vitamin D that are used only give physiological concentrations of 25-hydroxycholecalciferol, but quite quickly—within 48 h—supranormal concentrations of calcitriol are produced. This is the result of increased 1α-hydroxylase in the kidney, which has been induced by the hypocalcaemia (Fig. 7.15). This overactivity persists for many months, presumably as a consequence of persistent secondary hyperparathyroidism.

Other causes of rickets and osteomalacia. There are many causes of rickets and osteomalacia apart from a deficiency of vitamin D. Chronic renal failure is one cause, probably because there is a lack of the 1α-hydroxylase activity with the loss of functioning renal tissue. There is also a congenital disorder due to a lack of 1α-hydroxylase, which can be treated with small doses of calcitriol. Barbiturate and phenytoin therapy (for epilepsy) can cause rickets and osteomalacia; this may be related to the induction of enzyme systems by these drugs and interference with the normal metabolism of vitamin D.

Not all cases of rickets or osteomalacia are related to vitamin D. For example, phosphate depletion can be responsible, and this can arise in renal tubular disorders that result in excessive loss of phosphate and hypophosphataemia. Even this type of rickets can be treated with vitamin D, although the condition is resistant to vitamin D, and large doses are therefore needed. One cause for this hypophosphataemic rickets is a mutation on the X chromosome, which causes an X-linked dominant disorder.

Effects of excess vitamin D

Large doses of vitamin D can cause hypercalcaemia, and this is referred to as 'vitamin D intoxication'. This can result from excessive ingestion of any of the forms of vitamin D that are available for therapeutic purposes (such as cholecalciferol, ergocalciferol, 25-hydroxycholecalciferol and calcitriol). They can be used, for example, to correct hypocalcaemia due to hypoparathyroidism. Large amounts of vitamin D_2 or vitamin D_3 have to be given, e.g. 50 000–100 000 U (1.25–2.5 mg) daily. Much smaller amounts of calcitriol (0.5 μg/day) can be used; this increases calcium absorption and mobilizes calcium from bone. Intoxication of vitamin D causes nausea, vomiting and dehydration, because of hypercalcaemia. If the hypercalcaemia is prolonged, calcification can develop within the kidney, and renal function can be impaired. Thus, careful monitoring of therapy is needed to avoid overdosage. If hypercalcaemia is produced by calcitriol therapy, it is less prolonged when the treatment is stopped than if vitamin D has been given. One important reason for this is that vitamin D and 25-hydroxyvitamin D are fat-soluble; they accumulate in the body, while calcitriol does not. In addition, since calcitriol is not protein-bound, it is cleared rapidly, having a half-life in the circulation of only 6 h.

OUTLINE OF BIOCHEMICAL TESTS FOR DISORDERS OF CALCIUM REGULATION

The determination of calcium

Specific measurement of ionized calcium by ion-selective electrodes is becoming more available, but the determination of serum total calcium levels is adequate in the majority of cases of disordered calcium regulation. The observed total calcium values can be mathematically corrected to allow for disturbance in albumin concentrations. These corrected estimations should, however, be interpreted with caution, particularly if hydrogen ion concentrations are also abnormal. Although complexed calcium normally forms only a minor fraction, a significant decrease in ionized calcium may occur in hyperphosphataemia (e.g. in chronic renal failure), when increased calcium phosphate complexes form.

Despite large changes in the intake of calcium throughout the day, the endocrine regulators efficiently maintain calcium homoeostasis, with only minor diurnal variations being reported. In healthy individuals, calcium levels decline in older men, but not women; this may be associated with the age-related decrease in serum albumin in men. In pregnancy, serum total calcium decreases, together with serum albumin, but the ionized concentration is maintained.

Measurements of circulating concentrations of PTH and vitamin D (but not calcitonin) play a key role in the differential diagnosis of disorders of calcium regulation. Both 25-hydroxycalciferol and calcitriol estimations are routinely made to determine vitamin D status. Since 25-hydroxycalciferol is the predominant circulating form of vitamin D in the normal population, it is considered to be the most reliable index of vitamin D status. The values correlate with personal exposure to sunlight, and vary with season and skin colour.

Hypercalcaemia

Raised serum calcium levels are not infrequently detected as incidental findings before the appearance of any clinical symptoms. However, the most common pathological causes are malignant disease and primary hyperparathy-

Table 7.1 Causes of hypercalcaemia.

	Associated with
Commonest causes	
Primary hyperparathyroidism	Increased PTH; autonomous secretion
Malignancy	Increased osteoclast-activating factors due to PTH-related peptide
Less common causes	
Thyrotoxicosis	Increased osteoclast activity
Vitamin D intoxication	Increased osteoclast activity
Diet	Increased gut absorption of calcium
	Excessive milk consumption
	Excessive antacid
Acromegaly	Increased GH and therefore 1-alpha-hydroxylase

GH, growth hormone; PTH, parathyroid hormone.

roidism (Table 7.1). The relatively recent development of immunoassays for PTH in serum with the requisite sensitivity and specificity has resulted in a revolutionary change in laboratory investigation of hypercalcaemia. The direct use of these immunoassays in conjunction with calcium measurements is now increasingly employed to differentiate patients who will benefit from parathyroid surgery from those who require further evaluation to determine the cause of their hypercalcaemia.

Malignant disease

Hypercalcaemia is common in malignant disease. Malignant cells (metastases) in bone cause destruction of the bone itself and release calcium. Sometimes this is due to an 'osteoclast-activating factor', such as a prostaglandin (Fig. 7.3), being produced by the metastatic deposit. In the case of multiple myeloma, the osteoclasts are activated by lymphokines secreted by the tumour cells. In addition, tumours that have not metastasized to bone can cause hypercalcaemia by secreting a 'parathyroid hormone–related peptide'. This has a structural similarity, in its amino terminus, to the amino terminus of PTH, but the tumoral hypercalcaemic factor is larger. In the majority of cases, the levels of PTH itself will be decreased in this situation, when measured by immunoassay for the intact molecule. This is in response to the hypercalcaemia.

Primary hyperparathyroidism

This is caused by autonomous secretion of PTH. As previously outlined, this is usually due to a benign tumour of a parathyroid gland and is characterized by an inappropriately high level of PTH when measured by immunoassay. In normal circumstances, the PTH should be suppressed by the elevated calcium, but in primary hyperparathyroidism it will either be increased above the reference range or be readily detectable within the normal range.

The measurement of PTH by immunoassays has until recently proved technically difficult, and the results of a given immunoassay should still be interpreted with caution. This is largely because the hormone is rapidly metabolized in blood into a number of polypeptide fragments. Only the N-terminal fragments are biologically active. However, the inactive C-terminal fragments tend to be more immunogenic, and since they have half-lives that are 10–20-fold longer than the intact hormone, they accumulate preferentially in serum. Thus, serum contains a mixture of the intact PTH and much greater concentrations of fragments consisting of the middle and C-terminal portion of the hormone. The low concentration of the intact molecules makes it technically difficult to measure them. Determination of midregion and C-terminal fragments has in the recent past been surprisingly useful, even though these values are generally assumed only to reflect biologically inactive species. Immunoassays that are specific for the intact biologically active PTH are now available, and appear to quantify both the normal reference range and the elevated and suppressed ranges accurately. Samples should be handled with care, and frozen immediately if the assay cannot be completed within a few hours, to prevent proteolytic modifications of the intact polypeptide hormone.

Less common causes of hypercalcaemia

Excess thyroid hormone increases the turnover of bone, due to increased osteoclast activity, and hypercalcaemia may result. Overdosage with vitamin D can also raise calcium, partly by the physiological effect of vitamin D, which is to increase calcium absorption from the gut, and partly from a pharmacological effect in which stimulation of bone breakdown occurs (Fig. 7.3). Rarely, ingestion of large amounts of milk or of calcium-containing antacids taken for peptic ulceration can cause hypercalcaemia, even though the body's homeostatic mechanisms can normally control wide variations in calcium intake. Occasionally, hypercalcaemia is encountered in the acromegalic patient. This may be due to stimulation of 1α-hydroxylase in the kidney by the elevated growth hormone.

Hypocalcaemia

The causes include vitamin D deficiency, hypoparathyroidism and renal disease.

Vitamin D deficiency

If the cause is dietary or the condition is due to malabsorption or inadequate exposure to ultraviolet light, there will be a decrease of 25-hydroxycalciferol and hence reduced calcitriol synthesis. These decreases can be quantified by the appropriate immunoassays. There will be decreased gut absorption of calcium as a consequence. Even though, in compensation, 1α-hydroxylation will be stimulated with severe vitamin deficiency, lack of substrate will prevent the formation of sufficient calcitriol. PTH levels should be elevated in response to the lowered serum calcium (secondary hyperparathyroidism).

Hypoparathyroidism

Parathyroid insufficiency leads to hypocalcaemia. PTH immunoassays will distinguish between true hypoparathyroidism and pseudohypoparathyroidism. In the former, PTH levels will be low or even undetectable, while in the latter situation they are elevated, due to end-organ resistance to the action of the hormone. Confirmation of the diagnosis can be made by administration of PTH to the patient: in true hypoparathyroidism there will be an increase in excretion of cAMP in the plasma or urine, but this does not occur in pseudohypoparathyroidism (Figs 7.5 and 7.10).

Hypoparathyroidism may rarely be due to type 1 polyendocrine autoimmunity. This is usually first recognized in children aged about 5 years, and may be followed 5–10 years later by other autoimmune endocrinopathies, with Addison disease being prominent. Antibodies to both adrenal and parathyroid tissue have been reported, and hyperplastic parathyroiditis, analogous to Hashimoto thyroiditis, may occur. Although parathyroid autoantibodies may be important in the pathogenesis of this condition, causing cytotoxicity and inhibiting gland function, autoantibody measurement is not as routine as it is for autoimmune thyroiditis.

Renal disease

In patients with end-stage renal disease, there will be decreased synthesis of calcitriol, which causes hypocalcaemia. The latter will stimulate PTH secretion, giving rise to secondary hyperparathyroidism.

CHAPTER 8

The Pancreas, Gastrointestinal Hormones and Leptin

SUMMARY

Two pancreatic hormones, insulin and glucagon, play a major role in the endocrine control of blood glucose, which also requires the integrated action of epinephrine, cortisol, growth hormone, the thyroid hormones and the gastrointestinal hormones, secretin and cholecystokinin. Insulin is the only hormone with a hypoglycaemic action.

Insulin binds to a cell-surface receptor that has intrinsic tyrosine kinase activity (see Fig. 2.6). Glucagon and epinephrine bind to G-protein–linked cell surface receptors (see Figs 2.1, 2.12 and 2.13), which then stimulate the adenylate cyclase catalytic subunit. Intracellular control of metabolism of carbohydrates and fats by insulin, glucagon and epinephrine involves groups of protein kinase enzymes within the cell, some of which are cyclic adenosine 5′-monophosphate–dependent; some are activated by calcium ions. These protein kinases, together with phosphatases, regulate the activities of other key metabolic enzymes by a phosphorylation–dephosphorylation switching mechanism.

The hormones of the gastrointestinal tract regulate the activity of the stomach and the intestine. For example, gastrin controls acid production and secretin controls pancreatic exocrine secretion. Pancreatic endocrine function is also modulated by events in the stomach, via a hormone called glucose-dependent insulinotrophic peptide. Many of the hormones of the gastrointestinal tract and pancreas are also found in the central or peripheral nervous system, including somatostatin, gastrin, cholecystokinin and vasoactive intestinal peptide; the brain also contains insulin and calcitonin, but the function of these peptides in the nervous system is not clear. Some may be important for the transmission of nerve impulses at synapses, but unlike classic neurotransmitters such as acetylcholine or norepinephrine, they are made in the cell bodies and transported along the axons to the synapses, not synthesized in the nerve terminals. Even if the peptides are not essential for transmission at synapses, they may be important in modulating the process.

Over the last decade, a protein hormone named leptin has been characterized. This new hormone suppresses appetite and increases energy expenditure. It is an *OB* gene product and is secreted in particular by white, subcutaneous adipose tissue and also the placenta. It acts via receptors in the hypothalamus.

INTRODUCTION

Diabetes mellitus is the most commonly encountered endocrine disorder. The disease was vividly described by Areteus in the second century AD as 'a melting down of flesh and limbs into urine'. This referred to the passage of large volumes of urine (polyuria) and to the loss of weight that characterizes uncontrolled diabetes. Due to the 'unquenchable thirst' associated with the condition, he named it 'diabetes', from the Greek word meaning 'siphon'. It was later shown that the urine of these diabetics was sweet to the taste, and it was therefore called diabetes mellitus, *mellitus* being the Latin for sweet. This feature distinguishes diabetes mellitus from diabetes insipidus (see Chapter 3).

In 1889, Minkowski reported that total pancreatectomy in dogs resulted in a condition resembling diabetes mellitus in humans. At the beginning of the twentieth century, it was shown that it was the islet cells in the pancreas of a diabetic patient that were abnormal. In 1921, Banting and Best extracted insulin from the islet cells in the dog pancreas, and demonstrated that the extract lowered blood sugar. Thereafter, the administration of insulin revolutionized the treatment of diabetes. This success prompted a world-wide research effort to achieve a better understanding of the biochemistry of the structure and function of insulin, which culminated in 1955 when Sanger reported the primary structure of insulin. This was the first example of the sequencing of a polypeptide hormone. In 1969, Hodgkin established the three-dimensional structure of insulin from crystallographic studies, and later recombinant human insulin was produced by genetic engineering.

The pancreas secretes a number of other hormones besides insulin. Important among these are glucagon, which raises blood sugar, somatostatin and pancreatic polypeptide (PP).

Morphology of the pancreas

In humans, the head of the pancreas rests in the loop of the duodenum (Fig. 8.1) and its body extends towards the spleen, which is usually in contact with the tail of the

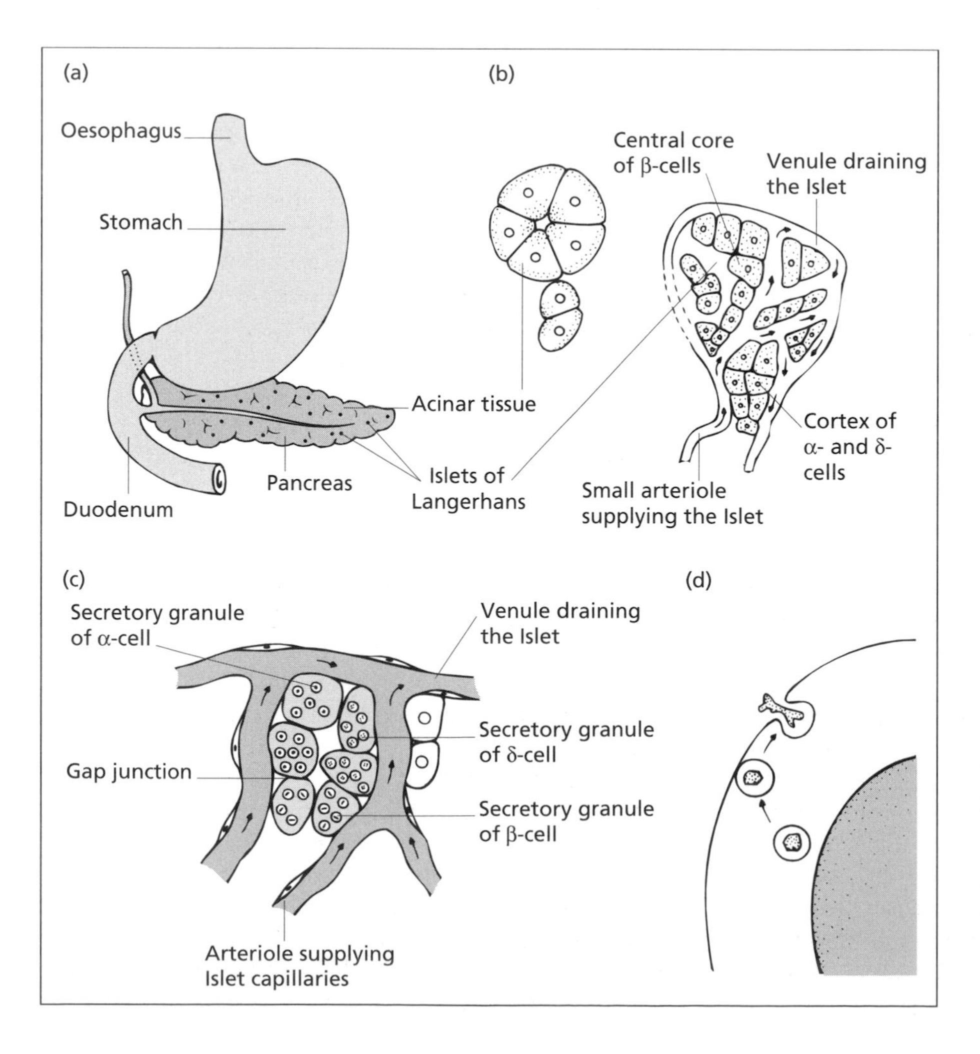

Figure 8.1 The endocrine pancreas. (a) This consists of small groups of cells, the islets of Langerhans, embedded in the exocrine acinar tissue. (b) Each islet consists of a core mainly of β-cells surrounded by a rim or cortex of α- and δ-cells. The islet is supplied with one or more small arterioles that penetrate to the centre of the islet and then break up into capillaries. These first supply the central β-cells and then flow to the periphery of the islet to supply the rim of α- and δ-cells. The capillaries leave the islet and form the draining venules. In this way, the circulation ensures that the β-rich core of islet cells is the first to be exposed to high glucose concentrations, and the peripheral α- and δ-cells are exposed to high insulin concentrations from the inner β-cells. (c) The three cell types of the islet have distinctive secretory granules, which enable them to be easily identified under the electron microscope. All three cell types have been shown to possess gap junctions, and thereby to be dye-coupled to one another. (d) Part of a β-cell, showing a secretory granule discharging its contents in the process of exocytosis, leading to the release of insulin.

pancreas. It is functionally and structurally segregated into two parts. The larger portion consists of exocrine cells arranged in acini; these produce digestive enzymes, which are secreted into the pancreatic duct and thence channelled into the duodenum. Scattered through the exocrine pancreas are aggregates of endocrine cells, forming what are known as the islets of Langerhans; these account for only about 2% of the pancreatic mass. In the islets, there are three major cell types; these are known as the α-, β- and δ-cells, each containing distinctive secretory granules. The islet cells can be distinguished from the acinar cells by a variety of histological techniques. They all have the cytological features that would be expected of cells that synthesize and secrete polypeptides—namely an extensive rough endoplasmic reticulum; a distinctive Golgi complex; and usually numerous secretory granules, which differ in size, form and electron density for each of the three islet-cell types (Fig. 8.1c). Immunocytochemically, the α-cells have been shown to contain glucagon, the β-cells insulin and the δ-cells somatostatin in their respective granules. The islet cells release their hormones by exocytosis (Fig. 8.1d), and the hormones then pass through two basement membranes into neighbouring blood capillaries and so into the circulation.

Developmentally, the pancreas arises from dorsal and ventral endodermal outgrowths from the foregut, close to its junction with the midgut. These outgrowths form a branching duct system, at the termini of which the exocrine acini develop. Other cells bud off from the ducts and form islets of cells, disconnected from their ductal origins. Eventually, the three cell types characteristic of the islets differentiate and become vascularized; sympathetic nerve terminals are found close to the islet cells.

Synthesis and secretion of insulin and glucagon

Insulin is a polypeptide with a molecular weight of 6 kDa, and it consists of two chains, called A and B, which are linked by two disulphide bonds (Fig. 8.2). A third disulphide bond links two cysteine residues within the A chain. There is a larger precursor form of insulin called proinsulin, in which there is a connecting peptide (the C-peptide) between the A and B chains. This has a molecular weight of 9 kDa. Proinsulin has the disulphide bonds of insulin, but instead of having two chains, it has only a single chain of 81–86 amino acids, depending on the species: proinsulin has only minimal insulin-like activity. When the C-peptide is removed, the single chain is broken, and the amino terminus of the A chain and the carboxy terminus of the B chain become separated.

In the β-cells of the islets, the peptide that is actually synthesized on the ribosomes is a still larger peptide, known as preproinsulin (Fig. 8.2). The gene for this is located on the short arm of chromosome 11 in humans, and there is polymorphism in the 5′ region flanking this gene that may be associated with type 2 diabetes. As the precursor molecule passes across the cisternal membrane of the rough endoplasmic reticulum, a chain of 24 amino acids is excised from the amino terminus, producing proinsulin. This is transported in microvesicles, which arise from the endoplasmic reticulum, to the Golgi complex of the cell, where it is packaged with specific proteolytic enzymes, which are not as yet activated, into so-called 'early' secretion granules. These granules subsequently mature into recognizable β-granules, during which time the proteases are activated and convert proinsulin into insulin by specific cleavage of the C-peptide.

Once the C-peptide is removed, the part of the insulin molecule that is important for biological activity becomes exposed. The newly formed insulin, a hexamer together with zinc atoms, constitutes the crystalline core of the β-granule; the C-peptide probably remains in the clear space surrounding the crystalline core (Fig. 8.2). Eventually, as a result of appropriate stimuli, the membranes of the mature β-granules fuse with the cell surface membrane, and insulin is released into the bloodstream.

Glucagon is a polypeptide with a molecular weight of ≈ 3.5 kDa, which has been highly conserved throughout evolution. Like insulin, biosynthesis of glucagon is via a larger precursor, preproglucagon, the gene for which is located in chromosome 2 in humans. Proteolytic degradation within the α-cells results in the release of the active hormone, which has 29 amino acid residues arranged as a single chain. Zinc is not required to complex glucagon in the secretory granules of the α-cells, but glucagon–metal complexes, such as glucagon–zinc, have been shown to have prolonged biological activity.

Human insulin

The primary structure of insulin has been conserved throughout evolution, but there are significant differences in the structures of insulin in different vertebrate species. Most mammalian insulins have similar biological potencies in humans, but nevertheless their structural differences are sufficient to render them antigenic in some patients. This can result in resistance to insulin derived from a particular species of animal.

The adult human pancreas contains about 5 mg of insulin (~300 U). Modified porcine insulin differs only at the carboxy terminus of the B chain, with threonine at B30 in the human insulin and alanine at B30 in porcine insulin, but most insulin in clinical use is synthesized using recombinant methodology. Deoxyribonucleic acid (DNA) sequences encoding the A and B chains of human insulin are inserted into separate plasmids and cloned in

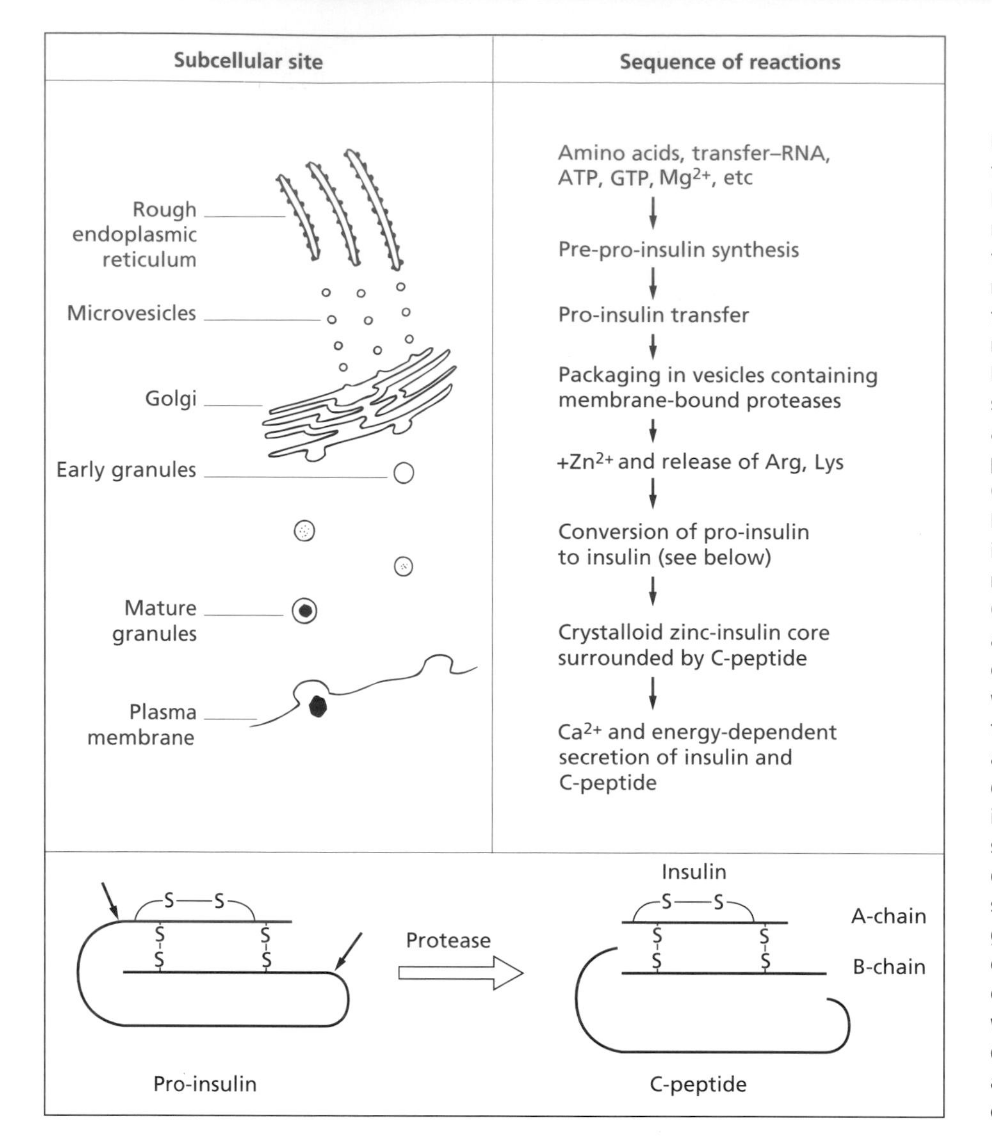

Figure 8.2 Insulin synthesis and secretion from the β-cells of pancreatic islets of Langerhans. Protein synthesis on the rough endoplasmic reticulum yields preproinsulin, which is transferred into the lumen of the endoplasmic reticulum. Hydrolysis yields proinsulin, which is then transferred to the Golgi apparatus, about 20 min after the initiation of protein synthesis. Proinsulin is enclosed in vesicles that carry specific proteases bound to the membrane. Over a period of about 30 min to 2 h, the specific proteases act on proinsulin to release the C-peptide and insulin within the granule. Progressive maturation and crystallization of zinc insulin takes place to yield a dense crystalloid region surrounded by a clear space containing C-peptide. When the cells are stimulated, e.g. by a rise in blood glucose, an energy-dependent and calcium ion–dependent fusion of the granules with the plasma membrane of the cell releases the contents into the bloodstream. Insulin and C-peptide are released in approximately equimolar amounts. The lower portion of the illustration shows a schematic diagram of the structures of proinsulin and insulin. Proinsulin, on the left, is cleaved at two points (arrows) by specific proteases packaged into early β-cell granules. The C-peptide is cleaved from a single-chain peptide to form insulin, which then has two chains, A and B, linked by two disulphide bridges, with the A chain also carrying an intrachain disulphide bridge. Proinsulin contains 86 amino acids, while insulin has 21 amino acids in the A chain and 30 in the B chain.

Escherichia coli. The proteins are then isolated, purified and joined together with the correct intrachain and interchain disulphide bonds. The final genetically engineered product is identical to insulin extracted from the human pancreas.

Regulation of insulin and glucagon release

The main regulator of insulin and glucagon release is the amount of glucose in the blood (Table 8.1). A rise in blood glucose stimulates release of insulin, while a fall in blood glucose suppresses it. Conversely, the secretion of glucagon is stimulated by a fall and suppressed by a rise in the concentration of glucose in the blood. Amino acids stimulate the release of both insulin and glucagon. The insulin ensures that the amino acids are taken up by the cells of the body, and the simultaneous release of glucagon protects against hypoglycaemia.

There is also a neural component controlling the secretion of pancreatic hormones (Table 8.1). Stimulation of the vagus or pancreatic nerve increases insulin release. This can be blocked by atropine, due to the parasympathetic, cholinergic innervation of the islets. Stimulation of the pancreatic nerve also induces glucagon release through a sympathetic, adrenergic innervation mediated by β-receptors, which can be blocked with phentolamine but not atropine. There is a sympathetic supply to the β-cells, and these cells possess both α- and β-adrenergic receptors. Low doses of norepinephrine increase insulin output via an α-adrenoreceptor. However, high doses of norepinephrine inhibit insulin release; this inhibition is also caused by epinephrine, and is mediated by β-adrenoreceptors. *In vivo*, the overall effect of sympathetic stimulation is to

Table 8.1 Some factors regulating insulin release from the β-cells of the pancreatic islets.

Increased by	Decreased by
Raised blood glucose	Low blood glucose
Amino acids	
Glucagon	Somatostatin
Gastrin, secretin	
Cholecystokinin	
GIP	
Sympathetic innervation (α-receptors)	Sympathetic innervation (β-receptors).
Parasympathetic (cholinergic) innervation	Stress (e.g. exercise, hypoxia, hypothermia, surgery, severe burns)

GIP, glucose-dependent insulinotrophic peptide.

depress insulin release. It seems likely that the main role of the sympathetic supply is to modulate cell responses to other stimulators. Epinephrine, which inhibits the secretion of insulin, also stimulates the secretion of glucagon. Thus it increases blood glucose indirectly, quite apart from the direct effect that it has in stimulating the mobilization of glucose from glycogen in the liver.

Several of the gastrointestinal hormones—secretin, gastrin, cholecystokinin (CCK) and glucose-dependent insulinotrophic peptide (GIP, also known as gastric inhibitory peptide)—stimulate insulin secretion. This release is stimulated by ingested food, and an oral glucose load thus increases insulin secretion much more than glucose given intravenously.

Regulation of blood glucose

The amount of glucose in the circulation depends on its absorption from the intestine, uptake by and release from the liver, and uptake by peripheral tissues (Fig. 8.3). Normally no glucose is lost in urine, since all that is filtered in the glomeruli is reabsorbed in the proximal renal tubule. In the fasting state, the concentration of glucose in blood normally lies between 3 and 5 mmol/L; it may rise to 7 mmol/L after a meal, but generally has to exceed 10 mmol/L to produce glycosuria.

Serum glucose concentrations rise following absorption of carbohydrate from the intestine. After a meal or an oral glucose load (Fig. 8.4), absorption occurs rapidly, and blood sugar reaches a peak within an hour. The glucose is converted to glycogen (in the liver and muscle) and to fat (in the liver and adipose tissue), as shown in Figs 8.3 and 8.5. Insulin and glucagon together control the metabolites required by peripheral tissues, and both are involved in maintaining glucose homoeostasis. Insulin is considered to be an anabolic hormone, in that it promotes the synthesis of protein, lipid and glycogen, and it inhibits the degradation of these compounds (Fig. 8.3). The key target tissues of insulin are liver, muscle and adipose tissue. Insulin promotes cell growth in many different cell types, and is an absolute requirement for normal growth in all immature animals. Glucagon acts largely to increase catabolic processes, particularly in the liver (Fig. 8.3).

Between meals or during a fast, the most tightly regulated process is the release of glucose from the liver. This is particularly important in maintaining the concentration of glucose in the circulation to supply tissues such as muscle and brain, which have very limited ability for using other fuels, except in the fetal and newborn periods. Major pathways involved in this process are highlighted in Fig. 8.5. During fasting, amino acids are released from muscle and are used to form pyruvate in liver, from which glucose is formed by the enzymes of the gluconeogenic pathway. At the same time, glucose is produced from glycogen by activation of the enzyme phosphorylase (Fig. 8.6). In addition, fatty acids are released from adipose tissue and metabolized in the liver, where they are converted to ketones (Fig. 8.3). Fatty acids, as well as ketones, are then used as an energy source in place of glucose by various tissues, especially muscle, thus reducing the amount of glucose that needs to be synthesized by metabolism of the amino acids from muscle cells. It should be noted that the synthesis of ketones in normal individuals does not usually exceed the rate at which tissues can utilize them.

Glucose normally provides a principal energy source for tissues of the body, and uptake by many peripheral tissues requires a minimal, though continuous, secretion of insulin. Thus, because of the dual and opposite actions of glucagon and insulin, hypoglycaemia does not normally develop, even in the fasting state, or during exercise, which can require the mobilization and utilization of many grams of glucose.

Glucose uptake

The initial step of glucose utilization requires the transport of glucose into the cell. This is followed by phosphorylation of glucose by adenosine 5′-triphosphate (ATP),

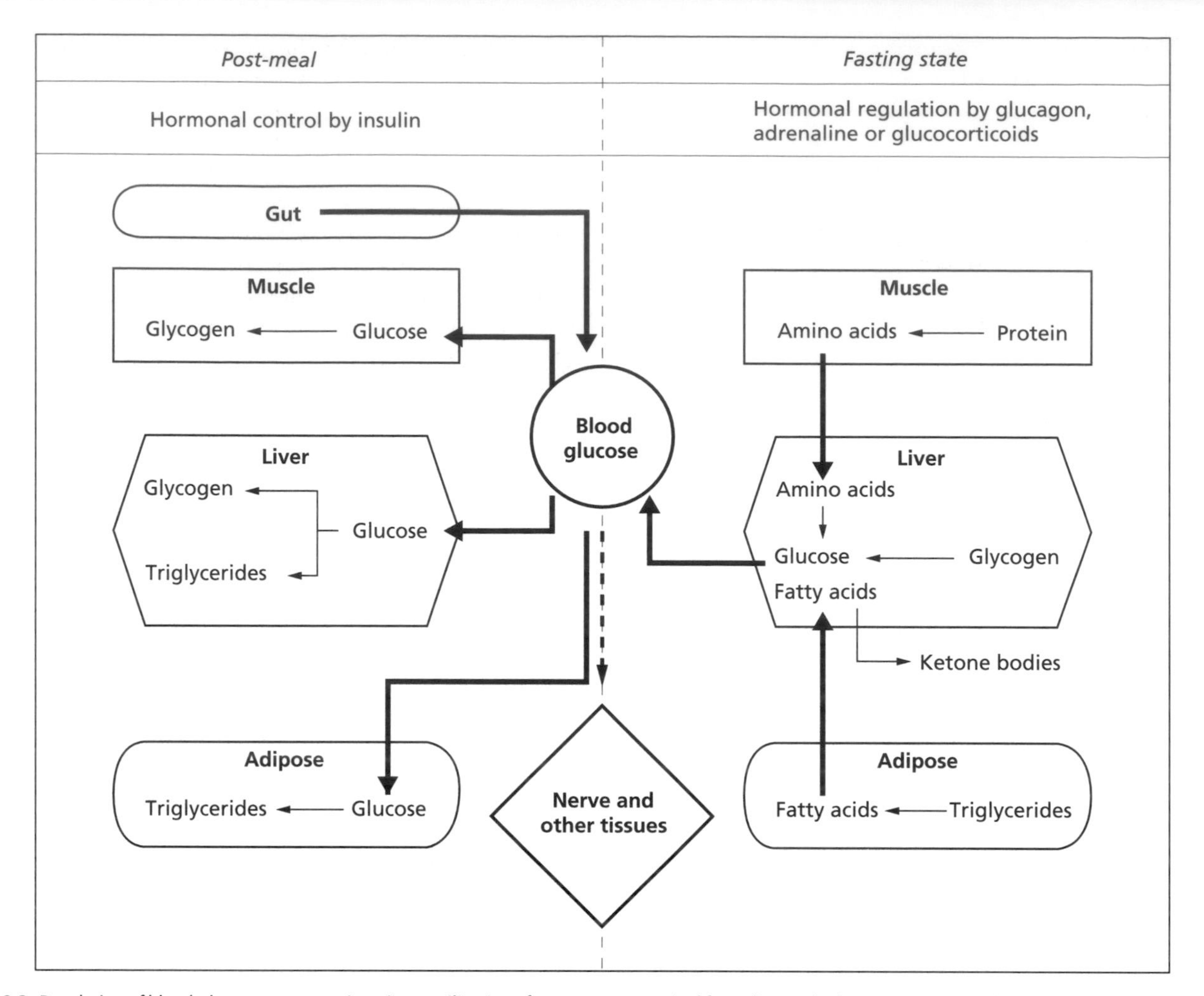

Figure 8.3 Regulation of blood-glucose concentration; tissue utilization of metabolites after a meal and in a fasting state are contrasted. Food is absorbed from the gut and increases the blood-glucose concentration. Insulin facilitates absorption and the control of the synthesis of glycogen and triglyceride storage depots in liver and adipose tissues. Approximately 90% of stored glucose is in the form of lipids. In the fasting state, amino acids are mobilized from muscle proteins to yield pyruvate in the liver, where gluconeogenesis and glycogenolysis are capable of maintaining the blood-glucose concentration required for utilization by brain, nerves and other tissues. Various hormones, including epinephrine, glucagon and glucocorticoids, exert a regulatory action at different sites in these tissues. Fatty acids, mobilized from adipose tissues under the control of a number of hormones (epinephrine, adrenocorticotrophin, glucagon, growth hormone), provide a substrate for liver and muscle metabolism. Ketone bodies produced in the liver provide an energy source for muscle and brain during long periods of fasting.

catalysed by hexokinase, to produce glucose-6-phosphate (Fig. 8.5). The glucose-6-phosphate is not able to leave the cell, because the plasma membrane is impermeable to phosphoric acid esters. The transport of glucose across certain cell membranes, such as muscle, adipose tissue, heart and some peripheral nerves, is regulated by insulin, and this process involves phosphorylation within the membrane. The insulin–receptor complex stimulates the cellular uptake of glucose, the latter then being taken into the cell by mobilization of the insulin-dependent glucose transporter protein GLUT4 (see Chapter 2).

Inside the cell, there are four isoenzymic forms of hexokinase: three (types I–III) have a low affinity constant (K_M) for glucose, and are markedly inhibited by glucose-6-phosphate. This direct feedback inhibition by the reaction product ensures that there is coupling between the rate of glucose phosphorylation and the rate of glucose utilization by the many pathways that rely on this metabolite. A characteristic of insulin-dependent tissues is the high proportion of hexokinase type II, the content of which decreases markedly in diabetic animals. Much of the hexokinase is bound to mitochondrial membranes, which is an advantageous site for the utilization of mitochondrial ATP. The enzyme can be displaced from mitochondria by glucose-6-phosphate and this displacement facilitates the inhibitory action of glucose-6-phosphate. Experimental

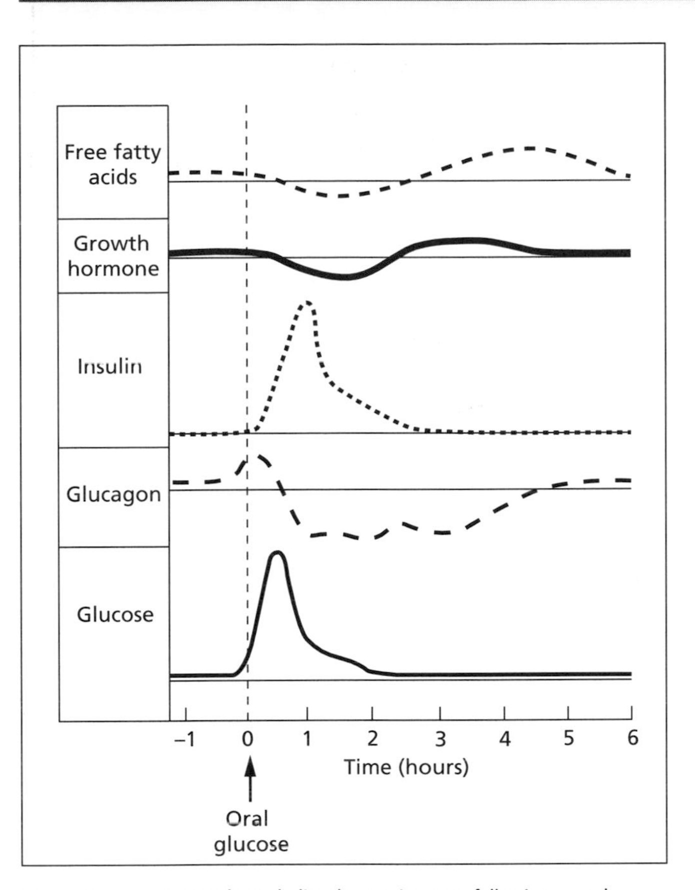

Figure 8.4 Hormone and metabolite changes in serum following an oral glucose load. In an oral glucose-tolerance test, a 50-g glucose load is administered to a normal adult at time zero, and the subsequent changes in serum concentrations of glucose, free fatty acids and three hormones are illustrated. Horizontal faint lines show the basal, fasting levels of the hormones or metabolites. Rapid absorption of glucose yields a peak in the serum concentration within the first hour, with a return to basal levels within 2 h. Neural, anticipatory stimulation initially increases the glucagon concentration, which is then suppressed by the increase in insulin. The rise in insulin slightly lags behind the glucose peak. High glucose concentrations suppress basal growth-hormone release initially, but a small surge of growth hormone can be observed after 2–3 h, which may be in response to the falling glucose concentrations. Elevated insulin concentrations stimulate lipogenesis, and hence cause a decrease in circulating free fatty acids. Growth hormone later causes a release of free fatty acids from adipose tissue for use by muscle and liver cells (see Figs 3.4 and 8.3; Table 3.4).

diabetes reduces the binding of hexokinase to mitochondria, especially in adipose tissue.

Hexokinase type IV, also called glucokinase, is found almost exclusively in the liver cytosol, where it is particularly important in the regulation of blood sugar. This isoenzyme may account for 80% of the normal capacity of liver for phosphorylation of glucose. The kinetic properties of glucokinase are important in glucose homoeostasis; it has a high K_M for glucose of approximately 10 mmol/L, i.e. twice the normal glucose concentration. The enzyme comes into action when the glucose load reaching the liver via the portal circulation is elevated, as would occur following a high dietary carbohydrate intake. The high K_M ensures that the enzyme is fully active only at high blood-glucose concentrations: the activity of the enzyme at normal blood-glucose concentrations is only a fraction of its maximum possible activity. Another important feature of glucokinase is that, unlike the other hexokinase isoenzymes, it is not inhibited by its product, glucose-6-phosphate. This feature highlights the importance of glucokinase in liver storage of glycogen and in the homeostasis and regulation of blood-glucose concentrations.

Hormonal regulation of carbohydrate, fat and protein metabolism

The flux of glucose to and from the liver is closely regulated by several endocrine factors acting in concert to alter the activity of important intracellular enzymes. Insulin and glucagon, being peptide hormones, must act primarily on the cell surface. Insulin activates tyrosine kinase, which is an integral part of its receptor (see Fig. 2.6). Glucagon, in contrast, binds to G-protein–linked cell-surface receptors and activates the adenylate cyclase catalytic subunit (see Figs 2.11–2.13). Indeed the very significance of cyclic adenosine 5′-monophosphate (cAMP) as a second messenger was first discovered through studies of glucagon action on glycogenolysis. A number of the enzymes important in carbohydrate and fat metabolism can exist *in vivo* in an active or inactive form; these two forms are interconvertible by phosphorylation and dephosphorylation mechanisms. This is what is known as 'covalent modification' of the enzymes, i.e. the chemical addition or removal of phosphate by protein kinase or phosphoprotein phosphatases, respectively. This mechanism provides a basis for the regulatory process of carbohydrate and fat metabolism, although not all the effects of insulin and glucagon can at present be explained in this way.

Many of the enzymes involved in catabolic processes are activated by phosphorylation, while others (which are generally involved in biosynthetic reactions) are more active in the dephosphorylated form. Phosphorylation itself is catalysed by a group of enzymes known as protein kinases, of which at least three classes exist. The first group is dependent on the presence of cAMP for activity (see Fig. 2.16), while the second is active in the absence of this nucleotide; a third class of calcium ion (Ca^{2+})-dependent protein kinases has been found, which are regulated by alterations in the intracellular concentration of Ca^{2+} (see Fig. 2.18). These kinases are reasonably specific, and phosphorylate either a single protein or a small group of structurally related proteins. The removal of phosphate

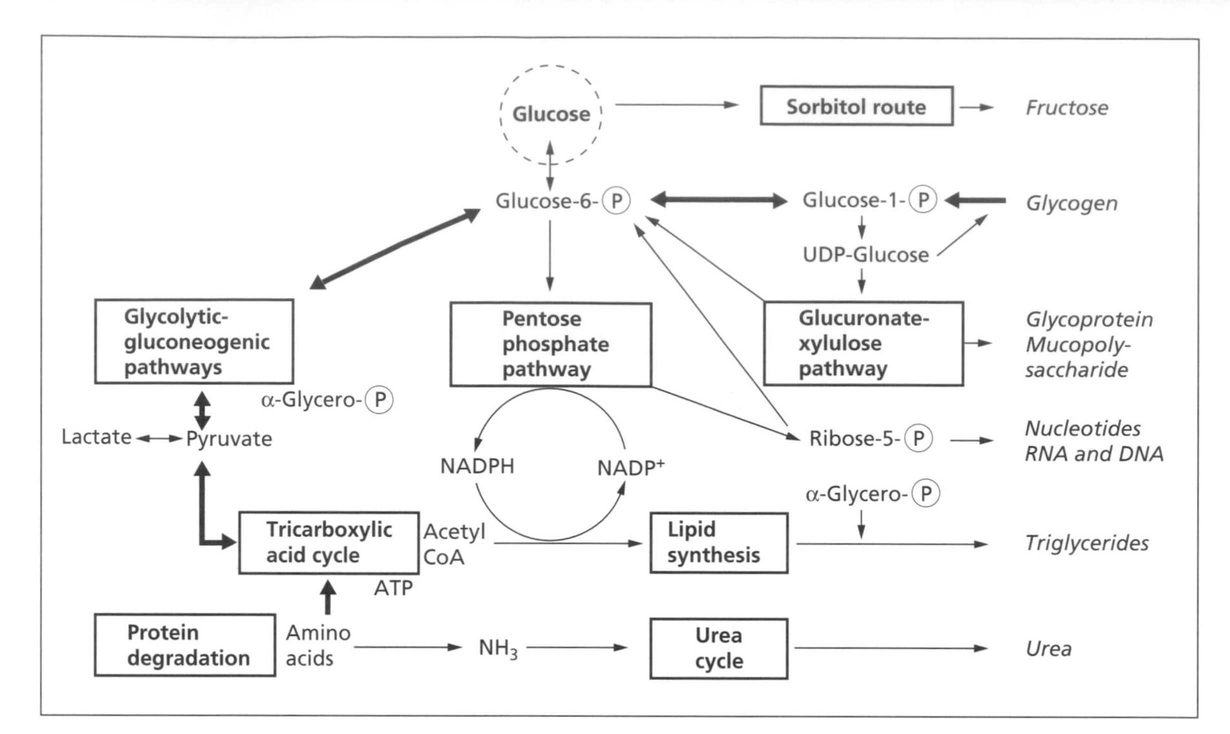

Figure 8.5 Interrelationships among alternative routes of glucose metabolism. The central role of glucose in carbohydrate, fat and protein metabolism is summarized. The principal metabolic pathways are shown enclosed in boxes in order to simplify the diagram; some key intermediates and products of metabolic interconversions are shown. The reversibility of certain reaction sequences implied by double-headed arrows is not necessarily intended to suggest that the same enzymes are involved in both the forward and reverse reactions. The principal reversible pathways that are activated during fasting are marked with heavy arrows.

is catalysed by phosphoprotein phosphatases, which are much less specific than the kinases.

Glycogen metabolism

The control of glycogen metabolism is dependent on the phosphorylation–dephosphorylation of the relevant enzymes. The rate-limiting enzymes of glycogen metabolism are the catabolic enzyme, phosphorylase (which is active in the phospho- form), and the anabolic enzyme, glycogen synthetase (which is active in the dephosphoform), as shown in Figs 8.6 and 8.7, respectively. These reciprocal effects can be interlinked; thus, both glucagon and epinephrine stimulate glycogenolysis, with mobilization of glucose from glycogen via a cAMP-dependent protein kinase (Fig. 2.16).

The converse process—that is, the switch from glycogenolysis to glycogen synthesis—may be triggered either by a fall in the tissue content of cAMP or by a rise in blood-glucose concentration. The fall in tissue concentration of cAMP may result from a switch from a glucagon-dominated to an insulin-dominated state (Fig. 8.7). In addition, the rise in blood glucose itself may be critical, since it is possible that the attachment of a glucose molecule to the active form of the relevant phosphorylase (phosphorylase *a*) (Fig. 8.6) may modify the conformation of this enzyme. This change favours dephosphorylation and consequent inactivation of the enzyme to phosphorylase *b*. With the removal of phosphorylase *a*, there is therefore a cessation of glycogen breakdown. In addition, phosphorylase *a* is also a potent inhibitor of glycogen synthetase phosphatase (Fig. 8.7). Thus when glucagon is low, the decrease in phosphorylase *a* (Fig. 8.6) leads to activation of glycogen synthetase phophatase. This then converts glycogen synthetase to its activated form, which leads to stimulation of glycogen synthesis.

Triglyceride metabolism

Insulin affects the rate of lipogenesis (triglyceride synthesis) in a number of ways, and thus regulates triglyceride metabolism. A critical step in lipogenesis is the activation of an insulin-sensitive lipoprotein lipase in the capillaries. Fatty acids are then released from circulating chylomicrons and very-low-density lipoproteins, and taken up into adipose tissue. Lipogenesis is also facilitated by uptake of glucose, because its metabolism via the pentose phosphate pathway provides reducing equivalents (i.e.

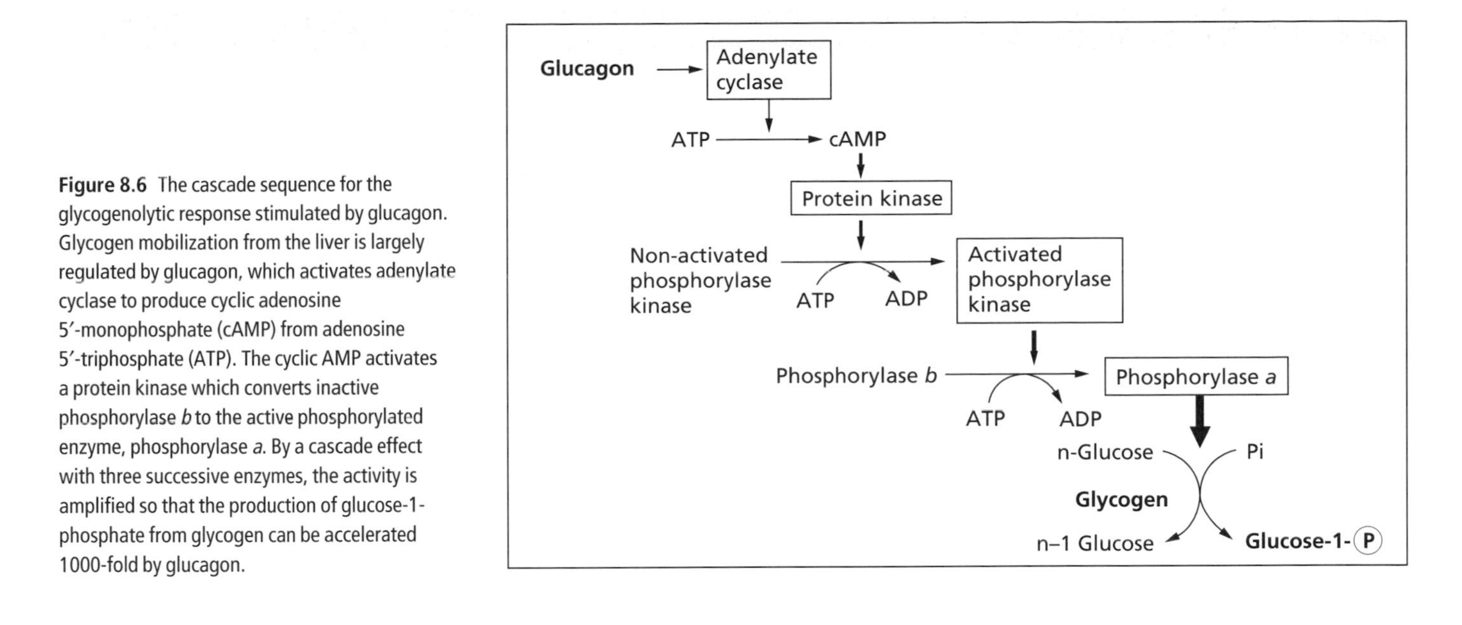

Figure 8.6 The cascade sequence for the glycogenolytic response stimulated by glucagon. Glycogen mobilization from the liver is largely regulated by glucagon, which activates adenylate cyclase to produce cyclic adenosine 5′-monophosphate (cAMP) from adenosine 5′-triphosphate (ATP). The cyclic AMP activates a protein kinase which converts inactive phosphorylase *b* to the active phosphorylated enzyme, phosphorylase *a*. By a cascade effect with three successive enzymes, the activity is amplified so that the production of glucose-1-phosphate from glycogen can be accelerated 1000-fold by glucagon.

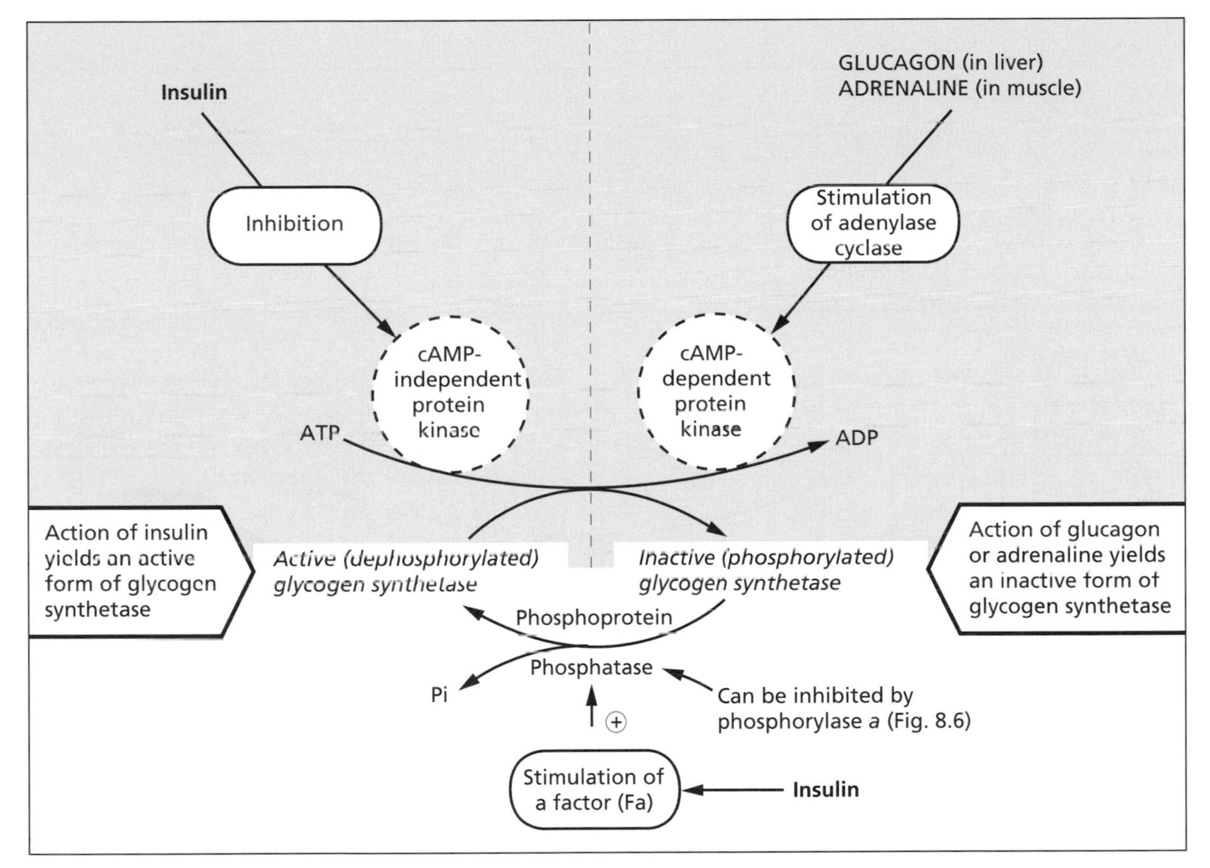

Figure 8.7 Regulation of glycogen synthetase activity by phosphorylation–dephosphorylation mechanisms. Glycogen synthetase is inactive in the phosphorylated form. Two protein kinases are capable of phosphorylating glycogen synthetase, one of which is cyclic adenosine 5′-monophosphate (cAMP)-dependent and the other cAMP-independent. Glucagon action on the liver or epinephrine action on muscle (top right of the illustration) stimulates adenylate cyclase. The increased concentrations of cAMP stimulate the cAMP-dependent protein kinase, which in turn inactivates glycogen synthetase; this reaction is required as part of the glycogenolytic action of these two hormones. The second protein kinase, which is cAMP-independent, is inhibited by insulin action (left of the illustration). The mechanism of inhibition is uncertain, but it may involve calcium ions or some other intracellular component that is produced by insulin action on the cell. Formation of inactive, phosphorylated glycogen synthetase is thus inhibited by insulin action, and glycogenesis is promoted. Insulin also activates a factor (Fa) that reacts with an inactive form of phosphoprotein phosphatase to produce the active form of the phosphatase. Insulin therefore acts on glycogen synthetase (a) by suppression of protein kinase activity and (b) by stimulation of phosphoprotein phosphatase activity, both of which favour the presence of the dephospho- form of the enzyme, and hence glycogenesis.

reduced nicotinamide adenine dinucleotide phosphate, NADPH) for fatty acid synthesis (Fig. 8.5). The availability of α-glycerophosphate for esterification is also important for triglyceride synthesis. Many of the actions of insulin in stimulating lipogenesis are opposed by glucagon. Triglycerides are stored as metabolic fuel depots in adipose tissue, and the maintenance and mobilization of these depots is under hormonal control. Mobilization of triglyceride from adipose tissue is dependent on an intracellular hormone-sensitive lipase, which can be activated by a number of hormones, including catecholamines, adrenocorticotrophin and glucagon. These hormones, via a cAMP-dependent protein kinase (see Fig. 2.16), convert the inactive form of the lipase to an active phosphorylated form. The enhanced release of free fatty acids from adipose tissue by this lipase can be reversed rapidly by insulin, although the mechanism of this antagonism is not yet clear.

Lipogenesis is also regulated by covalent modification, i.e. phosphorylation or dephosphorylation of the relevant enzymes, acetyl coenzyme A (CoA) carboxylase and fatty-acid synthetase. These two enzymes, which together constitute the lipogenic pathway, are also subject to allosteric modification; their activity is also dependent on the supply of precursors from the glycolytic pathway or in the pathway of lipogenesis itself. The first enzyme in the pathway, acetyl CoA carboxylase, is subject to phosphorylation–dephosphorylation interconversion, at least in adipose tissue and in the mammary gland (Fig. 8.8). The phosphorylation (inactivation) is catalysed by a cAMP-dependent protein kinase. Presumably, similar control mechanisms operate in the liver; phosphorylation of the carboxylase under the influence of a cAMP-dependent protein kinase could explain the very rapid inhibition of fatty-acid synthesis that occurs in liver

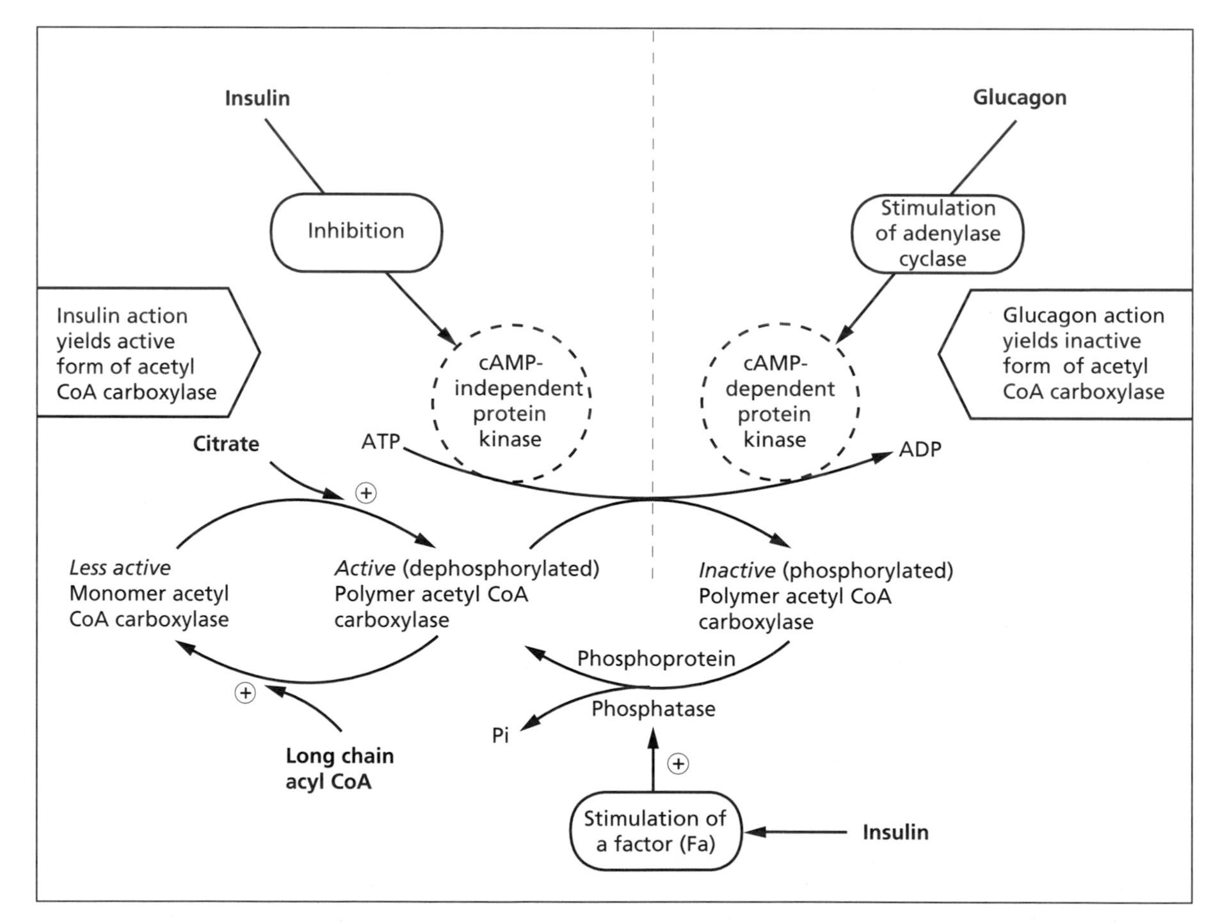

Figure 8.8 Regulation of acetyl coenzyme A (CoA) carboxylase by allosteric regulators and by phosphorylation–dephosphorylation mechanisms. Acetyl CoA carboxylase, which is involved in fatty-acid synthesis, exists as a monomer and in two polymeric forms, which are interconvertible by dephosphorylation. Citrate and long-chain acyl CoA control the relative proportions of the less active monomer and the active polymeric form of acetyl CoA carboxylase by allosteric mechanisms. As in the case of glycogen synthetase (see Fig. 8.7), two protein kinase enzymes are capable of regulating the conversion of active polymer acetyl CoA carboxylase to the inactive phosphorylated form of the enzyme. The cyclic adenosine 5′-monophosphate (cAMP)-dependent protein kinase may be activated by glucagon (top right of the illustration), while the cAMP-independent protein kinase is inhibited by insulin action on the target cell (top left of the illustration). Glucagon action on the cell hence decreases lipogenesis, while insulin stimulates fatty-acid synthesis.

following treatment with glucagon. A cAMP-independent protein kinase that can phosphorylate acetyl CoA carboxylase is also present, and this protein kinase may be the locus of control by insulin in stimulating fatty-acid synthesis. A second locus could be on the phosphoprotein phosphatase, with dephosphorylation of acetyl CoA carboxylase in a manner analogous to that described for insulin action on glycogen synthetase (Fig. 8.7).

As with glycogen synthesis (Fig. 8.7), the presence of both cAMP-dependent and cAMP-independent protein kinases controlling a single reaction provides an additional dimension to hormonal regulation of enzyme activity. When the concentration of glucagon is low and that of insulin is high (as can occur following a high carbohydrate load), both kinases could be inactive, and acetyl CoA carboxylase would be converted to the active form, with stimulation of lipogenesis. Regulation of the phosphatase by insulin can further accelerate this process, as could removal of long-chain acyl CoA derivatives (Fig. 8.8).

In diabetes, the activities of a group of enzymes involved in lipogenesis are reduced, but can be restored by the administration of insulin. These enzymes include acetyl CoA carboxylase, fatty-acid synthetase and enzymes of the pentose phosphate pathway. Not only is their activity reduced, but the amount present also falls because of a reduced rate of enzyme synthesis. The consequent decrease in lipogenesis and increased lipolysis yields free fatty acids, which are metabolized to ketones in the liver (Fig. 8.3).

Protein synthesis

Insulin stimulates the uptake of amino acids into cells, and in this way could stimulate protein synthesis. It may also regulate translation. The phosphorylation of ribosomal S6 protein is believed to be increased by insulin. Insulin can in addition increase polyamine synthesis, which appears to be involved in synthesis of ribosomal ribonucleic acid (RNA).

With insulin deficiency, amino acids are mobilized from muscle and transported to the liver, where they are deaminated (Fig. 8.3); this leads to increased urea production (Fig. 8.5). The carbon skeleton arising from amino acids will contribute not only to gluconeogenesis, but also to ketogenesis. Removal of the pituitary gland (hypophysectomy) in large measure restores the blood glucose of a diabetic animal towards normal, because of removal of growth hormone (GH) and adrenocorticotrophin, which are involved along with insulin in regulating glucose homoeostasis; while hypophysectomy can reduce the disturbance of carbohydrate metabolism in diabetic animals, protein synthesis remains disordered because of the absence of insulin. An advance in diabetic control may result from the development of pharmacological antagonists to GH secretion.

Conversely, the hormonal responses that occur after a protein-rich meal, or following the administration of an amino acid-rich mixture, will induce different changes from those of orally administered glucose (shown in Fig. 8.4). Amino acids cause the increased release of both insulin and glucagon, together with GH. These stimulate the uptake of amino acids into muscle cells, while maintaining the serum-glucose concentrations.

Ion transport

Insulin also modifies anion and cation transport into tissues. It counteracts the effects of glucagon and the cAMP-induced release of potassium ions (K^+) from perfused liver. Insulin may also alter Ca^{2+} flux and ion binding in a number of tissues. Increase in the concentration of Ca^{2+} within mitochondria could play an important part in regulating the activity of pyruvate dehydrogenase and altering the conversion of pyruvate to acetyl CoA, required for lipid synthesis, for ketone-body formation and for the tricarboxylic acid cycle (Fig. 8.5).

GLUCOSE OVERUTILIZATION IN DIABETES

The characteristic changes occurring in uncontrolled diabetes are a rise in blood glucose and increases in glycogen breakdown, gluconeogenesis, fatty-acid oxidation, ketone production and urea formation. There is depression in the synthesis of glycogen, lipid and protein in the cells of those tissues that are normally dependent on insulin.

Diabetes has classically been considered to be a disease with glucose overproduction by liver and underutilization by insulin-requiring tissues, such as muscle and adipose tissue. The cells of those tissues that have an insulin-dependent glucose transport system are relatively unaffected by the high blood-glucose concentrations in a diabetic, since the specific transport system for glucose into the cell is not active in the absence of insulin. This is not so, however, for the insulin-independent cells, in which glucose entry is largely governed by the concentration gradient between the exterior and interior of the cell. In consequence, overutilization of glucose can occur in these tissues. Thus, in diabetes there appears to be diversion of glucose from insulin-dependent pathways to those not requiring the hormone. The facilitation of many processes in such insulin-independent tissues by the raised levels of intracellular glucose results in some of

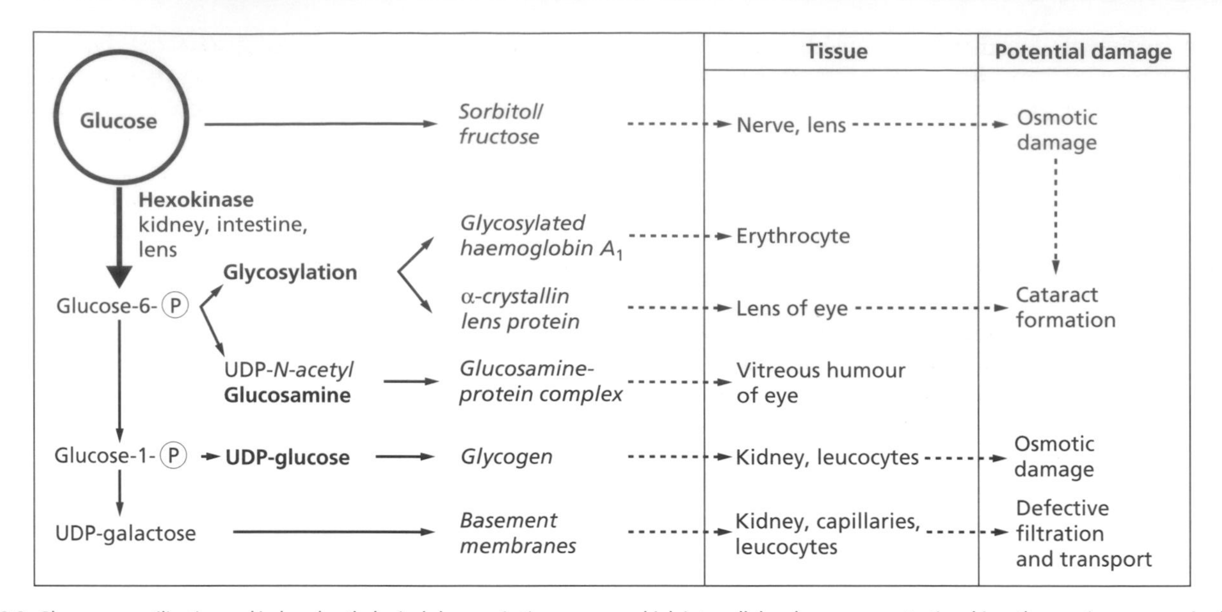

Figure 8.9 Glucose overutilization and induced pathological changes in tissues resulting from noninsulin-requiring pathways. Glucose movement into many cells, including those of the kidney, certain nerve tissues, the eye, the seminal vesicle, erythrocytes and leucocytes, is not dependent on insulin; in diabetes, the concentration gradient between the extracellular and intracellular compartments is sufficient to drive glucose into these cells. The mass effect of a high intracellular glucose concentration drives the reactions summarized above through some of the key intermediates shown. The increased activity of the sorbitol and glycogenic pathways yields osmotic damage, while glycosylation reactions lead to alterations in the eye and basement membranes of cells, which in turn affect permeability and transport mechanisms. These reactions may account for many of the pathological changes observed in severe diabetes.

the pathological phenomena associated with long-term diabetes (Fig. 8.9).

In uncontrolled or poorly controlled diabetes, there is increased glycosylation of a number of proteins, including haemoglobin and the α-crystallin of the lens in the eye. In long-term diabetes, the glycosylated form of haemoglobin, HbA_1, has altered affinity for oxygen, and this may be a factor in tissue anoxia; while the glycosylation of α-crystallin lens protein may lead to cataract formation. A glucosamine–protein complex is also formed in long-standing diabetes, resulting in biochemical and morphological alterations to the capillary system, and there is some evidence that increased glycosylation of collagen is related to basement-membrane thickening in the kidney.

Several factors tend to promote the diversion of glucose into the sorbitol pathway leading to fructose. In diabetes, the most important factors are first, the high level of intracellular glucose in tissues in which the glucose transport system is insulin-independent, such as lens, eye and kidney; and secondly, the high NADPH : $NADP^+$ ratio, which results from the decrease in the rate of other reductive synthetic reactions, such as fatty-acid synthesis. The accumulation of sorbitol could cause osmotic damage—which may be important, for example, in the aetiology of cataract formation. The peripheral neuropathy and altered motor-nerve conduction velocity that occurs in some diabetic patients may be linked to sorbitol accumulation and associated changes in myoinositol.

In some tissues, such as the kidney, which do not require insulin for glucose uptake but rely on maintenance of the higher serum-to-tissue concentration gradient of glucose, changes in the activity of a variety of enzymes occur that facilitate rates of glucose utilization along specific metabolic routes. In diabetes, the increased activity of hexokinase in renal cortex, intestinal mucosa and lens may lead to glucose overutilization; the concentration of glucose-6-phosphate rises, and this can lead in turn to an increase of glycogen and of components of basement membranes in these tissues (Fig. 8.9). An increase has also been observed in the activity of enzymes of the pathway that leads to uridine diphosphate (UDP)-glucose (used in glycosylation reactions), and of the glucuronate–xylulose pathway and the pentose phosphate pathway in kidney.

The activity of the kidney glucosyl transferase is increased; this enzyme transfers glucose residues from UDP-glucose on to the galactosyl hydroxylysine residues, which can thus be linked to the thickening of the filtration basement membrane that occurs in diabetes, but which is reduced following insulin treatment. Hence, the increase in hexokinase, which provides the precursor glucose-6-phosphate for these multiple pathways, could be an important determinant in the subsequent metabolic response to diabetes; its increased activity may lead to structural changes in the tissues, and excessive glucose utilization in certain tissues may in the longer term be more damaging than glucose underutilization in the body as a whole.

Effects of diabetes mellitus

The classical symptoms of diabetes mellitus are the passage of an increased volume of urine (polyuria) and thirst (polydipsia). Polyuria occurs because of the elevation of the glucose concentration in glomerular filtrate. This induces an osmotic diuresis, because the renal threshold for the reabsorption of glucose in the proximal tubule is exceeded in the proximal tubule. Thus glucose continues down the loop of Henle, distal tubule and collecting duct, exerting an osmotic force that reduces reabsorption of water. Glycosuria therefore entrains loss of water.

Loss of water causes thirst, which in turn stimulates the patient to drink more. Weight loss is common, and can be attributed to the combination of loss of calories as glucose in the urine and the increased breakdown of fat and protein. Urine containing large amounts of glucose can induce infection and soreness of the vulva in women and of the foreskin in men, and the presence of glycosuria predisposes to infections of the urinary tract. Testing for the presence of glucose in the urine is used as a screening procedure to identify diabetes; the diagnosis can then be confirmed by showing that the blood sugar is elevated. This may be due either to a lack of insulin (type 1, insulin-dependent diabetes mellitus, IDDM) or to insulin resistance (type 2, noninsulin-dependent diabetes mellitus, NIDDM).

Severe uncontrolled IDDM leads to diabetic ketosis or ketoacidosis. Rapid mobilization of triglycerides releases fatty acids into the circulation, where they are taken to the liver and metabolized. β-Hydroxybutyric acid and acetoacetic acid are produced far in excess of the ability of the tissues to use them, and their concentration in the circulation rises rapidly. They can cause nausea, vomiting and a serious metabolic acidosis. The respiratory centre is stimulated and this produces a characteristic deep sighing respiration (Kussmaul breathing).

Uncontrolled insulin-deficient diabetes leads to a very high blood-glucose concentration and a profuse osmotic diuresis, with loss of large amounts of water, sodium and other electrolytes in urine. This in turn depletes the extracellular fluid, and the plasma volume falls, leading to a reduction of blood pressure and of glomerular filtration. Breakdown of intracellular protein leads to a loss of cell water and electrolytes, and if the glomerular filtration rate is reduced because of the decreased extracellular fluid volume, the plasma K^+ may rise. At the same time, increased deamination of the amino acids released from the cells may contribute to a rise in blood urea and a serious negative nitrogen balance. Dehydration is caused by the passage of large volumes of urine, and contributes to the rise in blood urea. Total body water may fall by as much as 6 L, half of this coming from the extracellular and half from the intracellular compartments.

The main principles of treatment of diabetic ketoacidosis are based on an understanding of the pathophysiology of this condition. Fluid has to be given intravenously to restore extracellular fluid volume and maintain the circulation and blood pressure, and thus restore the glomerular filtration rate. This has to be given as saline in order to prevent rapid entry of water into the hyperosmolar cells, particularly brain cells. Cerebral oedema is the most feared complication of the management of diabetic ketoacidosis, and is the main cause of the continuing mortality in this condition.

It is necessary to give sufficient insulin to control the unrestrained gluconeogenesis by the liver and to restore glucose metabolism to insulin-dependent tissues; this will arrest lipolysis and ketone production. At an early stage, administration of K^+ is required to restore the intracellular losses of this ion; this can be done safely when glucose is entering cells under the influence of insulin and when renal function is satisfactory. Insulin is normally given by intravenous infusion in small amounts. The large boluses that used to be given down-regulate the insulin receptors, and this defeats the therapeutic intention.

Hormone imbalance and other factors in the genesis of diabetes mellitus

Overproduction of some hormones can give rise to the clinical syndrome of diabetes mellitus, because their actions are opposite to those of insulin. Examples are the elevated growth hormone concentrations associated with acromegaly, excessive production of epinephrine—for example, by a phaeochromocytoma in the adrenal medulla—and overproduction of cortisol from the adrenal cortex or the administration of large amounts of glucocorticoids. Overproduction of glucagon is very rare, but severe damage to the pancreas by disease or surgery can produce diabetes from a deficiency of insulin.

There are two principal types of diabetes. In the first, juvenile IDDM (type 1), there is progressive, and eventually total, failure to secrete insulin. It is in this group of diabetics that ketoacidosis can develop. The cause of the disorder is autoimmune destruction of the insulin-secreting cells by islet-cell antibodies.

The second major group of patients with diabetes mellitus develop a condition in which an inadequate amount of insulin is secreted relative to the blood-glucose concentration, even though the insulin-secreting cells are structurally intact. This condition, NIDDM (type 2), is often familial. This is the more common form of the disease and it usually develops between the ages of 40 and 70, so that it is also called late-onset or maturity-onset diabetes. It is most common in obese individuals, because obesity leads to resistance to the action of insulin.

Genetic factors are important in the causation of both types of diabetes. It has long been known that there is a tendency for diabetes to run in families, and analysis of the contribution of genetic factors has been helped by studying identical twins. These twins have the same genetic make-up, so that if one develops diabetes and the condition really is inherited, the other should develop it within a few years. In the older group of noninsulindependent diabetics, the condition is found to be concordant, i.e. both twins are affected, but in the insulin-dependent, usually younger diabetics, only half of the twins are concordant and the other half are discordant. This led to the suspicion that there were other factors that cause IDDM apart from heredity.

Viral infections may be important, due to an effect on the islets of Langerhans in the pancreas. Viruses may initiate the destruction of the islets by the antibodies, which are genetically determined and already present.

Studies of human leucocyte antigen (HLA) markers have indicated that there is a relationship between these antigenic determinants and type 1 diabetes. The class II antigens DR3 and DR4 are associated with an increased risk of developing IDDM. As with autoimmune thyroid disease, it is possible that the expression of the DR antigen by 'injured' β-cells may be one mechanism by which the autoimmunogen is presented to the T-lymphocytes and the autoimmune process is thus initiated.

Diagnosis and treatment of diabetes mellitus

The diagnosis of diabetes mellitus relies primarily on determination of the concentration of glucose and ketones in blood and urine. Direct immunoassay of the hormones that regulate glucose homeostasis, i.e. insulin and glucagon, together with GH and glucocorticoids, is rarely required. In addition to hyperglycaemia, glycosuria and ketonaemia, raised concentrations of K^+, urea, creatinine and hydrogen ion concentrations will be encountered in diabetic ketoacidosis.

Blood for glucose determination is collected in 'fluoride–oxalate' tubes. The fluoride inhibits glycolysis by red blood cells, which could occur during transport to the laboratory and subsequent storage; potassium oxalate is present as an anticoagulant. Plasma-glucose or serum-glucose levels are 10–15% higher than those in unseparated whole blood, since structural components of the blood cells are absent. There is therefore more glucose per unit fluid volume. While whole blood is used for spot-testing of glucose in an emergency and in self-monitoring of capillary-blood glucose, plasma-glucose or serum-glucose measurement is more frequently used clinically, since plasma and serum are suitable for autoanalysers.

Laboratory determination of glucose can be carried out by several methods. These include enzymatic methods, such as those based on glucose oxidase or hexokinase, or colorimetric methods, e.g. *o*-toluidine. In addition, automated methods frequently rely on reduction of copper or iron compounds by reducing sugars in dialysed serum.

Self-monitoring of capillary-blood glucose is carried out by the patients themselves, and this is important for long-term management of the diabetics. There are several variations in the paper-strip methods, which rely on glucose oxidase, but testing of urinary glucose is no longer generally undertaken, because negative glycosuria does not mean good blood-glucose control: it is this which is important in preventing the progress of the complications of diabetes.

If clinical symptoms of diabetes mellitus are present, a diagnosis is confirmed by a fasting plasma-glucose concentration exceeding 7.8 mmol/L or by a random value that is greater than 11.1 mmol/L; the normal range is 3–5 mmol/L. If no symptoms are present, either of these criteria should be observed on more than one occasion to establish a diagnosis. If the results are considered equivocal, an oral glucose-tolerance test (OGTT) should be carried out. The patient is given 75 g glucose/1.73 m^2 body surface area orally, and blood glucose is monitored at 30-minute intervals for up to 2 h. In a normal individual, the 2-h value is the same or less than the basal concentration (Fig. 8.4), and diabetes mellitus is diagnosed if venous plasma glucose at 2 h exceeds 10.0 mmol/L. Some patients will not meet these diagnostic criteria, although the blood glucose will be raised. They are classified as having 'impaired glucose tolerance', and should be monitored on an annual basis.

Glucose tolerance declines with age, and as a consequence the reference range of glucose in separated or unseparated blood should be corrected; 0.056 mmol/L should be added for each year after 60.

If a patient is completely deficient in insulin, there is no alternative but to treat the individual with injections of insulin, since the polypeptide would be degraded if given by mouth. However, if the patient is resistant to insulin, particularly if this is associated with marked obesity, then dietary advice and a reduction of body weight is the best treatment, and seems to lead to restoration of insulin sensitivity; diabetes many even disappear, as long as the patient remains thinner. Between these two extremes, there are patients who are partially insulin-deficient, and there are drugs available that stimulate the pancreatic islet cells to secrete more insulin. These drugs are helpful in avoiding the need for injections of insulin, particularly in a number of middle-aged diabetics who are not overweight. Sulphonylureas, such as tolbutamide, chlorpropamide and glibenclamide, stimulate secretion of insulin and may even cause hypoglycaemia. Biguanides, in contrast, act by increasing glucose uptake in tissues and reducing appetite.

When insulin was first isolated, it was hoped that diabetics would no longer die from infections and diabetic ketosis, and that they would be able to lead a normal life. It is now possible to relieve the symptoms of diabetes and to prevent ketosis by treating the disease. Nevertheless, long-standing diabetes may lead to a number of complications. Some of these are due to deposition of cholesterol in the arteries, causing atheroma of the coronary arteries or the large blood vessels of the legs. In addition, there may be damage to the nervous system, including the autonomic nervous system. The eyes and kidneys may also be affected, owing to changes in the lens and basement membrane of small blood vessels, respectively (Fig. 8.9): the development of some of these complications may be attributable to overutilization of glucose by some tissues, as discussed above. The risk of progression of these complications is much greater if the diabetes is poorly controlled. However, even so, some well-controlled diabetics still develop complications, whilst some poorly controlled ones paradoxically escape them.

As mentioned above, frequent measurement of blood-glucose concentration by the patient is valuable for monitoring treatment. However, these glucose levels may not be representative of overall long-term diabetic control. A better reflection of this is obtained by measurement of glycosylated haemoglobin, since glycosylation of haemoglobin is dependent on the mean concentration of glucose in blood. Total HbA_1, which is in fact the sum of three different glycohaemoglobins, once formed, remains in the red cell for the 120-day lifetime of that cell. Consequently, this reflects average glucose concentrations that have occurred over the preceding 6–8 weeks. Normally $< 7\%$ of total haemoglobin will be present as HbA_1, but in poorly controlled diabetics this can rise to $\approx 15\%$. Abnormal haemoglobins or haemolytic states complicate the interpretation of HbA_1 results.

Sensitive immunoassays are now available for urinary albumin, and one of the earliest biochemical markers of diabetic nephropathy may be the detection of microalbuminuria. Excretion of $> 20\ \mu g$ albumin/minute, as determined from timed overnight collections, is indicative of this condition; controls excrete $< 16\ \mu g$/minute.

As has already been described, the normal pattern of insulin release after a meal results in a very rapid rise, with a peak between 30 and 60 min and then a rapid fall until the next meal is taken (Fig. 8.4). Insulin is released into the portal vein, so that it can act directly on the liver, and blood glucose is controlled between very narrow limits, usually between about 3 and 5 mmol/L in normal individuals. Subcutaneous injections of insulin cannot mimic this pattern, since serum insulin rises and remains elevated longer than in the normal individual, and all tissues of the body are exposed to the same concentration; it is not yet possible to reproduce selectively the higher concentration in the portal vein. Insulin replacement therapy is therefore very different from the physiological release of insulin from the pancreas of the healthy subject, and this may contribute to the failure to achieve glucose homeostasis and to the onset of the complications.

Effects of excess insulin

Excess insulin causes a fall in the concentration of blood sugar. The brain is extremely sensitive to the lack of glucose, and this goes some way to explain the symptoms of hypoglycaemia, which include blurring of vision, slurring of speech and unsteadiness of gait: cerebral tissue may be irritated, and fits can result. If the blood-glucose concentration remains very low, the patient becomes unconscious. This combination of symptoms is sometimes referred to as 'neuroglycopenia' or a 'hypoglycaemic attack'. Sympathetic activity is increased, and the enhanced epinephrine concentrations will produce glycogenolysis and release glucose from the liver. At the same time, the patient sweats profusely, and there is tachycardia and often tremor. While the sympathetic nervous system can respond rapidly, other regulatory mechanisms, such as glucagon from the pancreas, cortisol from the adrenal cortex and GH from the pituitary contribute more slowly to glucose homeostasis.

Hypoglycaemic attacks can occur in diabetic patients who are being treated with insulin. Most commonly this occurs if they do not have enough food after an injection of insulin, or if they exercise excessively; if it is known that exercise is to be more vigorous than usual, the patient should either reduce the dose of insulin or take extra carbohydrate.

Hypoglycaemic attacks can be caused in previously normal individuals by a tumour of the islet cells of the pancreas, which secretes insulin; such a tumour is called an insulinoma. The symptoms may be precipitated by a prolonged fast or by exercise, and the blood glucose can fall to below 2 mmol/L. Investigation of a patient with an insulinoma will show that, even at a time when the blood sugar is low, insulin is still detectable in the circulation, whereas, if the blood sugar falls in a normal person, the secretion of insulin is suppressed. The blood sugar of a patient with an insulinoma is not continuously low, and it is important to measure the blood sugar and the concentration of insulin present during a period when the patient has hypoglycaemic symptoms. If this is not possible, it may be necessary to provoke hypoglycaemia and see whether the production of insulin by the pancreas is suppressed. This is best achieved by administration of insulin to provoke hypoglycaemia and then measure the amount of C-peptide in the circulation. If endogenous secretion of insulin from an insulinoma continues, there will be release of C-peptide into the circulation at the same time in the same proportion to the insulin released; C-peptide is not removed in the liver (as is the case for portal venous insulin), and can thus be measured to distinguish endogenously produced insulin from that administered exogenously.

Since the insulin-producing islet cells are more commonly located in the tail of the pancreas, an insulinoma is more likely to be found there. However, the islet cells are scattered through the pancreas, and there may be more than one tumour present. It is possible to locate the tumours before surgery by arteriography, by computer-assisted tomographic scanning, or by ultrasound. The tumours may be very small and difficult to find, and it may not be possible to remove them; occasionally they are malignant, and there may be metastases that secrete insulin. In either case, an alternative form of therapy is to administer the drug diazoxide orally; this inhibits insulin secretion and prevents the production of hypoglycaemia. Such treatment obviously does not cure the patient, which is the object of surgery.

OTHER HORMONES SECRETED BY THE PANCREAS

Somatostatin

This peptide, which consists of 14 amino acids arranged in a single chain, is secreted from the δ-cells of the islets of Langerhans, and is stored in the granules of the δ-cells (Fig. 8.1). Somatostatin inhibits the release of insulin and glucagon from the pancreas in a paracrine manner (see Fig. 1.2). In the pancreas, somatostatin secreted from the δ-cells probably acts mainly on its neighbouring α- and β-cells. Somatostatin from the hypothalamus is the well-recognized negative regulator of GH secretion from the anterior pituitary (Chapter 3), but it has also been localized in gut cells and in peripheral nerves; with such a distribution, it can be seen to act as an endocrine or paracrine peptide, or as a neurotransmitter.

Pharmacological doses of somatostatin inhibit virtually all gastrointestinal functions. Exocrine and endocrine secretions from the gastrointestinal tract and also intestinal absorption are reduced, even when stimulated by maximal doses of the appropriate hormones (e.g. gastrin and CCK). Synthetic somatostatin is now available, and infusions that yield plasma concentrations similar to those found after the ingestion of a meal induce several of the inhibitory effects noted above. In addition, somatostatin may physiologically inhibit the secretion of gastric acid, gastric emptying and the release of gastrin. The secretion of pancreatic bicarbonate and enzymes is reduced, as is gallbladder emptying. The release of PP, motilin and GIP is inhibited, as is the absorption of glucose, xylose and triglycerides.

A mixed meal elicits an increase in plasma somatostatin concentrations. The peptide is released from both the stomach and pancreas following the administration of proteins, fats, or carbohydrates, either intragastrically or intraduodenally. Acid in the duodenum is also a very potent stimulus, making somatostatin a strong candidate for a role in the 'bulbogastrone mechanism', in which there is a reduction in gastric-acid secretion during the acidification of the duodenal bulb. It would appear that the biological role for somatostatin is to prevent exaggerated responses following a meal.

As somatostatin has so many inhibitory effects, it is hardly surprising that its potential use as a therapeutic agent has been considered. However, a limitation is that somatostatin is cleared from the circulation in a matter of minutes. This has restricted the peptide's therapeutic use, and a synthetic octapeptide with two D-amino acid substitutions has been developed that provides therapeutic efficacy with only two daily subcutaneous injections (a situation comparable to the administration of insulin to a diabetic patient). Patients with life-threatening diarrhoea associated with gut or pancreatic tumours—e.g. gastrinoma or vasoactive intestinal peptide tumour (VIPoma)—can be treated with this analogue. The results can be dramatic: the peptide is well tolerated, the stool volumes are greatly reduced, and liquid excretions are replaced by semiformed and normal stools.

Pancreatic polypeptide

This peptide is produced by endocrine cells that are found in small clusters of PP cells located between cells of the islets of Langerhans and the acinar cells of the pancreas.

PP is a powerful inhibitor of the secretion of enzymes by the pancreas, and also blocks the contraction of the gallbladder and hence the secretion of bile. These effects might at first appear strange. However, PP concentrations remain high for several hours after a meal, long after other hormone concentrations have reverted to their basal levels observed during the interdigestive period. By this means, PP may help to conserve digestive enzymes and store bile for a subsequent meal.

As in the case of insulin, the secretion of PP increases after a meal, particularly of meat or fish. Unlike insulin, however, this stimulation is not dependent on the concentration of glucose in the circulation, and the regulation is partly under both neural and hormonal control.

Stimulation of the vagus nerve induces secretion of PP, and there is also an endocrine regulatory system in which hormones such as CCK, which is itself released by food, stimulate the release of PP. The role of PP remains uncertain; it is often produced in large amounts by pancreatic endocrine tumours, but there are no symptoms or metabolic disturbances that can be attributed to this overproduction.

HORMONES FROM THE GASTROINTESTINAL TRACT

It was possible at one time to argue that hormone control of the gastrointestinal tract could be accounted for by three hormones: secretin, gastrin and CCK (also called pancreozymin) (Table 8.2). Since 1970, however, a large number of hormones have been detected in the gastrointestinal tract, in which they have also been shown to exert effects. In many instances, though, it still remains to be determined whether these effects are physiological or pharmacological.

Hormones of the gastrointestinal tract are difficult to study, because they are not produced by discrete groups of cells organized into glands. Instead, they are released from single cells scattered along the digestive tract. Furthermore, as several of these peptides are found both in specific endocrine cells and in neurones and their nerve terminals, it is difficult to establish which effects are dependent on peptide release from nerve terminals and which represent endocrine activity. Because of this, many would prefer to group the biologically active peptides together as 'regulatory peptides', rather than describe, with uncertainty, an agent as having endocrine or neurotransmitter activity.

Hormones acting on the pancreas

Secretin

In 1902 Bayliss and Starling demonstrated that the pancreas responded to stimuli applied within the duodenum even when it had been denervated, and in this way they showed that Pavlov's theories had to be modified. Pavlov had established that the physiological responses of the body appeared purposive; for example, meat placed in the duodenum evoked enzyme secretions and acid produced an alkaline secretion. He proposed that nervous regulation was the most likely mechanism of control. However, the denervated pancreas still responded, and in addition, extracts of the duodenum were found to stimulate the pancreas. Bayliss and Starling deduced that the duodenal mucosa released an active principle, named secretin, into the blood that controlled pancreatic function. Eventually, secretin was isolated and shown to be a peptide with 27 amino acids arranged in a single chain. It is produced by endocrine cells in the duodenal and jejunal mucosa (Fig. 8.10), which appear to be replaced every 120 h.

Secretin stimulates the pancreas to elaborate a fluid rich in bicarbonate. Such a fluid contributes to the neutralization of acid chyme released from the stomach, and it provides a medium of suitable pH for digestion of food by pancreatic enzymes. The threshold for secretin release is pH 4.5, and it is maximally secreted in the range of pH 1–3, but only limited areas of the proximal small intestine are transiently exposed to such a low pH. Plasma concentrations of secretin are reduced when meal-induced acid secretion is prevented or inhibited from reaching the

Table 8.2 Actions of gut hormones on the gastrointestinal tract.

Hormone	Origin	Released by	Produces
Secretin	Proximal small intestine	Acid in duodenum	A bicarbonate-rich pancreatic secretion
Gastrin	Gastric antrum	Distension of stomach and by peptides	Stomach contractions and gastric secretion
Cholecystokinin (pancreozymin)	Proximal small intestine	Products of fat and protein digestion	Gall-bladder contractions An enzyme-rich pancreatic secretion

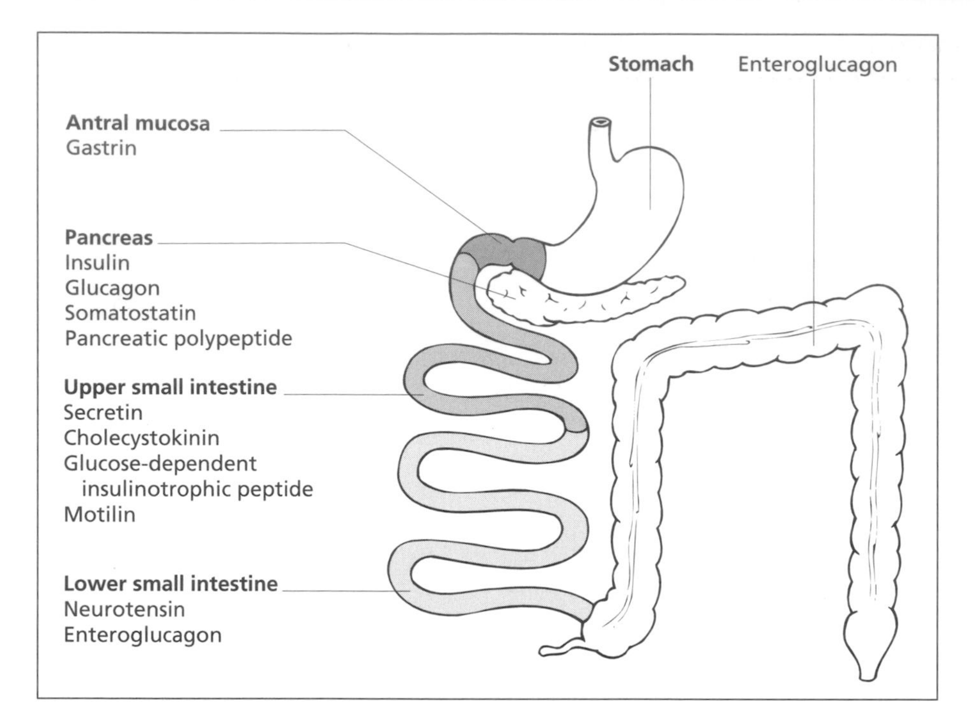

Figure 8.10 The distribution of the hormones of the pancreas and gastrointestinal tract. The approximate location of hormones is shown by shaded areas. Insulin, glucagon and somatostatin are synthesized in cells of the pancreatic islets of Langerhans, and pancreatic polypeptide is found in endocrine cells scattered throughout the pancreas. Gastrin is located in the antral mucosa of the stomach, while the other peptide hormones are found in endocrine cells in the upper or lower small intestine, as shown in the diagram. Enteroglucagon is quite widely distributed throughout the small intestine, as well as in the mucosa of the colon and rectum.

duodenum by aspiration, the use of antacids or the action of an H_2 histamine-receptor antagonist (which inhibits gastric-acid secretion). Postprandial changes of secretin concentrations in humans are small, but there is a positive correlation between the load of acid entering the duodenum and the circulating concentration of secretin. The most rapid rate of acid disappearance and the maximal secretin concentration occur 1.5–2 h after a liquid meal, suggesting that the peptide is important in the postprandial period. Antiserum against secretin reduces postprandial bicarbonate secretions by more than 80%.

Cholecystokinin (also called pancreozymin)

The name 'cholecystokinin' refers to the action of this hormone in causing contraction of the gallbladder. It is synthesized in the endocrine cells of the mucosa of the upper small intestine, and the peptide can also be detected in neurones of the small and large intestine. CCK exists in a number of forms: the largest has 39 amino acids arranged in a single chain, but there is another peptide, consisting of 33 amino acids, which was the first to be isolated. However, only the last eight amino acids, in the carboxy terminus of the peptide, are necessary for full activity, and this octapeptide also occurs naturally. All these peptides have the same spectrum of biological activity, although the smaller forms are more rapidly destroyed. A synthetic octapeptide can be used to test the ability of the pancreas to secrete enzymes. CCK is unstable in the circulation. Its release is stimulated by fat and protein present in a meal. CCK stimulates the release of pancreatic juice rich in enzymes, e.g. amylase, or inactive enzyme precursors, e.g. trypsinogen. These enzymes are the most versatile of those encountered along the digestive tract, in that they are capable of hydrolysing the two major classes of nutrients, carbohydrates and proteins. CCK induces the contraction and evacuation of the gall-bladder, with the release of bile into the duodenum. It may control the motility of the sphincter so as to prevent the emptying of bile into the duodenum from being too rapid.

CCK has other important properties. It appears to be the most powerful stimulator of pancreatic growth, causing increases in pancreatic weight, DNA and enzyme content. It may also produce a sensation indicating that enough food has been eaten, and so determine satiety and appetite. Finally, the peptide may have a role in intestinal transport; both sodium and water absorption have been found to increase in response to CCK.

Other hormones secreted by the stomach and gastrointestinal tract

Gastrin

Gastrin is secreted by the specialized endocrine G-cells, which are located in the antral part of the gastric mucosa (Fig. 8.10 and Table 8.3). In the fetus, but not in the adult,

Table 8.3 Actions of gut hormones on the gastrointestinal tract.

Hormone	Site of action	Effect
Secretin	Pancreatic acini Liver	↑ HCO_3-rich secretion ↑ Bile secretion
Cholecystokinin (pancreozymin)	Gall-bladder Pancreatic acini	↑ Contraction ↑ Enzyme secretion
Gastrin	Stomach (parietal cells)	↑ Gastric-acid secretion
Glucose-dependent insulinotrophic peptide	Pancreas (islets of Langerhans)	↑ Insulin secretion
Motilin	Stomach, duodenum, jejunum, oesophagus	↑ Smooth-muscle contractions
Enteroglucagon	Stomach and rest of GI tract	↑ Mucosal growth
Neurotensin	Stomach	↓ Gastric-acid secretion ↓ Smooth-muscle motility
Vasoactive intestinal peptide	Stomach Liver Pancreas	↓ Gastric-acid secretion ↑ Glucose release ↑ Insulin release ↑ HCO_3^--rich secretion

GI, gastrointestinal; HCO_3^-, bicarbonate.

gastrin cells are also found in the pancreas. The main action of gastrin is to stimulate the gastric parietal cells to secrete acid. Secretion of gastrin is stimulated by distension of the stomach and by the presence of small peptides and amino acids in the stomach. Gastrin increases the blood flow to the gastric mucosa, and has a direct effect on the gastric glands themselves. Presence of food in the stomach will release gastrin, as will also the thought, sight, smell and taste of food, as well as chewing and swallowing (the cephalic phase), through activation of the vagus. When the pH of the gastric contents falls below 2.5, the release of gastrin is inhibited. It is thought that acid acts directly on the G-cells and terminates the gastrin-stimulated phase of gastric digestion.

Gastrin also influences gastric peristalsis. The frequency of this event depends on rhythmic waves of depolarization and repolarization, which originate in smooth muscle on the superior curvature and pass towards the lesser curvature and pyloric region. The term 'basal electrical rhythm' (BER) has been used to describe these waves; they are not muscular contractions. These electrical changes do not necessarily lead to contractions, but they do set the frequency of gastric peristalsis (about two per minute), and hence they co-ordinate it. If the stomach is stimulated when the smooth muscle is in a state of maximal depolarization, a contraction is more likely to occur. Gastrin produces a greater force of contraction, and can also increase the frequency of the BER.

As in the case of CCK, gastrin can exist in a number of forms. The largest has 34 amino acids, but peptides with 17 and 14 amino acids are secreted as well. In fact, it is only the four amino acids at the carboxy terminus that are required for full biological activity, and a synthetic tetrapeptide is fully active. The only difference between these forms is that the larger ones are less rapidly degraded, and so their action persists for longer. The same four amino acids that constitute the active form of gastrin are also present in CCK; therefore, large amounts of CCK can stimulate acid production, and the enzyme-secreting cells of the pancreas can respond to large amounts of gastrin.

The concentration of gastrin is normal in patients who have duodenal ulcers, but if attempts are made to neutralize gastric acid by administration of antacids, the secretion of gastrin increases. The gastrin-secreting cells may be removed by surgical excision of the gastric antrum, which thereby diminishes not only the production of acid, but also the secretion of gastrin. Overproduction of gastrin is found in patients with tumours of the G-cells. This syndrome was first described by Zollinger and Ellison, and is associated with severe ulceration of the stomach and duodenum. The condition can be treated by removal of the tumour, but if this is not possible, removal of all acid-producing cells by total gastrectomy may be required. However, it is often possible to treat the condition satisfactorily by giving large oral doses of a histamine-blocking agent, such as cimetidine or ranitidine, both of which are H_2 antagonists.

Glucose-dependent insulinotrophic peptide (gastric inhibitory peptide)

This hormone is found in the endocrine cells of the upper small intestine, and it can stimulate the release of insulin, but only if blood glucose is raised; the latter feature obviously provides a safety mechanism, since stimulation of insulin secretion when blood glucose is low would be undesirable. Glucose and fat in the lumen of the intestine can stimulate release of GIP. It has been known for some time that glucose given by mouth produces a far greater rise in the secretion of insulin than the same quantity of glucose infused intravenously. GIP is not an insulin secretagogue, but it augments glucose-stimulated insulin release when the plasma glucose concentration is about 20% above the fasting level. The correlation between GIP and insulin release has been convincingly demonstrated in humans, using a 'glucose-clamp' technique, in which constant hyperglycaemia is created by continuous intravenous glucose infusion. This produces a typical biphasic insulin response. Glucose at a dose of 40 g/m^2 of body surface area is then ingested. Although plasma concentrations of immunoreactive GIP change little before glucose ingestion, there is a pronounced increase following an oral glucose load. Insulin concentrations also rise strikingly above the elevated levels induced by hyperglycaemia alone. The time-courses for the rises in concentrations of GIP and insulin are nearly identical. GIP therefore has an important role in signalling to the pancreas that a significant carbohydrate or fat load is present in the gut that will require metabolic disposal.

Motilin

This is a peptide that can stimulate the smooth muscle of the stomach and upper small intestine. It is secreted by specific endocrine cells found in the mucosa of the duodenum and jejunum (Fig. 8.10), and the hormone is present in the circulation even in the fasting state. Administration of motilin increases the contractions of the stomach and small intestine, even in the fasting state, when it is thought that it acts to keep the lumen of the bowel free of secretions and debris. Motilin also increases the rate of gastric emptying after a meal. It may stimulate the lower oesophageal sphincter to prevent reflux of acid into the oesophagus. The concentration of motilin increases only slightly after a meal, however. In older people, there may be inadequate secretion of motilin, and this may contribute to stasis and the development of bacterial overgrowth in the lumen of the bowel; this may damage the mucosa and cause malabsorption. Intravenous infusion of glucose or amino acids suppresses the release of motilin, and it may therefore have a role in regulating contractions of the gut and adjusting them to the rate of absorption of the food.

Enteroglucagon

Extracts of the small intestine contain enteroglucagon, a peptide that is similar, although not identical, to pancreatic glucagon. The similarities are sufficient for immunological assays for glucagon to be used in measurement of enteroglucagon. The properties of enteroglucagon are different from those of pancreatic glucagon, and it does not, for example, stimulate the release of glucose from the liver. Moreover, the enteroglucagon is released by ingestion of fat and glucose, two substances that depress the release of glucagon from the pancreas. Enteroglucagon is secreted from the endocrine mucosal cells, which are found throughout the small intestine and also in the mucosa of the colon and rectum (Fig. 8.10); it is therefore the most distal of the gastrointestinal hormones. The secretion of enteroglucagon rises quite rapidly after a meal and is continued for many hours; fasting for several days is necessary to obtain a truly basal state.

Hormones that occur in both the gastrointestinal and the nervous system

A number of hormones have been found in both the gastrointestinal system and the nervous system. CCK, for example, has been found in the neurones and the fine nerves of the brain and in the peripheral nervous system. In the nervous system, the major form of CCK appears to be the octapeptide; it is rapidly destroyed, and this form is therefore appropriate to a role as a neurotransmitter. It may well be that the function of neural CCK is quite different from that of the larger peptide released from the intestinal endocrine cells. Injection of CCK into the brain indicates that it may be important in the control of appetite, and this may link its function in the nervous system with its role in the intestine.

Somatostatin was first isolated from the hypothalamus, as described above, in studies of the regulation of the secretion of GH, and only subsequently was it shown that it could inhibit the release of almost all the gastrointestinal hormones, in addition to blocking the effects on their target organs, such as enzyme secretions. In the brain, somatostatin is localized in neurones of the central nervous system, but in the periphery it is mostly found in endocrine cells.

Neurotensin

This peptide was first discovered in extracts of brain that were found to affect blood pressure. However, when the heads of rats and the rest of the body were extracted separately and assayed for their neurotensin content, it was found that most of the neurotensin occurred in the body, and it was then identified in the intestinal mucosa.

Intravenous infusions of neurotensin inhibit the secretion of gastric acid and the emptying of the stomach; vasodilatation also occurs in the mucosa. Thus, absorption of food may be enhanced by delaying internal transport, so that more time is available for mucosal transport to occur; a steep lumen-to-blood concentration gradient is maintained for the digested nutrients. The peptide consists of 14 amino acids, and is produced by specialized neurotensin endocrine cells in the ileum (Fig. 8.10). It is released into the bloodstream after a meal, and the amount secreted depends on the size of the meal; the larger the meal, the greater the release of the peptide. Neurotensin may be important in regulating the release of food from the stomach and hence the passage of food along the small intestine, thus avoiding an overload to the system. The release of neurotensin is disturbed after gastric surgery for duodenal ulcer; in this situation, the remnants of the stomach may empty rapidly, and the food may be 'dumped' too quickly into the intestine.

Substance P

This was the first peptide to be located both in the brain and in the gut. In the brain, it is synthesized in neurones, stored in axonal synapses and acts as a neuromodulator or a neurotransmitter. Its function in the brain and spinal cord appears to be closely related with the sensation of pain. In the periphery, particularly in the gut, substance P is found in neurones and occasionally in endocrine-type cells. It is not clear yet whether it is released only locally or also into the circulation—i.e. whether it is part of the paracrine or endocrine system. Substance P may also be the excitatory transmitter for neurones in the gut. In addition, it stimulates nitric oxide synthesis in endothelial cells. This gaseous messenger then diffuses into adjacent cells and activates guanylate cyclase, leading to smooth-muscle contraction.

Vasoactive intestinal peptide

Vasoactive intestinal peptide (VIP) was originally found in the gut, but was later also isolated in considerable quantities in the central nervous system. In both gut and brain, this peptide is found mainly in neurones and their synapses. In the gut, these neurones are found between the muscle layers, in the myenteric or Auerbach plexus and in the submucosa, the Meissner plexus. Pharmacologically, VIP can cause release of glucose from the liver and inhibit gastric-acid production, while stimulating pancreatic bicarbonate production and insulin secretion. These actions are normally expressed by the hormones glucagon, secretin and GIP. As the amino acid sequence of these peptides is similar, it has been suggested that they have evolved from a single precursor hormonal peptide, and there may therefore be an evolutionary relationship between these hormones and the neurotransmitters. VIP is present in many other tissues apart from the gut, and like acetylcholine, its role at each anatomical location is quite different. The general capacities of VIP for stimulating hormone secretion and relaxing blood vessels and smooth muscle give some indication of the possible diversity of its roles.

It seems likely that VIP released from postganglionic neurones produces salivary vasodilatation. It also has a role in relaxing the so-called 'cardio-oesophageal' sphincter and the stomach during gastric filling. VIP also affects intestinal blood flow during digestion. Mechanical stimulation of the mucosa results in the release of 5-hydroxytryptamine from enterochromaffin cells, which activates a VIP-dependent process whereby vasodilatation occurs. Overproduction of VIP occurs in the presence of a neural tumour, a ganglioneuroma. This causes severe watery diarrhoea, with low blood pressure and flushing attacks. The diarrhoea can be so severe that the patient can die of hypokalaemic paralysis (due to K^+ deficiency) or renal failure. This syndrome was first described by Verner and Morrison; resection of the tumour cures the symptoms.

Bombesin and related peptides

In 1971, bombesin was isolated from frog skin. Surprisingly, it was found to be a powerful stimulant of gastric-acid secretion. In addition, it elicited a flow of pancreatic juice rich in protein and it caused the gall-bladder to contract. Interest increased when bombesin-like immunoreactivity was discovered in nerves throughout the human gastrointestinal tract. The agent responsible appears to be a neuropeptide, and it is regarded as a strong candidate for a role in the release of gastrin by the vagus.

Enkephalin

Enkephalins are present in the nerve fibres of the myenteric and submucous plexuses of the gastrointestinal tract. Presumably, endorphins can exert local effects, and this may explain why morphine derivatives are so effective in the treatment of diarrhoea, since there must be receptors there.

LEPTIN

It has long been recognized that experimental manipulation of neural circuits in specific regions of the hypothalamus strikingly influences the desire to eat. For example, electrical stimulation of the lateral hypothalamus stimulates feeding, whereas medial stimulation leads to a loss of appetite. Over the last decade, a major mediator of these neuronal networks, named leptin (from the Greek word meaning 'thin'), has been characterized. The most salient features of this new hormone are listed in Table 8.4. Leptin is an *OB* gene product. It is a helix-bundle protein that is secreted from adipose tissue and interacts with receptors in the hypothalamus. In adequately fed individuals, it has two main physiological actions. First, it decreases the appetite and secondly, it increases energy expenditure. It is therefore sometimes referred to as the hormone of satiety. However, it is probably more correct to view leptin as a hormone that evolved to protect us against the adverse effects of starvation. Under fasting conditions, its circulating levels are low so that the appetite is stimulated and, crucially, stored energy is conserved.

Table 8.4 Major characteristics of leptin.

- 16 kDa protein hormone
- Synthesized and secreted by adipose tissue and the placenta
- Product of the *OB* gene, on chromosome 7q31.3–32
- Main target tissue: hypothalamus
- Receptor: a member of the cytokine-receptor group of cell surface receptors (see Table 2.1)
- Intracellular signalling: JAK–STAT pathway predominates (see Chapter 2)
- Leptin binding protein: as with GH, a soluble isoform of the ectodomain of the leptin receptor forms a binding protein in the circulation.
- Main actions: suppresses the appetite and increases energy expenditure
- Fasting: plasma leptin is very low, so stored energy is conserved
- Nonfasting leptin: circulating leptin increases with adiposity
- Circulating leptin exhibits a circadian rhythm—highest around midnight, with a nadir around midday
- Relative levels of plasma leptin throughout life:
  - —Newborn child: high
  - —Childhood: low
  - —Puberty: leptin increases early in puberty. In boys, the increase is only transient; in girls it is sustained
  - —Adulthood: leptin higher in women than men

JAK, Janus-associated kinase; STAT, signal transduction/activation of transcription.

Leptin deficiency is a rare cause of obesity. There have been reports of dramatic reversals of obesity in morbidly obese patients who have rare mutations in the *OB* gene, after treatment with recombinant therapeutic leptin. The administration of leptin resulted in normalization of the patient's otherwise voracious appetite and a consequent weight loss. In contrast, it is thought that leptin resistance is a major cause of the more frequently encountered forms of human obesity. This hormone resistance may lead to an endocrine resetting analogous to that encountered in insulin resistance, whereby a suboptimal metabolic state is maintained by a raised level of the hormone to which resistance is encountered. With insulin resistance, a hyperglycaemic state is maintained in the presence of increased insulin, whereas with leptin resistance there is an inappropriate setting of the lipostat despite the elevated levels of leptin in the circulation. Given the serious health-care problems that derive from the ever-increasing incidence of obesity in the Western world, the mechanisms of leptin resistance are currently the subject of major endocrine research efforts.

Measurement of the Concentrations of Hormones in Blood

Hormones are generally measured by immunoassays. However, other techniques, particularly bioassays, also play significant roles. All assays rely on a comparison between responses produced in the assay system by the sample and those produced by different known concentrations of a reference preparation. For immunoassays and bioassays, a calibration curve is generated with the reference preparation, and the unknown concentration of the hormone in the sample can then be interpolated from this.

Bioassays, which measure the potency of a hormone by quantifying a biological effect produced by the hormone, usually suffer from many practical problems. As a consequence, their use is limited to fundamental research. Immunoassays, which rely on the recognition of a hormone by an antibody, are technically manageable and capable of high sample throughputs. This has resulted in their widespread use throughout the world since their introduction in the 1960s. Four main attributes account for their successful application in diagnostic services: their sensitivity, specificity, precision and convenience.

IMMUNOASSAYS

Immunoassays take one of two different forms. Although they are collectively referred to as immunoassays, a somewhat confusing convention has arisen whereby one of the two alternative forms is itself referred to as the 'immunoassay' system, as in radioimmunoassays (RIAs). The other is the 'immunometric' assay system as encountered in immunoradiometric assays (IRMAs). Both RIAs and IRMAs employ a radioactive isotope as a 'label' or 'tracer', which generates the final quantitative signal for the assay; however, alternative nonisotopic labelling systems are being increasingly used. The assays that employ these other labelling systems have been given similar names, so that when fluorescence is used, for example, the two types of immunoassay are referred to as fluoroimmunoassays (FIAs) and immunofluoroimmunometric assays (IFMAs). Although different labels are used, producing an apparently diverse assortment of assays, they are all based on the same principles and fall into one of the two categories listed above.

Principles of immunoassays

Both forms of immunoassay are based on the interaction between an antibody and its antigen, the latter being the hormone to be measured. Thus, for an assay for a hormone such as human growth hormone (hGH), the basic reaction can be represented as:

Antigen and antibody $\rightarrow$ antigen–antibody complex, e.g.:

hGH + anti-hGH $\rightarrow$ antibody-bound hGH

In other words, if hGH is incubated with anti-hGH antibodies, the latter will bind to the hormone and form the complex shown. In reality, the reaction is reversible, and the antigen and its antibody are continuously dissociating and associating.

To set up a calibration or standard curve for an immunoassay for a hormone such as hGH, a constant amount of antibody is added to a series of tubes, while increasing and known amounts of a reference preparation of hGH are added to each tube in succession (Fig. A1.1). This reference preparation is also referred to as the 'standard'. After incubation, the equilibrium depicted in the equation will take place, and the tubes with the greater amount of hGH will form more of the bound complex. Measurement of the amount of the bound complex can thus be related to the quantity of hGH that was originally added, and a calibration curve can be plotted. The

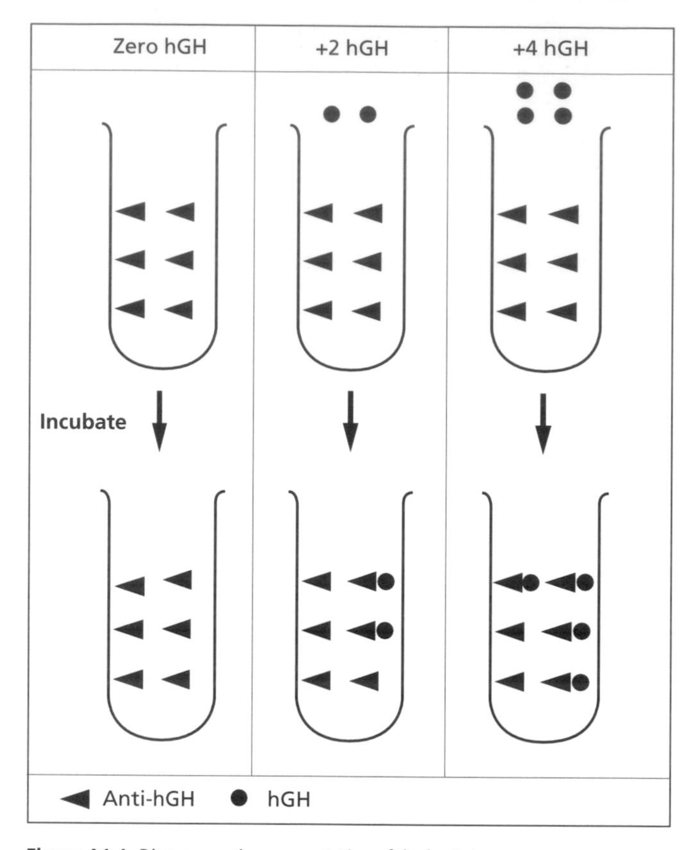

Figure A1.1 Diagrammatic representation of the basic immunoassay system for human growth hormone (hGH). Note: for the sake of clarity, in Figs A1.1–A1.3 only small numbers are shown for the numbers of molecules of hormones and antibodies. In practice, the numbers of molecules of a given reagent present in a given tube will be of the order of 10^8–10^{13}.

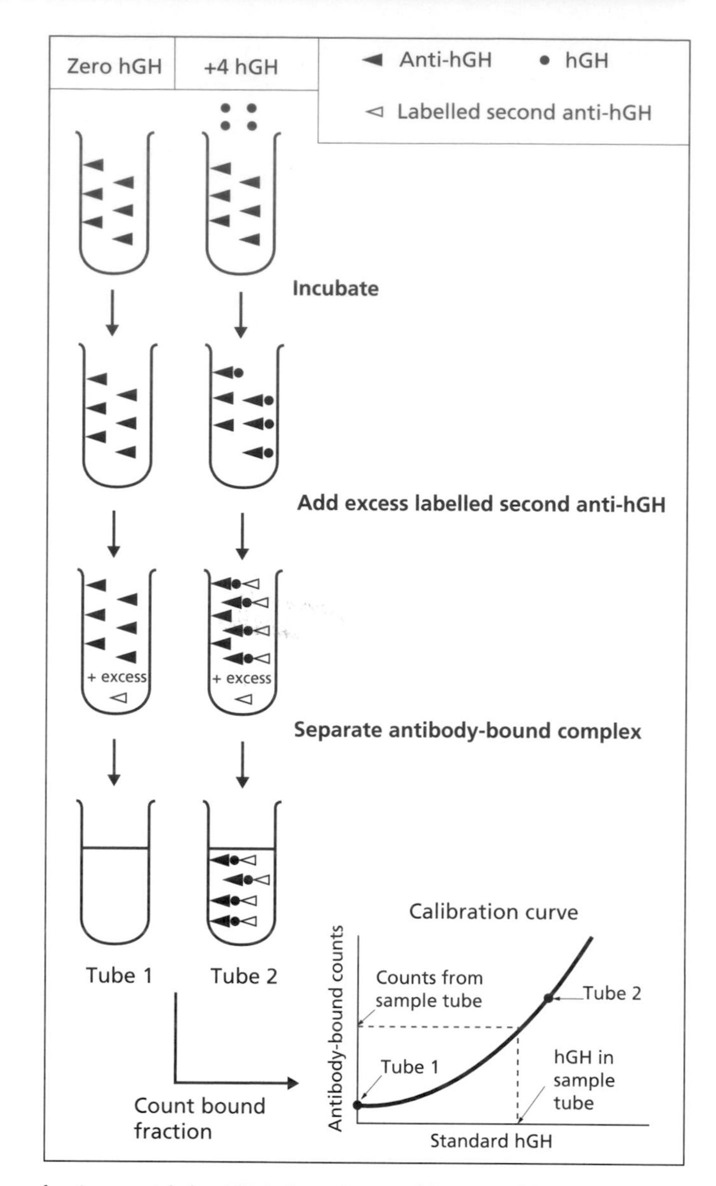

Figure A1.2 Diagram illustrating how to set up a two-point calibration curve for an immunoradiometric assay (IRMA) for human growth hormone (hGH). See the text for a full description. In practice, the incubation steps with the first and second antibodies are usually combined, with both antibodies being added simultaneously. They are shown separately here to aid the visual representation. Because of the formation of the triple complex (◀●◁) with the hormone 'sandwiched' between the two antibodies, this type of immunoassay system is sometimes referred to as a sandwich assay. Separation of the complex from the excess labelled second antibody is usually achieved by a physical method. For example, the complex can be selectively precipitated so that after centrifugation, the supernatant, which contains the unbound labelled second antibody, can be aspirated and the bound labelled second antibody can then be quantified by counting the pellet. The low counts from tube 1 and the higher count from tube 2 have been plotted on the calibration curve. Tube 1, the 'zero tube', might have been expected to contain no counts. In practice, a small amount of label will be found in this tube, due to the inherent 'stickiness' of most reagents such as labelled antibodies. This is referred to as the 'nonspecific' binding. In addition, the calibration curve will be curved as shown, rather than forming a straight line. This is due to the reversible nature of the basic interaction between antibodies and their antigens. Thus, a more accurate representation of the reaction would be:

$$\text{hGH} + \text{anti-hGH} \rightleftharpoons \text{antibody-bound hGH}$$

which indicates that the hGH and the antibody are continually associating and dissociating. An equilibrium situation will be reached when the rates of association and dissociation become equal. The dynamic equilibrium is governed by the law of mass action that forms the basis of the mathematical modelling of immunoassay systems, which has been important in their development. For the high-affinity antibodies used for immunoassays, this equilibrium will lie well to the right, as is depicted in the reversible reaction shown above. A helpful analogy for didactic purposes is the dynamic equilibrium that exists in society between marriage (association) and divorce (dissociation). This situation may hopefully be represented as:

$$\text{M} + \text{F} \rightleftharpoons \text{MF}.$$

substitution of the reference preparation of hGH by a patient sample will lead to the formation of an appropriate amount of bound complex. Measurement of this can then be used to deduce the concentration of hGH standard which was equivalent to that in the sample by interpolation from the calibration curve.

Immunometric assays: the sandwich assays

The principle of an immunometric assay for hGH is shown in Fig. A1.2. A constant amount of anti-hGH antibody is added to each tube, together with increasing known amounts of the reference preparation of hGH in each successive tube. After incubation, the amount of hGH bound to the antibody is detected by adding a second labelled anti-hGH antibody to all the tubes. The second antibody is directed against an antigenic site on hGH sterically remote from the binding site of the first antibody. Thus, a triple complex is formed, with the hGH being sandwiched between the two antibodies. The second antibody is also added at a constant amount to each tube, and is added as an excess. Since it carries a label (e.g. ^{125}I), the amount of complex formed can be measured by separating the complex from the excess unbound labelled second antibody and quantifying the bound label present in each tube—e.g. counting the radioactivity emitted by the ^{125}I associated with the separated complex, which is retained in the tubes.

This radioactivity is measured and plotted against the increasing but known amount of hGH standard initially added, and a calibration curve can be generated, as shown in Fig. A1.2. In practice, this curve is of the form shown in Fig. A1.2 and not a straight line passing through the origin, as might have been expected from the equation shown above. The reason for this is explained in the legend to Fig. A1.2. In addition, to determine the curve with precision, more than two concentrations of the standards are required, and usually between five and eight different concentrations of hGH will be used.

If a sample that contains an unknown concentration of hGH, but is identical in all other relevant respects, is also run, the amount of hGH present in the sample can be determined by interpolating from the calibration curve in the manner shown (Fig. A1.2).

Immunometric assays use relatively large quantities of antibodies, and the development of systems for producing monoclonal antibodies was therefore important for the adoption of these methods on a large scale. It should be noted that the immunometric assay system is suitable only when the hormone to be measured is relatively large. The hormone hGH has a molecular weight of 22 kDa, and this is a sufficiently large molecular structure to permit the binding of two antibody molecules and form the triple complex. This would not apply to molecules such as the thyroid hormones thyroxine (T_4) or triiodothyronine (T_3), for which the competitive-binding immunoassay system must be used.

Immunoassays: the competitive-binding assays

The principle underlying this alternative immunoassay system is shown in Fig. A1.3, which illustrates how a two-point calibration curve can be generated for the RIA of a hormone such as T_4. As with the immunometric assay (Fig. A1.2), constant amounts of antibody are added to each tube. In addition, a constant amount of labelled antigen is also added to each tube; for the RIA of T_4, this would be ^{125}I-labelled T_4. In the example shown, a 'zero' tube is set up that contains no unlabelled standard T_4, as well as a tube containing a known amount of standard T_4. For ease of illustration, the amount of standard in tube 2 has been selected to be equal to the number of molecules of the labelled T_4. A suitable incubation period follows, to allow the antigen–antibody complex to form. Since tube 1 contains twice as much ^{125}I-T_4 as anti-T_4 antibody, half of the ^{125}I-labelled T_4 will be bound by the antibody, but the other half will be unable to bind and will be present as an 'excess'. In tube 2, unlabelled standard T_4 has been added, which will compete with the ^{125}I-labelled T_4 for the limited number of binding sites available. In this way, the radioactivity bound to the antibody will be reduced in tube 2. This decrease in bound radioactivity is the assay signal that is measured. Clearly, it is a function of the amount of unlabelled T_4 added, and the antibody-bound counts decrease as the amount of unlabelled T_4 increases.

The bound T_4 (both labelled and unlabelled) is separated, e.g. by precipitation, and the radioactivity associated with the bound fraction is counted. If this radioactivity is plotted against the increasing known amounts of standard T_4 initially added, a calibration curve can be generated, as is illustrated in Fig. A1.3. It should be noted that the antibody-bound radioactivity decreases with increasing amounts of the unlabelled standard in a 'competitive-binding' type of immunoassay, in contrast to the immunometric assay system represented in Fig. A1.2.

To measure T_4 in a sample, it is necessary merely to replace the standard T_4 added with the sample, while keeping all other assay conditions identical. The T_4 present in the sample can then be interpolated from the calibration curve in the manner shown in Fig. A1.3.

This assay system can be adapted to measure the free or total concentrations of hormones such as T_4 and T_3. Measurement of the free concentrations, which are 100-fold to 15 000-fold lower than those of the bound hormone

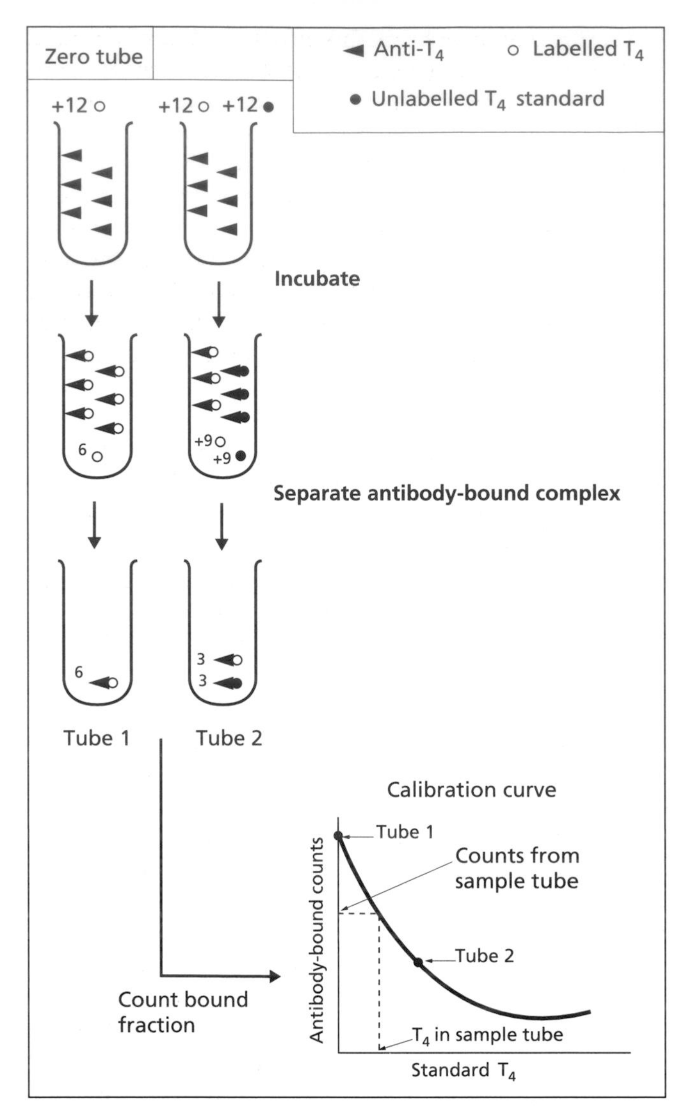

Figure A1.3 Diagram illustrating how to set up a two-point calibration curve for a radioimmunoassay for thyroxine (T_4). See the text for a full description. As stated in the legend to Fig. A1.1, in practice large numbers of molecules of each reagent are present in each tube. Under these conditions, the competition between labelled and unlabelled T_4 in tube 2 in this figure will be such that on 'average', in statistical terms, 50% of the antibody-binding sites will be occupied by labelled T_4 when it is competing with an equal amount of unlabelled T_4. Because of this apparent 'competition' between the labelled and unlabelled hormone for a limited amount of antibody, this type of immunoassay is sometimes referred to as a 'competitive-binding' assay.

(Table A1.1), has until recently proved a theoretical and technical challenge. This is because of the potential for disturbing the equilibrium between the bound and free hormone in a sample when it is introduced into an assay, when a high-affinity antibody will be present. The latter may induce dissociation of the large pool of hormone that is bound to the binding proteins, and this would result in a misleadingly high value for the concentration of the free

Table A1.1 Examples of typical adult reference ranges for plasma hormone concentrations. Note that these will vary depending on the method used* and the local population studied.

Hormone	Adult reference range	Units†
Adrenocorticotrophic hormone (ACTH)	< 10–80	ng/L
Aldosterone		
Recumbent	100–500	pmol/L
After 4 h standing	600–1200	pmol/L
Cortisol (at 9 a.m.)	140–700	nmol/L
Follicle-stimulating hormone (FSH)		
Males	1.0–12.0	U/L
Females		
Follicular phase	3.0–8.0	U/L
Postmenopausal	> 15	U/L
Glucagon (fasting)	< 50	pmol/L
Gastrin (fasting)	< 40	pmol/L
Growth hormone		
After a glucose load	< 2	mU/L
Stress-induced	> 20	mU/L
Insulin		
Fasting	< 15	mU/L
During hypoglycaemia	< 2	mU/L
Luteinizing hormone (LH)		
Males	2.0–12	U/L
Females		
Follicular phase	3.0–12	U/L
Postmenopausal	> 20	U/L
Oestradiol		
Males	37–130	pmol/L
Females		
Follicular phase	110–440	pmol/L
Luteal phase	370–770	pmol/L
Pre-ovulation	550–1290	pmol/L
Post-ovulation	37–130	pmol/L
Parathyroid hormone (PTH)	1.0–6.5	pmol/L
Prolactin	0–660	mu/L
Progesterone: luteal phase (indicates ovulation)	> 32	nmol/L
Renin: recumbent (plasma renin activity)	1.1–2.7	nmol/h/L
Testosterone		
Male	11–33	nmol/L
Female	0.5–2.5	nmol/L
Thyroid-stimulating hormone (TSH)	0.3–5.0	mU/L
Thyroxine (T_4)		
Total	60–150	nmol/L
Free	9.1–24	pmol/L
Triiodothyronine (T_3)		
Total	1.2–2.9	nmol/L
Free	4.7–8.2	pmol/L
Vitamin D (25-OH-cholecalciferol)	15–120	nmol/L

* Method-related bias can be ascertained by consulting reports from independent quality-control schemes, in which all immunoassay laboratories should participate.

† Whenever possible, concentrations are expressed as molarities and in SI units. However, this is not possible for complex hormones such as the glycoproteins TSH, LH and FSH, because these circulate in a range of slightly different forms. These structural variants are referred to by using an international reference preparation for a given hormone, which has a potency expressed in 'units' (U). This potency is assigned after large-scale collaborative trials involving many laboratories world-wide, which use a range of bioassays and immunoassays, together with physical analytical techniques. All patient results are then expressed relative to this reference preparation.

hormone. A range of techniques have now been developed for the determination of free T_3 and free T_4 concentrations. These are satisfactory in most clinical settings, and greater reliance is being placed on free concentrations as indicators of patient thyroid status. However, when interpreting the results of these assays, it should be borne in mind that the methods are liable to distortion by a number of artefacts, such as those that occur when there are extreme abnormalities in the concentration or nature of the binding proteins for a given patient. In some areas, such as the immunoassay of insulin-like growth factors I (IGF-I) and II in serum, the problem of binding proteins remains to be completely resolved.

In Table A1.1 we list typical adult reference ranges for a number of hormones, as determined by immunoassays. These will vary between laboratories, due to differences in the methods employed and also the local populations studied.

There are still situations in which satisfactorily specific and sensitive immunoassays have yet to be developed. For example, immunoassays can lack specificity for specific steroid hormones. Other techniques, such as high-performance liquid chromatography (HPLC) or gas chromatography followed by mass spectrometric analysis (GC/MS), have been used successfully in conjunction with a relatively nonspecific immunoassay, or in some cases in place of the latter.

BIOASSAYS

Bioassays compare the bioactivity of a hormone with that of a reference preparation. They are no longer required for analytical purposes for low molecular weight hormones that have well-defined and unique chemical structures, such as the thyroid or steroid hormones. A different situation exists with the more complex polypeptide hormones, such as the glycoprotein thyrotrophin (thyroid-stimulating hormone, TSH). The biological effectiveness of such complex molecules may be due to the interaction of one or more specific regions with a cell-surface receptor. These regions are referred to as 'bioactive sites' on the molecule.

Antibodies recognize discrete antigenic sites that are formed by just a few amino acids. Problems may then arise because the antigenic site may not coincide with the bioactive site or sites. Thus, for example, an antibody may recognize a mutated hormone that has a compromised bioactive site. Clearly, under this circumstance, a 'structural' assay, such as an immunoassay, would give a misleadingly high result. This may be revealed if an appropriate bioassay is run in parallel, when this 'functional' assay would register the compromised hormone structure as a poor or even absent response in the bioassay. The complexity of this problem is compounded by the microheterogeneity of hormones such as TSH, such that a range of slightly different structural forms will be present in the circulation.

In practice, antibodies that are used in immunoassays are usually selected to minimize these problems, and as a consequence, the immunoassay of a complex hormone such as TSH is clinically very valuable and used on large scale. However, bioassays may be resorted to in specialized centres if it is suspected that results from these structural assays are distorted due to the types of problem discussed above.

There are two forms of bioassays. The *in vivo* bioassays investigate the biological potency of a hormone following its administration to an animal and quantification of a specific response. *In vitro* bioassays are based on the biological effects produced by the hormone when it is added to an *in vitro* preparation of the target tissue. Examples of both of these types of bioassays are listed in Table A1.2. *In vivo* bioassays are typically used in conjunction with other assay techniques to establish the potency of new preparations of the complex polypeptide hormones, which may be tissue extracts or products of recombinant technology. The potency may then be assigned in terms of 'units' of bioactivity in a particular bioassay per unit weight of the preparation used, as discussed in Table A1.1. *In vivo* bioassays are also used for investigations of the effects of site-directed mutagenesis on the potencies of recombinant preparations. In this way, they may be invaluable in mapping a bioactive site. Results from *in vivo* bioassays uniquely reflect both the efficacy of the hormone preparation when acting on its specific target receptors and the *in vivo* clearance rate of the active molecules. Thus, for example, they may demonstrate that a circulating binding protein increases the potency of a hormone *in vivo* by prolonging its clearance—even though, when tested *in vitro*, the binding protein may appear to inhibit the hormone.

In vivo bioassays are not only laborious, technically demanding and expensive, but they can also be insensitive and imprecise due to inherent between-animal variation. They may also be subject to artefacts due to species specificity of the hormone being tested. Nowadays, *in vitro* bioassays can usually be designed to overcome many of these problems. With the coupling of microtitre-plate technology and advances in the culture of immortalized target cells that have been transformed to express appropriate human receptors for hormones, colorimetric and luminescent *in vitro* bioassays—e.g. microculture tetrazolium assay (MTA) and microculture reporter gene assay (MRGA)—are available that rival immunoassays in terms of many of their advantageous performance characteristics (Table A1.2).

Table A1.2 Examples of *in vivo* and *in vitro* systems for the bioassay of hormones.

Hormone	Experimental system	Response
In vivo bioassays		
Growth hormone	Hypophysectomized rats or hypopituitary strain of dwarf mice	Body weight gain or increase in the width of tibial epiphyseal cartilage
Prolactin	Pigeon crop sac	Crop weight or thickening
Parathyroid hormone	Parathyroidectomized rats	Increase in serum calcium
Insulin	Rabbits and mice	Lowering blood glucose
FSH	Hypophysectomized female rats	Increased ovarian weight
LH	Hypophysectomized male rats	Increased prostate weight
TSH	Mice: thyroids prelabelled with ^{131}I	Discharge of ^{131}I into the circulation
In vitro bioassays		
Growth hormone	Nb2 rat lymphoma cell line	Increases in cell number and metabolic activation, MTA*
Prolactin	As for growth hormone	As for growth hormone
Parathyroid hormone	Renal plasma membranes	Increased adenylate cyclase
Insulin	Rat diaphragm muscle	Increased glucose uptake and glycogen synthesis
FSH	Cultured ovarian granulosa cells or CHO cells that express the human FSH receptor	Aromatase activity, MRGA†
LH	Cultured Leydig cells	Increased testosterone production, MRGA
TSH	Immortalized rat thyroid cells (FRTL-5 cells) or CHO cells that express the human TSH receptor	Increases in adenylate cyclase or ^{131}I uptake, MTA and MRGA

* MTA: microculture tetrazolium assays, which are colorimetric microtitre-plate bioassays based on the bioreduction of a yellow tetrazolium salt to its purple formazan by hormone-activated target cells maintained as microcultures in microtitre plates.

† MRGA: microculture reporter gene assays, which are microtitre-plate bioassays based on the generation of a signal by reporter-gene activation, e.g. the cAMP-responsive luciferase reporter gene.

cAMP, cyclic adenosine 5′-monophosphate; CHO, Chinese hamster ovary; FSH, follicle-stimulating hormone; LH, luteinizing hormone; TSH, thyroid-stimulating hormone (thyrotrophin).

RECEPTOR ASSAYS

It is possible to use alternative hormone-binding reagents for a range of ligand-binding assays. The binding reagent replaces the antibodies used in the immunoassays, but otherwise the same principles and similar assay designs are employed. Receptor assays form an important example of ligand-binding assays, in which a hormone-receptor preparation is used as the binding reagent. Generally, the competitive-binding system (Fig. A1.3) with labelled hormone is used. Receptors may be either in solubilized form or, in the case of cell-surface receptors, used while still attached to isolated plasma membranes. Receptor assays exploit the high affinity and hormone specificity of hormone receptors, and often have the favourable performance characteristics of immunoassays in terms of their sensitivity, precision and high sample capacities. In addition, they have the advantage that they are based on a direct interaction between the binding reagent and the relevant bioactive site on the structure of a complex hormone, such as TSH. However, the ability to bind to the receptor does not completely identify molecules that will also activate the subsequent intracellular receptor–second messenger systems. Receptor assays may therefore be thought of as forming a compromise between bioassays and immunoassays, and they have remained important research techniques, although they have had limited impact as hormone-measurement systems. They are also used to measure receptor numbers in specific tissues. For example, oestrogen-receptor and progesterone-receptor assays may be useful in the management of breast cancer, where a hormone-dependent tumour may be present that cannot thrive in the absence of the hormone. Tumours with receptors for both of these steroid hormones respond particularly well to tamoxifen, which blocks receptor activation.

Hormone–Receptor Interactions

The interaction between a hormone and a receptor located in or on the target cell is the mechanism that forms the first step in an endocrine response. Thus, characterization of these interactions has formed an important area for understanding the molecular processes that govern the responses of target cells to hormones. The receptors have been shown to exhibit several characteristics. First, since hormones are present in the circulation at low concentrations, the receptors, which may be thought of as 'capture systems', should have high affinities for the hormones. Secondly, binding should be reversible, to allow for the transient nature of endocrine responses. Thirdly, receptors must be able to distinguish between closely related molecular structures and thereby confer hormonal specificity on the system.

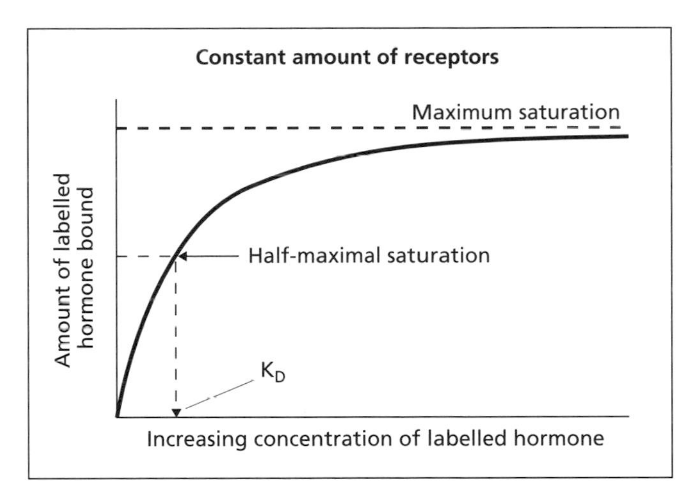

Figure A2.1 Demonstration of the saturability of a hormone–receptor system. Increasing concentrations of labelled hormone are incubated with a constant amount of receptors. The bound hormone is then separated; for example, if the receptors are in the form of a suspension of isolated plasma membranes, separation can be effected by centrifugation. The amount of labelled hormone bound is then seen to increase as shown, such that it approaches an asymptote. The asymptote will represent the number of receptors added to the system expressed in terms of the amount of hormone required to saturate them. In addition, the concentration of hormone that is required for half-maximal saturation of the receptors in this experiment is equal to the dissociation constant (K_D) of this hormone–receptor interaction (see Fig. A2.3 for further discussion).

Characterization of hormone–receptor interactions has relied on simple experiments that use radiolabelled hormones, together with preparations of the receptors. The latter may be in the form of subcellular fractions enriched in hormone receptors (e.g. suspensions of isolated plasma membranes with attached cell-surface receptors), detergent-solubilized receptors, or receptors prepared by recombinant technology. The reversible interactions can then be investigated by incubating the hormones and receptors together under carefully controlled conditions, and finally separating and quantifying the bound hormone.

Often, an initial experiment is performed to establish that the interaction forms a 'saturation system'. For this, a constant amount of the receptor preparation is incubated with increasing amounts of the labelled hormone. Saturation is indicated when the amount of the bound hormone is found to approach an asymptote, as shown in Fig. A2.1. This indicates that relatively high concentrations of the

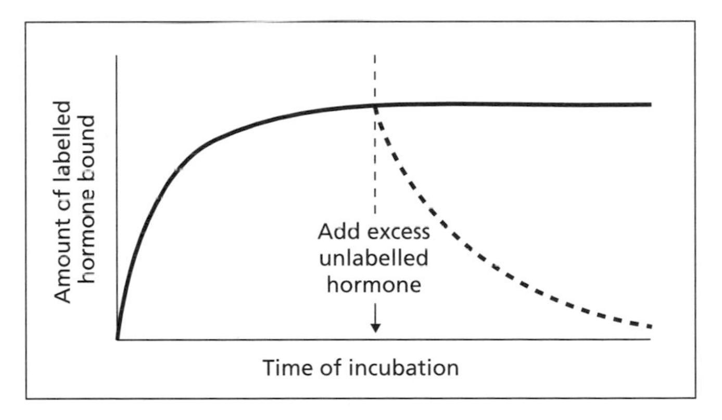

Figure A2.2 Demonstration of the reversibility of a hormone–receptor interaction. Constant amounts of labelled hormone and receptor preparation are incubated together for different times. The bound label is separated after selected incubation periods, and will be found to increase with time until it reaches a plateau. At this time, the bound and free hormone have reached a dynamic equilibrium. The reversibility of the hormone–receptor interaction can be demonstrated by adding excess unlabelled hormone at a specific time, as shown. This will compete with the labelled hormone for the receptors, since in the dynamic equilibrium the hormone continually associates with and dissociates from the receptors. As a consequence, the amount of labelled hormone bound will decrease with the extended incubation period, as shown (----).

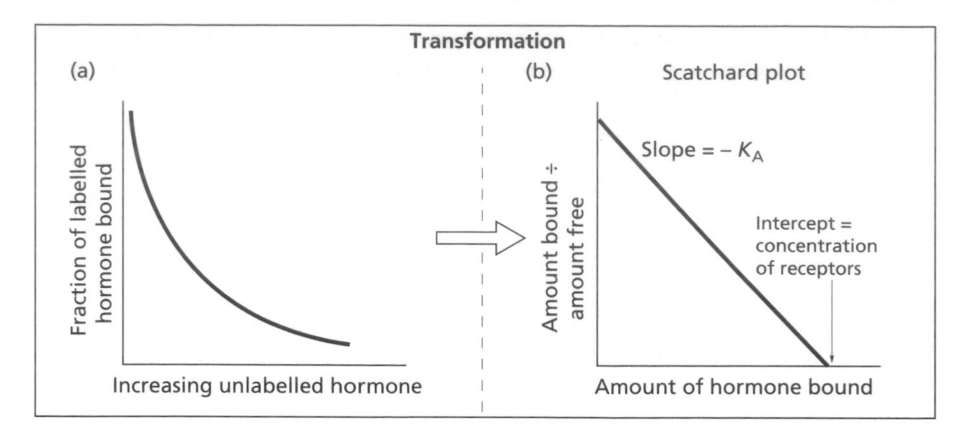

Figure A2.3 The Scatchard plot. This illustrates the transformation of results obtained from a competitive-displacement study, which has been set up as described in Fig. A1.3, into a Scatchard plot (b). This allows one to determine the affinity of the receptor for the hormone (or, alternatively, as described in Fig. A1.3, the affinity of an antibody for a hormone). This is calculated as the slope of the plot that equals $-K_A$, where K_A is the affinity constant. This is derived as follows. The basic reaction may be described as

$H + R \rightleftharpoons HR$

where H is the hormone and R the receptor. This reversible reaction is governed by the law of mass action, so that the rate of the forward reaction (complex formation) and backward reaction (complex dissociation) will be as follows:

Rate of forward reaction $= K_{+1} \cdot [H] \cdot [R]$

Rate of backward reaction $= K_{-1} \cdot [HR]$

where K_{+1} is the association rate constant and K_{-1} is the dissociation rate constant. Both of these are physical constants that are a unique characteristic of each hormone–receptor reaction. The square brackets in the above equations denote concentrations. At equilibrium, the rates of these two reactions will be equal, and the situation can be represented as:

$K_{+1} \cdot [H] \cdot [R] = K_{-1} \cdot [HR]$

thus

$K_{+1}/K_{-1} = [HR]/[H] \cdot [R] = K_A$ (1)

The affinity constant, which can also be termed the association constant, is a ratio of the two rate constants, and hence is also a physical constant that is a unique characteristic of each hormone–receptor interaction. The affinity constant is commonly determined by the transformation of the results from the competitive-displacement study, using Scatchard's transformation of equation 1, such that:

$[HR]/[H] = K_A \cdot [R]_T - K_A \cdot [HR]$

where $[R]_T$ is the total concentration of receptors added to each tube, which has been kept constant for all of the tubes in the displacement study. Since $[R]_T = [R] + [HR]$, the transformation is achieved by using this to substitute for [HR] in equation 1. Clearly, this has the form of the linear relationship $y = mx + c$, so that when [HR]/[H] is plotted against [HR], a straight line should be obtained, the slope of which (m) $= -K_A$ (Fig. 2.3b). As can be seen from equation 1, the affinity constant (K_A) has the dimensions of concentration^{-1}, and would typically be 10^7–10^{12} L/mol. It is frequently expressed as its reciprocal, which is then the dissociation constant (K_D). Clearly, a typical value for this would be $10^{-12} - 10^{-7}$ mol/L. Using the approach commonly encountered in Michaelian analysis of enzyme kinetics, it can readily be shown that K_D is the concentration of hormone that is required for half-maximal saturation of the receptors in the original competitive-displacement experiment (see Figs A1.3 and A2.1). Alternatively, it is the concentration of hormone that is required for half-maximal saturation of the antibodies used in an immunoassay. As one might anticipate, this is of the same order as the concentrations of hormones in the circulation, i.e. $10^{-12} - 10^{-7}$ mol/L (see Table A1.1).

hormone are 'saturating' the limited quantity of receptors that have been added. A second experiment is designed to demonstrate the reversible nature of the hormone binding. In this, constant amounts of labelled hormone and receptor are incubated together, and the increase in binding is followed as a function of time of incubation (Fig. A2.2). Often, incubation is allowed to proceed until equilibrium has been attained, as shown in the time-course in Fig. A2.2. This is followed by the addition of a relatively large amount of unlabelled hormone. If the system is reversible, the unlabelled hormone will compete with the labelled hormone, which is continually associating and dissociating from the receptor, such that the amount of labelled hormone bound will decrease with time. This demonstrates the dynamic nature of the equilibrium of the hormone–receptor interaction.

Further characterization will then use the competitive-binding system, illustrated in Appendix 1 for immunoassays (see Fig. A1.3). Constant amounts of labelled hormone and receptor preparations are incubated with increasing but known amounts of unlabelled hormone for a specified time. Clearly, in this experiment, the receptor preparation is replacing the antibody used for the immunoassay illustrated in Fig. A1.3. After separation of the bound label, a 'competitive-displacement' curve is plotted, such as those shown in Figs A1.3 and A2.3a. In addition, these results may be mathematically transformed into a Scatchard plot (Fig. A2.3b), which allows critical evaluation of whether the hormone–receptor interaction is governed by the law of mass action, as applied to a reaction described by the equation $H + R \rightleftharpoons HR$. This is satisfied if a linear relationship is established between the ratio of bound : free hormone and the amount of hormone added, as shown in the Scatchard plot in Fig. A2.3b. If this criterion is established, both the affinity of the receptor for the hormone and the number of hormone-receptor molecules added to the experiment can be determined. The latter, which is then calculated from the intercept on the x axis in Fig. A2.3b, can then be used to estimate the number of hormone receptors per target cell.

Many hormone receptors have been found to interact with the hormone according to this system, although ambiguities sometimes arise, with the Scatchard plot being curved rather than linear. This can sometimes be accounted for by difficulties in excluding a nonspecific binding component from the experimental system, which is due to the inherent 'stickiness' of hormones such as the glycoprotein thyrotrophin (thyroid-stimulating hormone, TSH). Alternatively, curvilinear Scatchard plots can indicate that more than one type of receptor–hormone interaction is operative in the system. An example of this is provided by the receptor-dimerization model, which appears to apply to the interaction between growth hormone and its receptors, as discussed in Chapter 2 (see Fig. 2.7).

Hormonal specificity of receptors is usually demonstrated by the inability of unlabelled related hormones to displace a labelled hormone in a competitive-displacement experiment such as that illustrated in Figs A1.3 and A2.3a. Typically, a number of unlabelled related hormones are added at very high concentrations, together with the labelled specific hormone and its receptors, and are shown to be without effect on the binding of the labelled hormone.

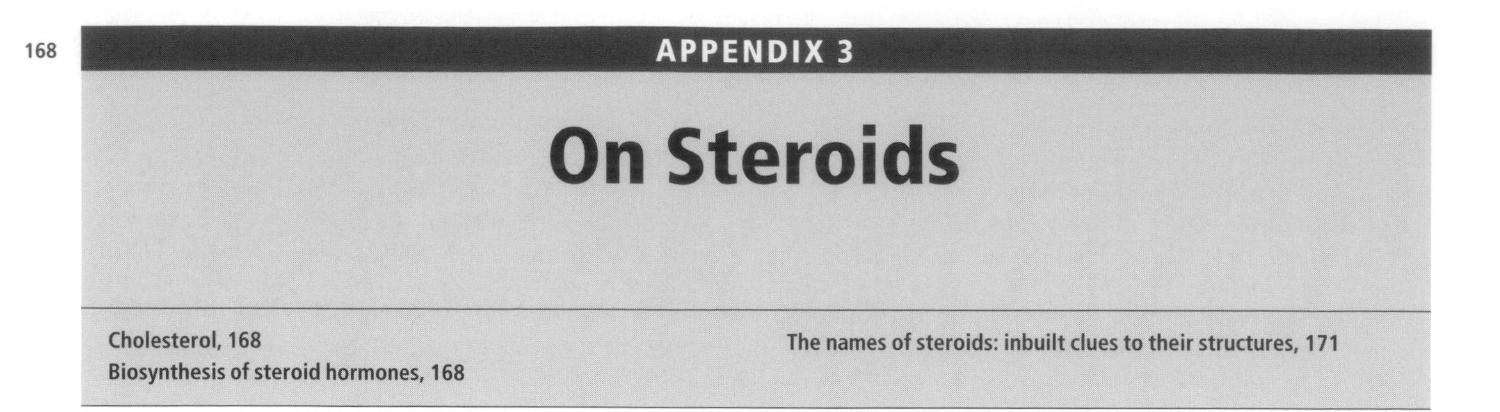

APPENDIX 3

On Steroids

CHOLESTEROL

Cholesterol is the starting material for the biosynthesis of steroid hormones. Its structure is shown in Fig. A3.1.

Cells can synthesize cholesterol from carbohydrate or fatty acid precursors, but the favoured route is to obtain cholesterol from dietary sources. Once in the circulation, cholesterol is complexed as low-density lipoproteins. The latter are taken up from the blood by receptor-mediated endocytosis. Steroid-producing cells are characterized by the presence of large lipid-filled vesicles (see Fig. 1.6). These are the cellular stores of cholesterol, largely in the form of fatty acid esters.

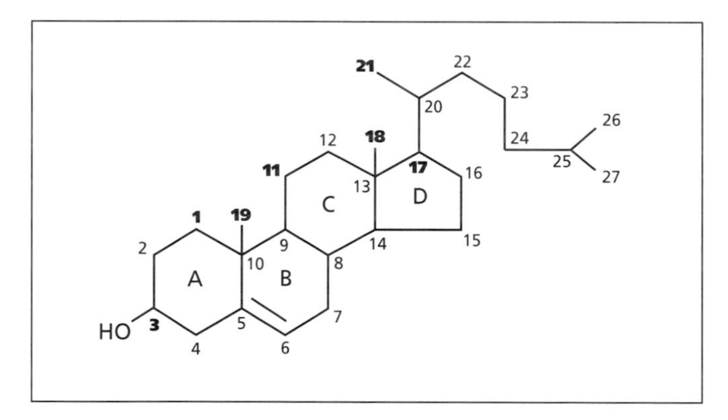

Figure A3.1 The structure of cholesterol is based on the steroid nucleus, with rings A to D lettered as shown. Cholesterol has a substantial side-chain attached at C-17, making it a C-27 molecule. This is progressively removed during the biosynthesis of the classical steroid hormones, but is retained by the pathway responsible for the biosynthesis of vitamin D, which is another important cholesterol derivative (see Fig. 7.13). The particularly significant C-atoms in the 27-carbon structure are highlighted. Note: although cholesterol is represented here as a flat molecule, steroid hormones do have complex three-dimensional structures. In particular, the prefixes α- and β-denote the orientation of specific substituent groups. 'Alpha' indicates that a substituent projects towards the reader, whilst conversely 'beta' indicates a group that projects away.

BIOSYNTHESIS OF STEROID HORMONES

Cholesterol is converted into the different steroid hormones by the major steroidogenic endocrine organs, namely the adrenal gland, testis and ovary. These use the biosynthetic pathways depicted in Fig. A3.2. The placenta also synthesizes steroids during pregnancy, but this process is significantly different, as is described in Chapter 6.

Tissue-specific and cell-specific synthesis of a given steroid is achieved by the expression of the appropriate sequence of enzymes by the cells of the tissue in question. The pathways in Fig. A3.2 are grouped to indicate the tissue-specific expression of the enzymes. For example, the adrenal cells in the zona glomerulosa are differentiated to express the enzymes along the pathway that culminates in the biosynthesis of aldosterone; these steps are highlighted in the illustration (↓). The first two enzymes, namely side-chain cleavage enzyme (SCCE) and 3β-hydroxysteroid dehydrogenase (3β-HSD), are expressed in steroidogenic cells in both the gonads and the adrenal, but 21-hydroxylase is restricted to the adrenal cortex, where it is expressed in the cells of the zona glomerulosa and fasciculata. However, aldosterone synthase is solely expressed in the zona glomerulosa. Here it is responsible for the final steps in the pathway, namely hydroxylation at C-11 and conversion of C-18 to the aldehyde group, which is unique to aldosterone. The zona glomerulosa does not express 17-α hydroxylation activity, and consequently cannot synthesize steroids such as cortisol or the sex steroids. Further details of the individual enzymes are given in Table A3.1.

The subcellular locations of the enzymes are shown in Table A3.1. Although the pathways use a sequence of enzymes, some of these are mitochondrial, whilst others are microsomal. Consequently, a given steroid shuttles between these two subcellular compartments as it progresses along a biosynthetic pathway.

Cholesterol is taken into mitochondria by a process which is mediated by the so-called StAR protein (Fig.

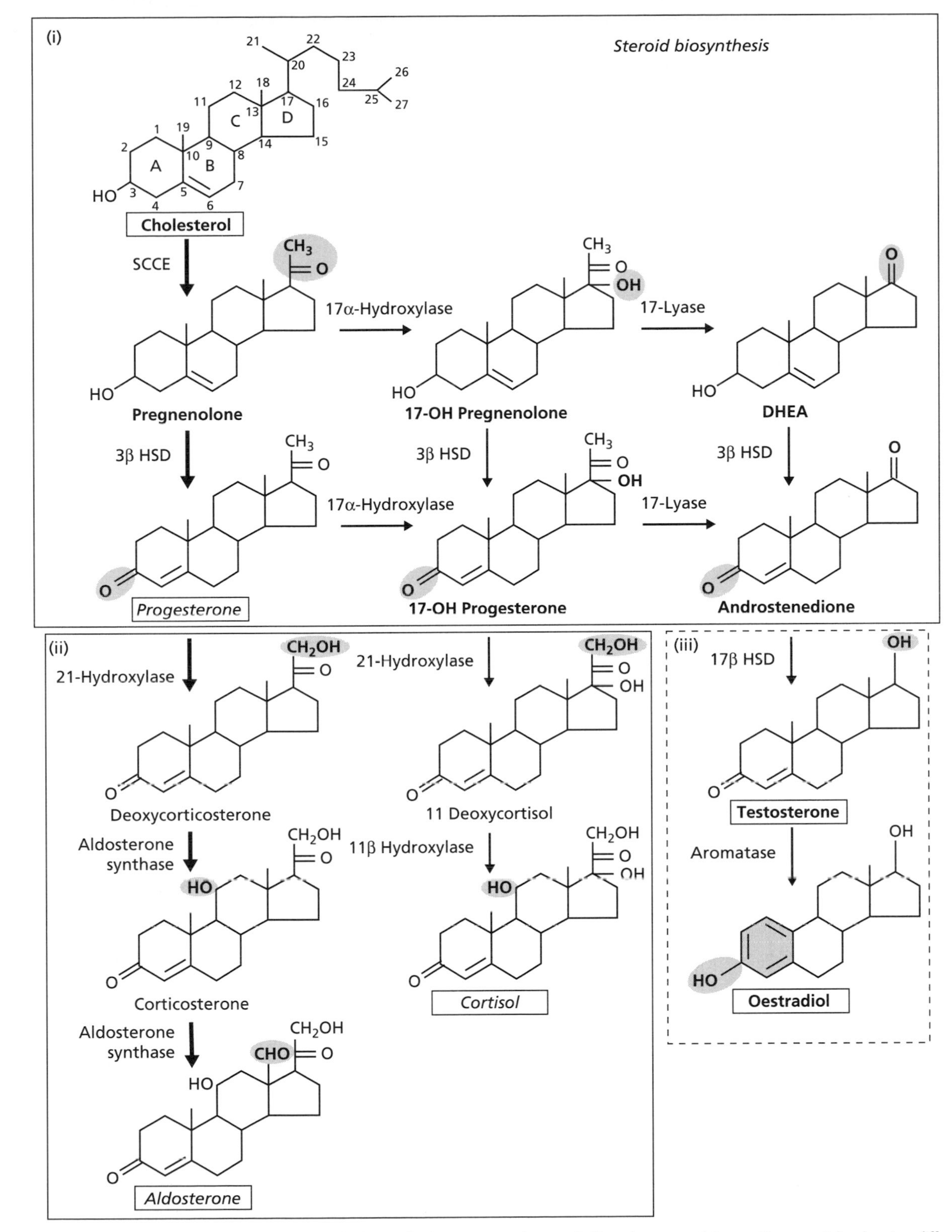

Figure A3.2 The major biosynthetic pathways responsible for the production of progesterone, aldosterone, cortisol, testosterone and oestradiol. The highlighted substituents on the structures indicate the chemical change that has occurred at a particular step. The enzymes responsible for each step are shown. The pathways are grouped into three blocks: (i) encompasses those that are found in both the adrenals and the gonads; (ii) shows the enzymes expressed in the cells of the adrenal cortex; and (iii) shows the enzymes largely restricted to the gonads. Note that some of the reactions may take place in a different sequence to that shown in this figure, and minor alternative pathways are also available. These are not shown in this diagram for the sake of clarity, but are discussed in specialist chapters. (DHEA, dehydroepiandrosterone; SCCE, side-chain cleavage enzyme; 3β-HSD, 3-β-hydroxysteroid dehydrogenase; 17-β-HSD, 17-β-hydroxysteroid dehydrogenase.)

Table A3.1 Nomenclature and chromosomal location of genes coding for the 9 enzymes shown on Fig. A3.2.

Alternative common names and abbreviations	Convention for naming the P450 enzymes	Chromosomal location	Subcellular location
Side-chain cleavage enzyme (SCCE) Desmolase	CYP11A1*	15	IMM
3β-hydroxysteroid dehydrogenase (3β-HSD)	—	1	ER
21-hydroxylase	CYP21	6	ER
11β-hydroxylase†	CYP11B1	8	IMM
Aldosterone synthase†	CYP11B2	8	IMM
17-hydroxylase‡	CYP17	10	ER
17-lyase‡	CYP17	10	ER
17β-hydroxysteroid dehydrogenase (17β-HSD) 17 ketosteroid reductase 4 tissue-specific isoforms	—	9,16,17§	ER
Aromatase	CYP19	15	ER

ER, endoplasmic reticulum; IMM, inner mitochondrial membrane.
* The root CYP is used to denote human cytochrome P450. 3β-HSD and 17β-HSD are not P450 enzymes.
† Isozymes: note that aldosterone synthase catalyses both hydroxylation at C-11 and the conversion of C-18 to an aldehyde group.
‡ CYP17 catalyses both 17-hydroxylation and 17,20-lyase activity at C-17.
§ Tissue-specific isoforms.

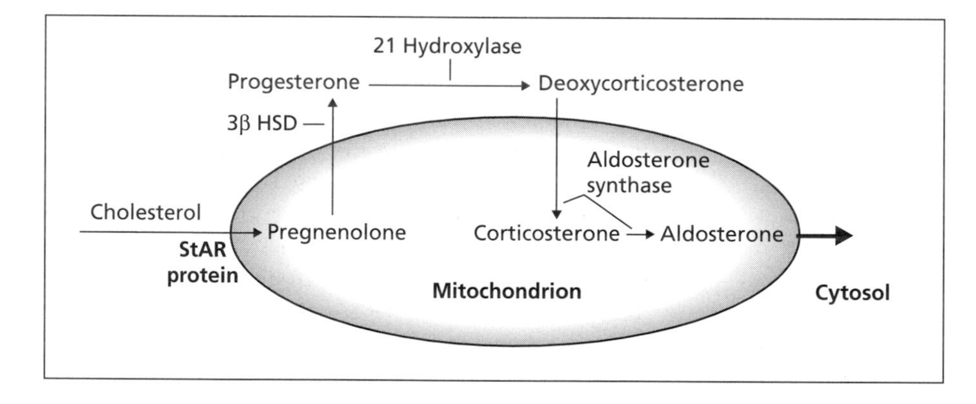

Figure A3.3 The biosynthesis of aldosterone from cholesterol, showing the shuttling of the intermediates between mitochondrial enzymes and those located in the endoplasmic reticulum.

A3.3). This is the *st*eroid *a*cute *r*egulatory protein, the gene for which has been mapped to chromosome 8. The synthesis of this 30 kDa protein is cAMP-inducible, and hence increases in response to trophic hormones such as adrenocorticotrophic hormone (ACTH) and the gonadotrophins. The dependence of steroidogenesis on the synthesis of StAR protein is demonstrable by the observation that inhibitors of protein synthesis, such as cycloheximide, block steroidogenic responses to trophic hormones such as ACTH. Although the molecular mechanism responsible for StAR-mediated transport of cholesterol into mitochondria is yet to be identified, it is appreciated that the rate-limiting step in steroidogenesis lies between cholesterol release from its storage droplets and the synthesis of pregnenolone in the mitochondria. Whereas StAR is found in the adrenal, ovary and testis, the regulatory protein responsible for facilitating delivery of cholesterol to the side-chain cleavage enzyme in the placenta is different from StAR, and is known as the MLN-64 protein. The tissue-specific existence of two separate cholesterol-delivery proteins accounts for the experience that in congenital lipoid adrenal hyperplasia (p70), the actual pregnancy is relatively normal.

As can be seen from Fig. A3.3, after StAR protein–mediated transport of cholesterol into a mitochondrion, the side-chain cleavage enzyme removes most of the C-27 cholesterol side-chain to give C-21 pregnenolone. The latter is translocated to the endoplasmic reticulum, where 3β-hydroxysteroid dehydrogenase changes the –OH group at C-3 to a ketone group and 21-hydroxylase substitutes an –OH group at C-21. The resulting deoxycorticosterone then shuttles back into the mitochondrion, where the enzyme aldosterone synthase adds a crucial –OH group at C-11, which is characteristic of all major adrenal steroids. Aldosterone synthase also substitutes an aldehyde group at C-18, yielding the potent mineralocorticoid, aldosterone. Aldehyde groups are not found in any of the other steroids shown in Fig. A3.2, being unique to aldosterone, as the name of this steroid indicates. Steroid-producing cells do not store their hormones, and once synthesized, aldosterone rapidly enters the circulation.

THE NAMES OF STEROIDS: INBUILT CLUES TO THEIR STRUCTURES

The sheer number of steroids and their structural similarities can be a baffling hurdle to a nonspecialist. However, careful inspection of Fig. A3.2 will reveal key structural features that define both the origin and character of a given steroid. This diagram, which assigns individual steroids to specific groups, provides a plan that is as helpful a guide as the periodic table is in inorganic chemistry. The prime structural feature of a given steroid is simply the number of its carbon atoms. Thus, C-27 cholesterol can be converted to C-21 steroids, which—apart from progesterone—are characteristic of adrenal steroids (e.g. aldosterone or cortisol) and all appear at the bottom left in Fig. A3.2. Alternatively, further clipping of the side-chain by 17-lyase activity produces the C-19 steroids—dehydroepiandrosterone (DHEA), androstenedione and testosterone—which appear at the upper right in Fig. A3.2. These can be grouped as androgens. Finally, the radical change in structure to the A ring brought about by aromatase results in the C-18 steroid oestradiol. Appreciation of the significance of the C-21, C-19 and C-18 categories is a helpful start to relating the structure of a given steroid to its tissue of origin and biological action. For example, if one is shown the C-21 structure of aldosterone, it is then easy to predict that it is an adrenal steroid and unlikely to be secreted from either the ovary or the testis.

Another help with steroid structures is the realization that there are relatively few C-atoms for which the substituent group defines the origin and actions of a particular steroid. These have been highlighted in Fig. A3.1. For example, all major adrenal steroids in Fig. A3.2 have a ketone group at C-3 and hydroxyl groups at C-11 and C21. C-17 is important for cortisol, since there is a hydroxyl group here that distinguishes it from a mineralocorticoid such as aldosterone. The latter, however, has a defining aldehyde group at C-18. The C-19 androgens, androstenedione and testosterone, both have a ketone group at C-3, but differ from each other by the ketone/hydroxyl group at C-17.

Finally, the common names used for steroids adhere to a loose convention, which is also a useful guide to their structures and/or actions. The suffix -ol indicates an important –OH group, as in cholesterol or cortisol. The suffix -diol, as in oestradiol, reminds one that there are two defining –OH groups in this C-18 structure. The suffix -one indicates an important ketone group, as in pregnenolone, progesterone, corticosterone, aldosterone, dehydroepiandrosterone and testosterone; whereas androstene*dione* indicates the two significant ketone groups in its structure. The inclusion of -ene- in a name, as in pregnenolone, indicates the presence of a significant double bond in the steroid nucleus.

These systematic conventions, which have been developed over the past few decades and applied with imagination, if not rigour, should provide a good basis for deducing, rather than memorizing, steroid structures. For example, the name oestradiol contains two vital clues as to its structure: (i) being an oestrogen, it must be based on a C-18 structure, with an aromatic A ring and the absence of any vestigial cholesterol side chain at C-17; and (ii) the suffix -diol indicates that there must be two significant –OH groups. Since it is not an adrenal steroid, C-11 will not be hydroxylated, and it is reasonable therefore to position these –OH groups at the two other particularly significant C-atoms, namely C-3 and C-17. The reader is now invited to *deduce* the structure of aldosterone.

A familiarity with these features of steroid endocrinology underpins any in-depth understanding of the functions of the major steroid-producing endocrine systems, and forms a particularly useful foundation for explaining a complex constellation of clinical signs, as encountered in a condition such as congenital adrenal hyperplasia (see Chapter 4).

Index